Specialist Training in:
CARDIOLOGY

D1408502

Commissioning Editor: Timothy Horne
Project Development Manager: Clive Hewat
Project Manager: Frances Affleck
Designer: George Ajayi

Specialist Training in
CARDIOLOGY

Edited by

Henry J Purcell MB PhD

Senior Fellow in Cardiology
Royal Brompton Hospital
London

Paul R Kalra MA MB BChir MRCP

Consultant Cardiologist
Portsmouth Hospitals NHS Trust
Portsmouth

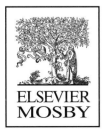

ELSEVIER
MOSBY

Edinburgh London New York Oxford Philadelphia St Louis Sydney Toronto 2005

ELSEVIER
MOSBY

An imprint of Elsevier Limited

First published 2005

ISBN 0723433216

British Library Cataloguing in Publication Data
A catalogue record for this book is available from the British Library

Library of Congress Cataloging in Publication Data
A catalog record for this book is available from the Library of Congress

Notice
Knowledge and best practice in this field are constantly changing. As new research and experience broaden our knowledge, changes in practice, treatment and drug therapy may become necessary or appropriate. Readers are advised to check the most current information provided (i) on procedures featured or (ii) by the manufacturer of each product to be administered, to verify the recommended dose or formula, the method and duration of administration, and contraindications. It is the responsibility of the practitioner, relying on their own experience and knowledge of the patient, to make diagnoses, to determine dosages and the best treatment for each individual patient, and to take all appropriate safety precautions. To the fullest extent of the law, neither the Publisher nor the Authors assume any liability for any injury and/or damage to persons or property arising out or related to any use of the material contained in this book.

The Publisher

Working together to grow
libraries in developing countries

www.elsevier.com | www.bookaid.org | www.sabre.org

ELSEVIER BOOK AID International Sabre Foundation

ELSEVIER your source for books, journals and multimedia in the health sciences
www.elsevierhealth.com

The publisher's policy is to use **paper manufactured from sustainable forests**

Printed in China

Contents

Contributors

Constandinos Anagnostopoulos MD PHD
FRCP FESC
Consultant in Nuclear Medicine
Royal Brompton Hospital
London, UK

Timothy R Betts MD MBChB MRCP
Consultant Cardiologist and
Electrophysiologist
Oxford Radcliffe Hospitals NHS Trust
Oxford, UK

Lucy Blows BM MRCP
Specialist Registrar in Cardiology
Guy's and St Thomas' Hospital
London, UK

Anna Brackenridge MB ChB MRCP
Specialist Registrar in Diabetes and
Endocrinology
Royal Surrey County Hospital
Guildford, UK

Stephen J Brecker MD FRCP FESC FACC
Consultant Cardiologist
St George's Hospital
London, UK

David Brull MBBS BSc MRCP MD
Consultant Cardiologist
The Whittington Hospital and the Heart
Hospital UCLH
London, UK

Alison Calver MA MBBS MD FRCP
Consultant Cardiologist
Wessex Cardiothoracic Unit
Southampton University Hospital
Southampton, UK

John P Carpenter MRCP
Specialist Registrar in Cardiology
Portsmouth Hospitals NHS Trust
Portsmouth, UK

Paul O Collinson MD FRCPath FACB
Consultant Chemical Pathologist
St Georges Hospital
London, UK

James Coutts MA BMBCh MRCP
Consultant Cardiologist
St Thomas Hospital
London, UK

Caroline Daly MB MRCPI
Cardiology Research Registrar
Royal Brompton Hospital
London, UK

Mark Dayer MBBS BSc MRCP
Clinical Research Fellow
National Heart Lung Institute
London, UK

Andrew Elkington BSc MRCP
Specialist Registrar in Cardiology
Taunton and Somerset Hospital
Taunton, UK

Perry Elliott MD MRCP FACC
Senior Lecturer and Honorary Consultant
in Cardiology
The Heart Hospital UCLH
London, UK

Kevin F Fox MD MRCP
Consultant Cardiologist
Hammersmith Hospitals NHS Trust
London, UK

Darryl Francis MB BChir MRCP MD
Specialist Registrar in Cardiology
St Mary's Hospital
London, UK

Patrick Gallagher MD PhD FRCPath
Consultant Cardiac Pathologist
Southampton General Hospital
Southampton, UK

John Greenwood MB ChB PhD MRCP
Lecturer in Cardiology
The General Infirmary
Leeds, UK

Diana Holdright MD FRCP MBBS DA BSc
Consultant Cardiologist
The Heart Hospital UCLH
London, UK

Paul Kalra MA MB BChir MRCP
Consultant Cardiologist
Portsmouth Hospitals NHS Trust
Portsmouth, UK

Philip Kalra MB BChir FRCP MD
Consultant Nephrologist
Hope Hospital
Salford, UK

John Kurian MBBS MRCP
Specialist Registrar in Cardiology
The General Infirmary
Leeds, UK

Chee Yee Loong BSc(Hons) MBBS MRCP
Cardiology Fellow
National Heart and Lung Institute
London, UK

Richard Mansfield BSc(Hons) MB ChB MRCP
Consultant Cardiologist
Royal United Hospital
Bath, UK

Gharda Mikhail BSc MD MRCP
Consultant Cardiologist
Central Middlesex Hospital and St Mary's
Hospital
London, UK

Sundip J Patel MB BCh MRCP
Specialist Registrar in Cardiology
Guy's and St Thomas' Hospital
London, UK

Sophie Petersen BA MSc
Senior Researcher
BHF Health Promotion Group
Oxford, UK

Mark Popplestone MB ChB MFOM
Consultant Occupational Physician
British Airways Waterside (HMAG)
Harmondsworth, UK

Henry Purcell MB PhD
Senior Fellow in Cardiology
Royal Brompton Hospital
London, UK

Simon Redwood MD FRCP FACC
Consultant Cardiologist
Guy's and St Thomas' Hospital
London, UK

Paul Roberts MRCP MD
Consultant Cardiologist
Wessex Cardiac Unit
Southampton General Hospital
Southampton, UK

David Russell-Jones MB ChB FRCP
Professor of Diabetes and Endocrinology
Royal Surrey County Hospital
Guildford, UK

Tushar Salukhe BSc MB BS MRCP
Clinical Research Fellow
National Heart Lung Institute
London, UK

Mike Seddon MBBS MA MRCP
Specialist Registrar in Cardiology
North Hampshire Hospitals NHS Trust
Basingstoke, UK

Rajan Sharma BSc(Hons) MRCP
Specialist Registrar in Cardiology
Wessex Cardiac Unit
Southampton General Hospital
Southampton, UK

Rakesh Sharma PhD MRCP
Specialist Registrar in Cardiology
Royal Brompton Hospital
London, UK

Ala'A Eldeen Shurrab MD MRCP
Specialist Registrar in Nephrology
Hope Hospital
Salford, UK

Mike Stewart MB ChB MRCP
Consultant Cardiologist
Portsmouth Hospitals NHS Trust
Portsmouth, UK

Rajesh Thaman MBBS MRCP
Specialist Registrar in Cardiology
The Heart Hospital UCLH
London, UK

Niels Velstrup MD MPhil
Research Fellow in Cardiology
The Heart Hospital UCLH
London, UK

Fiona Walker BM MRCP
Consultant Cardiologist
The Heart Hospital UCLH
London, UK

Claire Way BSc MB ChB MRCPath
Specialist Registrar in Histopathology
Southampton General Hospital
Southampton, UK

Julian R Wright MB ChB MRCP
Specialist Registrar in Nephrology
Hope Hospital
Salford, UK

Arthur Yue MA BM MCh MRCP
Specialist Registrar in Cardiology
Wessex Cardiothoracic Unit
Southampton University Hospital
Southampton, UK

Preface

With perhaps the exception of the Bible and the Complete Works of Shakespeare, no one book can be considered 'all things to all men or women'. This is particularly true in the case of this current text. We have, however, taken 'soundings' from people at various stages of training, as well as the good and the great of cardiology, in order to compile a logical list of clinical topics which might be regarded as a 'must-know' menu. The bread and butter of cardiology, such as the contemporary management of ischaemic heart disease, valvular heart disease, chronic heart failure and arrhythmias, are discussed in detail. Yet we have also included, important frequently encountered clinical scenarios commonly excluded from standard textbooks. These include the often difficult management of patients with cardiovascular disease and co-morbidities such as diabetes, renal and cerebrovascular disease. Since the aim of the book is to assist in the management of patients both in the outpatient setting and during acute presentation, further topics range from fitness to fly and secondary prevention of ischaemic heart disease to the assessment and treatment of aortic dissection and indications for thrombolysis in acute pulmonary embolism.

We have asked the contributors to try and adhere to a structured formula, ending in either frequently asked questions (and answers) or setting out typical cases which will help to reinforce the key messages. A succinct style of presentation is used, incorporating bullet points, tables and multiple figures. The latter is particularly evident in the form of a 'pictionary of grown-up congenital heart disease' which we believe will help demystify many aspects of this subject. Where relevant we will present some very recent clinical trial data at the end of chapters to bring the reader as up to date as possible. A detailed list of further reading is also provided.

Our book does not seek to follow any formal training protocols, either in the UK or elsewhere; rather it is designed to provide the reader with a comprehensive but not exhaustive review of diagnostic and treatment strategies. While the book is primarily written with the needs of the specialist registrar in mind (for both those pursuing a career in cardiology and those with continued involvement in the management of general medical patients), we believe that it will also prove to be invaluable for all professionals (doctors, nurses and students alike) with an interest in cardiology, whether based in primary or secondary care. The contributors have provided key information to satisfy those in need of immediate and succinct advice, while the editors have attempted to present this information in a consistent and comprehensive format. We hope that both objectives have been achieved. We look forward to feedback from readers in an effort to build on and improve future editions.

Henry J Purcell
Paul R Kalra
2005

Foreword

Cardiology is a fascinating discipline, both elegant and exciting. It combines the excitement of intellectual stimulation and the satisfaction of achieving worthwhile outcomes of prevention of death and disability. More than any specialist area cardiology has seen the development and adoption of major life-saving treatments become everyday practice. What is now taught to cardiology trainees was unthought of or even contra-indicated a decade ago. At the same time the need for specialist cardiologists has grown at a prodigious rate. This approachable and yet authoritative guide will help cardiology and general internal medicine trainees through the specialist registrar years and beyond as it introduces up-to-date concepts with a practical and relevant style.

Henry Purcell and Paul Kalra have done a superb job in distilling modern cardiology into a readable and enjoyable text. Each chapter is supplemented by frequently asked questions and model answers that reflect the current state of knowledge which are up to the minute despite the pace of new trial evidence coming in. The book can be recommended as highly relevant to practising trainees in cardiology and general medicine in the United Kingdom and elsewhere over the next few years. As for any specialist guide, it is important for any reader to check the date of their edition and appreciate that a particular section may include time limited information. This will necessitate regular revised editions.

The textbook comprehensively covers manifestations of atherosclerotic heart disease and includes the major clinical complications of myocardial dysfunction, chronic heart failure, angina and acute coronary syndromes. In addition, there are very practical chapters reviewing conventional investigations and their interpretation, use, value and limitations. These include echocardiography, nuclear imaging, cardiac magnetic resonance and computed tomography, as well as sophisticated tests of exercise physiology. A further chapter demonstrates a novel and interesting approach to cardiovascular disease management with a systematic review of biomarkers. As little as five years ago such a review would not have reached any textbook. Other important clinical conditions and presentations are not neglected. These include electrophysiolology and arrhythmias, hypertension, grown-up congenital heart disease as well as rarer but important cardiovascular conditions that practising specialists and registrars will encounter, such as aortic dissection, pulmonary embolism and pulmonary hypertension.

There is a timely inclusion of other sections covering major disease processes the cardiologist does not primarily investigate or manage, i.e. those of the renal patient, the cerebrovascular patient and the endocrine patient, with particular emphasis on the diabetic. There is increasing overlap between these conditions and classical cardiology practice and it is important that cardiologists understand advances in these disciplines. These chapters go some considerable way to redressing this balance. One hopes that our fellow specialists in these other areas of renal disease/medicine and rehabilitation and endocrinology and diabetes have an equal understanding of the major pace of advances in cardiology.

Professor Andrew Coats, MA, DM, FRACP, FRCP, FACC, FESC, FAHA, MBA
Dean, Faculty of Medicine, University of Sydney, NSW, 2006, Australia.
Formerly Professor of Clinical Cardiology, National Heart and Lung Institute, Imperial College and Director of Cardiology, Royal Brompton Hospital, London, UK

2005

Acknowledgements

We particularly want to thank all of our friends and colleagues who gave their time so readily to the project, and to Timothy Horne and Clive Hewat at Elsevier. We also want to acknowledge the great patience and encouragement from our wives, Sian and Kate, throughout the project.

Dr Greenwood and Dr Kurian would like to thank Gill Warton, Senior Chief Cardiac Physiologist, Leeds General Infirmary, UK, for providing the echocardiographic figures in Chapter 11.

Dr Dayer would like to acknowledge the help of Dr Mary Sheppard, Consultant Histopathologist; Dr Michael Henein, Consultant Cardiologist; and Dr Raad Mohiaddin, Consultant and Clinical Senior Lecturer from the Royal Brompton Hospital in preparation of Chapter 17.

Dr Ghada Mikhail would like to acknowledge the help of Dr Margaret Burke, Consultant Histopathologist at the Royal Brompton and Harefield NHS Trust, in providing Figure 19.1

Dr Elkington would like to thank Dr James Moon, Dr Sanjay Prasad, and Dr Michael Rubins for their contribution of images for Chapter 7.

Cardiovascular disease epidemiology

1

H. Purcell, C. Daly and S. Petersen

INTRODUCTION

Epidemiology is the study of disease in defined populations. This chapter focuses on the epidemiology of cardiovascular disease, with particular reference to the compilation of statistics, observation and explanation of geographical and temporal trends, and the emerging challenges from a global perspective. We will review some of the key data on the prevalence (total number of cases of the disease in a specified population at a given time) and the incidence (number of new cases that develop over a specified time span, e.g. a year) of cardiovascular diseases in the UK as compared to other parts of Europe and the USA. Accordingly, we will mainly restrict our comments to mortality and morbidity from angina, myocardial infarction (MI), coronary heart disease (CHD), heart failure, and stroke.

The aetiology of atherothrombotic cardiovascular disease is multi-factorial, and several 'risk factors' are recognized to predispose an individual to develop the disease. These cardiovascular risk factors, which were initially characterized in the Framingham Heart Study, include: age, family history of premature cardiovascular disease, smoking, hypertension, hyperlipidaemia, diabetes, obesity and sedentary lifestyle (reviewed in detail in Ch. 3). Although a family history of cardiovascular disease is a recognized risk factor, it is important to emphasize that cardiovascular disease is polygenic and numerous genetic abnormalities have been implicated in the development of the final common disease state. Furthermore, expression of disease is often closely linked to environmental risk factors such as smoking, diet and physical inactivity. In addition, the disease does not present until middle age, or later, in most cases. Clearly, therefore, the 'burden of disease' in a population is strongly associated with the prevalence of recognized risk factors within that population. Incidence and prevalence rates for cardiovascular diseases depend to a large extent on the age profile of the population, socio-economic, dietary and other lifestyle patterns; although other influences, including genetic differences influenced by ethnicity, are also important.

AGEING POPULATIONS AND DISEASE BURDEN

Amongst developed countries, the Japanese and the Swedes have the greatest life expectancy, but, indeed, among almost all developed countries there has been a progressive prolongation of life expectancy. The population of the UK is currently estimated to be 58 836 700 and in those born in the year 2000, life expectancy in males is 75 years and in females 80 years.[1] This increase in life expectancy has a potent effect on the population age profile of the developed nations. For example, in 1940, 6.8% of the American population were over the age of 65 years, but by 1999, this proportion had almost doubled to 12.7%. This is projected to rise to 20.5% by 2040.[2] As cardiovascular disease morbidity and mortality peaks in the latter decades of life, such increases in lifespan have already had considerable impact on the burden of cardiovascular illness, and are set to increase the burden even further in the years to come.

Although the developing countries lag behind considerably in life-expectancy ranking, e.g. there is a gap of more than 51 years between the highest life expectancy among Japanese women (84.3 years) and the life expectancy of men in Sierra Leone (33.2 years), the numbers are distorted somewhat by the tragic toll of infectious diseases, such as from HIV/AIDS in sub-Saharan Africa. Unfortunately, however, cardiovascular disease is in the ascendancy in many African and other developing populations, and is likely to become a significant problem in the decades to come; this will be discussed later.

DATA COLLECTION

According to Benjamin Franklin: '…in this world nothing can be said to be certain, except death and taxes.' Certainly, information on cardiovascular mortality can be obtained from the centralized recording of death certification. However, the quality of this mortality data is heavily dependent on the accurate recording of cause of death on the death certificate, which is rarely confirmed by post-mortem. There is considerable variability both within and between countries in recording deaths from MI. The compilation of accurate information on the numbers of non-fatal MIs in a population is even more difficult, and numbers may be underestimated for a variety of reasons as we shall discuss.

There is no single definitive source for health statistics. In the UK we are well served by the British Heart Foundation (BHF) Health Promotion Research Group at the Department of Public Health University of Oxford, who compile the BHF coronary heart disease statistics publications and website (www.heartstats.org). This provides statistics related to the prevalence, incidence, causes and treatment of cardiovascular disease in the UK.

Similar data are published in the USA by the American Heart Association based on a comprehensive range of sources, including the National Center for Health Statistics, and National Heart, Lung and Blood Institute. Yearly nationwide health examinations are not conducted to count exact numbers of individuals with medical conditions, but rather periodic surveys, conducted by governmental, international, or other agencies form the basis for specific disease rates. These rates are applied for several years as the population changes until new reliable survey rates are available.

In the USA the National Heart, Lung and Blood Institute's Framingham Heart Study,[2] which began in 1948, is the world's longest-running comprehensive prospective cardiovascular survey, and has now been joined by numerous others including Atherosclerosis Risk in Community (ARIC), the Physician's Health Study (PHS) and the Lipid Clinics Research Programme, to mention but a few.

Studies throughout Europe are co-ordinated by the World Health Organization (WHO) and the European Society of Cardiology (ESC) in the European registry of Cardiovascular Diseases and Patient Management, which draws on national databases. WHO's Monitoring Trends and Determinants in Cardiovascular Disease (MONICA) project monitored CHD trends across 37 populations in 21 countries over a decade between the mid-1980s and the mid-1990s.

In 1999, the ESC launched the Euro Heart Survey Programme, a series of systematic surveys designed to collect detailed cross-sectional and prospective information on large samples of patients (4500–13 000 per survey). It will provide quantitative information on the prevalence and incidence of cardiovascular diseases amongst patient-based populations and on methods of patient management. In addition to the Euro Heart surveys of secondary prevention, heart failure, acute coronary syndromes, valvular heart disease and coronary revascularization, which have already been completed, the Euro Heart survey on angina will be completed by the end of 2002 with a 1-year follow up at the end of 2003. Further surveys are planned for 2003/4 and include diabetes and the heart, congenital heart disease and cardiomyopathy and atrial fibrillation.

UK DATA SOURCES

A number of sources of demographic data are available, most notably the Office of National Statistics (ONS) (www.statistics.gov.uk) who publish mortality and population data for England and Wales. Demographic data for Scotland are available from the General Register Office, and for Northern Ireland from the Northern Ireland Statistics and Research Agency, as well as the BHF coronary heart disease statistics publications (www.heartstats.org). Prevalence estimates for CHD, angina, MI and heart failure are also available from the BHF coronary heart disease website. These are derived from population-based studies rather than patient-based data sources, such as Hospital Episode Statistics. In contrast to the US system of data collection, incidence figures for these conditions are similarly drawn from population-based studies rather than from hospital-based statistics, as there are significant concerns about the quality of data collection.

BHF prevalence estimates for CHD, angina and MI, are largely based on data from the Health Survey for England (HSE). This is an annual household survey of around 15 000 respondants, a stratified random sample of adults in England who are socio-demographically representative of the population. The annual response rate is about 78% overall, although slightly lower among men in inner cities.

The British Regional Heart Study (BRHS) (www.ucl.ac.uk/primcare-popsci/brhs) is a prospective study of middle-aged men drawn from general practices in 24 British towns. The study commenced in 1980 and has followed almost 8000 middle-aged men drawn at random from one general practice in each of the 24 towns in England, Scotland and Wales. It continues to follow-up these men, now aged 62–83 years, and has become a valuable resource for research into the cardiovascular health status of elderly men. More recently, a team from Bristol has recruited a cohort of women from the same 24 towns to match in age the current cohort of men and will follow them in the British Women's Heart and Health Study (http://www.epi.bris.ac.uk/bwhhs/).

GEOGRAPHIC AND TEMPORAL TRENDS: CORONARY HEART DISEASE LEAGUE TABLES

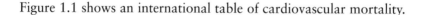

Figure 1.1 shows an international table of cardiovascular mortality.

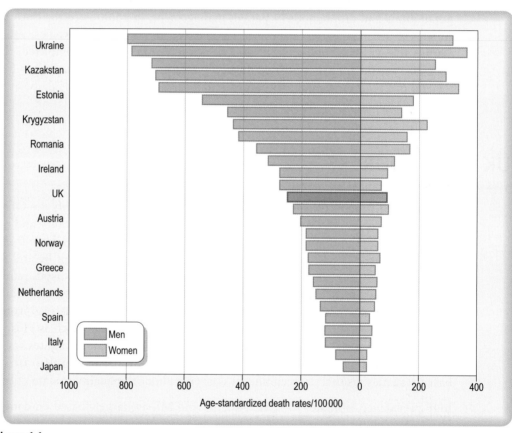

Figure 1.1
Death rates from coronary heart disease, men and women aged 35–74 years, 1999, selected countries (With permission from Petersen S, Peto V, Rayner M 2004: Coronary heart disease statistics. British Heart Foundation, London)

CHD deaths have been falling in some, but not all, industrialized countries since the early 1970s. In the UK, for example, CHD mortality has declined by more than 50% over the past 30 years, and the downward trend is continuing.[3] The scale of decline has been even greater in the USA and Australia. The explanations for these declines are controversial. Some have attributed it to reductions in the major cardiovascular risk factors, while others attribute it to the increasingly widespread use of thrombolysis, aspirin, ACE inhibitors and, more recently, statins. In England and Wales it has been estimated that 58% of the fall of CHD mortality between 1981 and 2000 was due to reductions in major risk factors, principally smoking. Treatments to individuals, including secondary prevention, explained the remaining 42% of the mortality decline.[4] While dramatic declines in CHD death rates in Finland (1972–1992) have been ascribed to risk-factor reduction, a similar analysis of the fall in CHD mortality rate in Auckland, New Zealand suggests that approximately half is due to medical therapies and half to risk-factor reductions.[5] The MONICA project concluded that two-thirds of the decline in coronary mortality in their study populations was due to the decline in coronary events (that is to improvements of risk factors) and one-third was due to a decline in case fatality (i.e. to improvements in treatment).[6]

The decline in coronary disease mortality has not been universal. There is huge variability in cardiovascular disease (CVD) rates throughout Europe (see Ch. 3) and a 'mortality crisis' has emerged among the newly independent states (NIS), where CVD causes well over half of all deaths, and an individual is four times more likely to die prematurely of CVD than their counterpart in Western Europe. Reasons for this will not be reviewed here, but include dramatic increases in prevalence of cardiovascular risk factors (especially smoking, poor nutrition and adverse socio-economic factors). Of equal concern is the observation that CVD, of which CHD, cerebrovascular disease and peripheral vascular disease comprise the greatest part, is the commonest cause of deaths worldwide and the main risk factors, traditionally linked to the affluent lifestyle, are now being seen in middle-income and poorer countries.

By 2010 CVD is estimated to be the leading cause of death in developing countries. This has been recently highlighted by the identification of high blood pressure, tobacco and high cholesterol as major contributors to the disease burden in developing countries, as well as in the developed world. In some developing countries an interesting paradox is seen with malnutrition and obesity competing for joint fourth position as a contributor to the overall burden of disease.[7] (To review 'the impending global epidemic of cardiovascular diseases' see reference 8 and information from the Harvard School of Public Health's Global Burden of Disease project [www.hsph.harvard.edu/organisations/bdu/summary.html].)

Information on the global distribution of cardiovascular risk factors and their impact on development of disease have potentially huge public health and treatment implications. In the recent WHO World Health Report,[9] it was suggested that if individuals at high cardiovascular risk were treated with a statin, antihypertensive and aspirin, it would be possible to cut worldwide annual cardiovascular deaths by 50%.

CARDIOVASCULAR AND CORONARY HEART DISEASE MORTALITY

CVD includes all diseases of the heart and circulatory system, thus encompassing heart failure, congenital heart disease, primary arrhythmias, rheumatic and other less common forms of heart disease, as well as the manifestations of atherosclerosis. However, it is atherosclerotic CVD that has the greatest effect on mortality rates because of the large number of individuals affected. According to WHO almost 17 million people die per annum of CVD worldwide. 7.2 million people died of heart disease and 5.5 million of stroke in 2001. Diseases of the heart, including CHD represent about three-quarters of total CVD mortality.

Deaths are attributed to CHD based on the information on the death certificate, which is classified in accordance with the International Classification of Diseases (ICD). These are revised periodically (every 9–10 years) to reflect changes in diagnostic advances. Revisions in the ICD occurred with ICD10 in 1999, giving CHD a broader definition. In the USA this change in coding practice was reflected in an increase in the number of deaths classified as due to CHD, from 459 841 in 1998 to 529 659 in 1999.[10]

MI or heart attack remains the single largest killer of men and women in the USA compared with other circulatory/CVDs (see Fig. 1.2).

In Europe, CVDs cause nearly one-half of all deaths throughout the 49 countries with reliable mortality data. This represents 4 million deaths annually in Europe and over

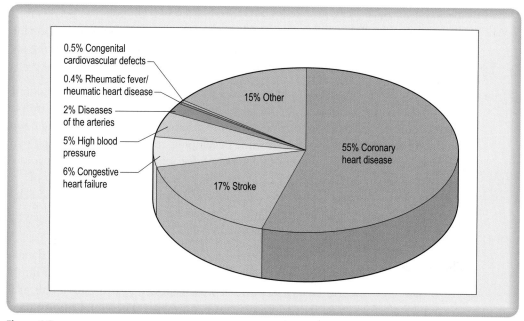

Figure 1.2
Percentage breakdown of deaths from cardiovascular disease (US 1999). From CDS/NCHS and the American Heart Association

1.5 million annually in the European Union (EU), CHD by itself is the most common cause of death, accounting for nearly 2 million deaths in Europe (over 600 000 in the EU) each year.[11]

CVD is also the main cause of death in the UK, accounting for just under 240 000 deaths annually. About one-half of all cardiovascular deaths are from CHD and one-quarter from stroke. There are around 120 000 CHD deaths per year, i.e. more than one in five men and one in six women dying from the disease. CHD is the most common cause of premature death, causing 22% of deaths in men under 75 and 13% of deaths in women under 75 in the UK.[3]

CHD death rates have been falling in the UK since the late 1970s. For people under 75 years, they have fallen by 36% in the last 10 years. However, the overall decline is not as rapid as in some other countries, and there are still huge regional and socio-economic differences in mortality. For example, premature mortality from CHD in men is 50% higher in Scotland than in the South West of England, and around 90% higher in women. Premature death rates are 58% higher for manual compared to non-manual workers. There are also large ethnic differences, for example mortality is about 50% higher in South Asians living in the UK compared to the general population.[3]

NON-FATAL MYOCARDIAL INFARCTION

In round figures, there are an estimated 1.5 million MIs annually in the USA, and about one-third of these result in death (one-half within 1 month of the heart attack). Comparable morbidity data are not recorded on a countrywide basis throughout Europe, however, data from the MONICA project show that the incidence of coronary events is higher in MONICA populations in Northern, Central and Eastern Europe compared to Southern and Western Europe. The pattern of incidence rates is similar to the geographical pattern of CHD mortality.

There were an estimated 268 000 MIs in the UK in 2002.[3] It is possible that between 20 and 25% of individuals who suffer MI have a history of angina pectoris.

Current estimates of the prevalence of MI are, however, limited and do not include unrecognized or 'clinically silent' MI. Such events, first described by Herrick in 1912, represent a significant proportion of all MIs. The Framingham Study suggests that they may represent between 26% and 34% of all MIs in men and women respectively.[12] Elderly and diabetic patients are more prone to suffer unrecognized events.

The new definition of MI, which is to include all troponin-positive patients (Ch. 8), is likely to significantly increase the numbers of MIs recorded, and pose considerable problems over the coming years until diagnostic capabilities between hospitals are standardized. It will also mean comparisons of event rates over time will become increasingly difficult.

ANGINA PECTORIS

The compilation of incidence and prevalence data for angina in the population is an even more difficult task. It is often regarded as a 'softer' diagnosis than MI, and diagnostic stringency varies. Overall, numbers tend to be extrapolated from small cohort population surveys. About 6 400 000 of the US population (2.4 million males and 4 million females) have angina,[10] defined as 'chest pain or discomfort' due to coronary insufficiency, with about 400 000 new cases of stable angina and 150 000 cases of unstable angina occurring each year.

In Europe, the same wide variation in angina rates exists as with non-fatal MI. More robust figures will emerge once the Euro Heart Survey on angina reports (see above).

In the UK there are an estimated 1.5–2 million individuals with angina. The incidence of new angina cases is conservatively estimated as 22 600 per annum; this figure is taken from a key study of 110 consecutive patients with typical angina referred to an open-access chest-pain clinic,[13] on which cohort 8-year follow-up prognostic data are now available.[14] Data from Morbidity Statistics from General Practice suggest a more generous estimate of 338 000 new cases per year.[15]

HEART FAILURE

There are an estimated 287 200 heart-failure deaths in the USA annually, with 4 790 000 Americans (2.36 million women and 2.44 million men) currently living with heart failure. Approximately 550 000 new cases occur each year.

Estimates of the prevalence of symptomatic heart failure in the general European population range from 0.4 to 2%, and prevalence increases rapidly with age, with the mean age of onset being 74 years. The ESC represents countries with a total population of 900 million, which suggests that there are at least 10 million patients with heart failure in those countries.

In the UK it is estimated that there are about 892 000 individuals with definite or probable heart failure (489 000 men and 403 000 women).[3] There are an estimated 63 500 new cases annually. Just under 40% of cases die within a year of diagnosis, and it is estimated that at least 4% of all deaths in the UK are due to heart failure.[15]

A recent publication from the Framingham study is the first to suggest a decrease in the incidence of heart failure, but confirms previous reports of improvements in survival. However, the observed decrease in incidence (among women) is modest in comparison to the increase in the proportion of the population over 65 years who are at increased risk of heart failure, so the 'heart failure epidemic' is set to continue as the prevalence increases.[15]

STROKE

When considered separately from other cardiovascular diseases, stroke ranks as the third leading cause of death in many developed countries. In the USA, stroke killed over 167 000 people in 1996 (around 1 in every 14 deaths). Each year 600 000 Americans suffer a new or recurrent stroke – half a million of these are first strokes and 100 000 are recurrent attacks. About 4 600 000 stroke survivors are alive today.[10]

Of the 4 million cardiovascular deaths in Europe annually, nearly one-third are from stroke, accounting for 1.5 million years of life lost per year.

In the UK stroke rates have been falling but this has slowed in recent years, particularly in those aged under 65 years. In the UK there were over 67 000 deaths from stroke in 2002. Each year, in the UK, approximately 110 000 patients experience a first stroke and 30 000 suffer a recurrent stroke. The incidence of strokes rises from 2/1000/year in the 55–64 age group to 20/1000/year in those aged 85 years and over. Stroke is responsible for 11% of all deaths in the UK and is the commonest cause of severe adult disability. Stroke prevalence is estimated to be approximately 5–7/1000, of whom at least 50% are disabled (see www.leedsstrokedatabase.net/strokensf.htm).

References

1. Office of National Statistics 2002 Census 2001 First results on population for England and Wales. Office of National Statistics, London (www.statistics.gov.uk)
2. Census Bureau 2002 National population projections. Census Bureau, Washington, DC (www.census.gov/population/www/projections/natproj.html.)
3. Petersen S, Peto V, Rayner M 2004 Coronary heart disease statistics. British Heart Foundation, London (www.heartstats.org)
4. Unal B, Critchley JA, Capewell S 2004 Explaining the decline in coronary heart disease mortality in England and Wales between 1981 and 2000. Circulation 109: 1101–1107
5. Capewell S, Beaglehole R, Seddon M, McMurray J 2000 Explanation for the decline in coronary heart disease mortality rates in Auckland, New Zealand, between 1982 and 1993. Circulation 102: 1511–1516
6. Tunstall-Pedoe H, Kuulasmaa K, Mahonen M, Tolonen H, Ruokokoski E, Amouyel P for the WHO MONICA project 1999 Contribution of trends in survival and coronary-event rates to changes in coronary heart disease mortality: 10 year results from 37 WHO MONICA Project populations. Lancet 353: 1547–1557
7. Ezzati M, Lopez AD, Rodgers A, Vander Hoorn S, Murray CJ 2002 Comparative Risk Assessment Collaborating Group. Selected major risk factors and global and regional burden of disease. Lancet 360 (9343): 1347–1360
8. Ounpuu S, Anand S, Yusuf S 2000 The impending global epidemic of cardiovascular diseases. Eur Heart J 21: 880–883
9. World Health Report 2002 Reducing risks, promoting healthy life. WHO, Geneva
10. American Heart Association 2002 Heart and stroke statistical update. American Heart Association, Dallas, TX
11. Rayner M, Petersen S 2000 European cardiovascular disease statistics. British Heart Foundation, London (www.heartstats.org)
12. Sheifer SE, Manolio TA, Gersh B 2001 Unrecognised myocardial infarction. Ann Intern Med 135: 801–811
13. Gandhi MM, Lampe FC, Wood DA 1995 Incidence, clinical characteristics, and short-term prognosis of angina pectoris. Br Heart J 73: 193–198
14. Gandhi MM, Lampe F, Scantlebury AM, Wood DA 2002 New exertional angina referred to a rapid access chest pain clinic: prospective eight-year follow-up compared with asymptomatic controls. Heart 87 (suppl II): 12
15. Royal College of General Practitioners, the Office of Population Censuses and Surveys, and the Department of Health 1995 Morbidity statistics from General Practice. Fourth National Study. 1991–1992. HMSO, London
16. Jackson G 2002 Hormone replacement therapy and cardiovascular disease: are the cardiovascular benefits established? In: Jackson G (ed.) Cardiology current perspectives. Martin Dunitz, London

SELF-ASSESSMENT

Questions

a. Are there large gender differences in cardiovascular disease rates?

b. Is prognosis different in unrecognized myocardial infarction (MI)?

Answers

a. As a generalization, women live longer than men and they present with heart disease 10 years later than men. The incidence of coronary heart disease (CHD) in women begins to increase after the menopause and increases with age, although the rate of developing heart disease is less in women at any age. Over the age of 60 years the incidence of CHD in women is equal to men but the greater number of older women explains the similar absolute numbers.[16]

b. No. Mortality rates after unrecognized and recognized MI are similar.

Basic cardiac pathophysiology

C. Way and P. Gallagher

INTRODUCTION

Coronary artery disease owing to atherosclerosis and its complications is a leading cause of death in the Western world and in some Asian communities, especially those with a high prevalence of diabetes. In this chapter we summarize significant recent advances in our understanding of the pathology (Box 2.1) of atherosclerosis concentrating on:

- new methods of classifying atheromatous lesions
- the role of disordered immunity and infection in the development of atherosclerosis
- the correlation of clinical events with the underlying morphology of lesions
- how lesions lead to arterial obstruction.

CLINICAL APPLICATIONS OF NEW NOMENCLATURE

The macroscopic and microscopic appearance of atherosclerotic lesions vary considerably. Detailed cross-sectional studies have identified a pattern of progression from the earliest intimal disease (intimal thickenings and fatty streaks), through atheromatous plaques with fibrous caps, to complicated lesions that cause arterial obstruction (Figs 2.1 & 2.2). The American Heart Association (AHA) classification system was developed from these studies and has recently been refined by Virmani and colleagues (Table 2.1).[1-3] These have proved invaluable as research tools and are increasingly used in surgical pathology and post-mortem reports. Classic well-developed atheromatous plaques appear white to yellow and protrude into the lumen of the artery. They are predominantly intimal lesions that consist of a core of lipid covered by a fibrous cap. The fibrous cap is composed of smooth muscle

---

Box 2.1: Important advances in the pathology of atherosclerosis

- A working classification system for atherosclerotic lesions and their precursors has been devised and refined.
- Inflammation and disordered immunity are important underlying mechanisms in the development of atherosclerosis. The role of infection is still debated.
- Plaque erosion and plaque rupture are important causes of the acute coronary syndromes.
- The pathology of stable angina is less clearly defined but arterial remodelling may be important here.

11

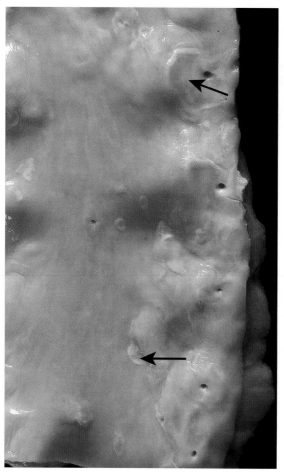

Figure 2.1
Early aortic atherosclerosis. A segment of the thoracic aorta from a middle-aged adult. Note the many linear fatty streaks in the background. Arrows indicate discrete areas of pathological intimal thickening. These would have, at the most, only very small lipid cores

cells (SMCs), leukocytes and dense connective tissue (Fig. 2.3). The shoulder area consists of macrophages, SMCs and T-lymphocytes. The core is a mass of extracellular lipid and lipid-laden foam cells, derived from SMCs and macrophages. In larger lesions, the core may be necrotic. There is usually evidence of neovascularization around the periphery of the plaque, and some lesions show extensive calcium hydroxyapatite deposition. The quantity of SMCs, macrophages, T-lymphocytes, lipid, fibrous tissue and calcium varies greatly between lesions and has a baring on how individual lesions are classified.

PATHOGENESIS: A DISEASE OF DISORDERED IMMUNITY

Although the cause of atherosclerosis is not known, numerous risk factors have been identified. The strongest of these are increasing age, male gender, raised serum cholesterol,

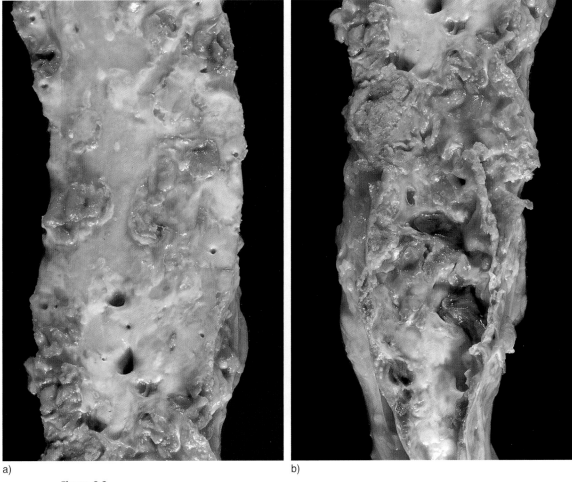

a)   b)

Figure 2.2
Advanced aortic atherosclerosis in an elderly female. (a) From the lower thoracic and upper abdominal
aorta and (b) from the lower abdominal. There is overlap between the two photographs at the level of
the superior mesenteric artery. These show the typical pattern of progression of atherosclerosis from
proximal to distal aorta. There are some fibrous cap atheromas that are unruptured, especially in the
thoracic aorta. In the lower abdominal aorta many have ruptured and thrombosed. These large masses of
thrombus can be dislodged during intra-aortic instrumentation. It is surprising that clinical consequences
are not more common

Table 2.1: The Modified AHA Classification System for atheromatous lesions and their precursors

Lesion	Description	Clinical/comment
Non-atherosclerotic intimal lesions		
Intimal thickening	Accumulation of SMCs in the intima in the absence of lipid or macrophage foam cells	First decade of life. Clinically silent. No thrombus
Intimal xanthoma	Fatty dot or fatty streak. Accumulation of foam cells without a necrotic core or fibrous cap.	*(continued overleaf)*

Table 2.1: (Cont'd) The Modified AHA Classification System for atheromatous lesions and their precursors

Lesion	Description	Clinical/comment
Progressive atherosclerotic lesions		
Pathological intimal thickening	Extracellular lipid beneath SMCs and macrophages. Poorly formed fibrous cap. No necrotic core.	Develop after puberty, clinically silent No thrombus
– erosion	Plaque as above with luminal thrombosis	Thrombus mostly mural and infrequently occlusive
Fibrous cap atheroma	Necrotic fatty core with overlying fibrous cap	Develop from third decade. May be clinically overt. Thrombus absent.
– erosion	Plaque as above with luminal thrombus No communication between thrombus and necrotic core	Thrombus mostly mural and infrequently occlusive
Thin fibrous cap atheroma	Thin cap infiltrated by macrophages and lymphocytes with reduced SMCs and an underlying necrotic core	Thrombus absent, but prone to plaque rupture
– plaque rupture	Plaque as above with cap disruption Communication between thrombus and necrotic core	Thrombus often occlusive if fatal, non-occlusive if silent
Calcified nodule	Eruptive nodular calcification with underlying fibrocalcific plaque	Possibly associated with healed plaque ruptures. Often found in mid-right coronary artery, infrequent cause of thrombosis without plaque rupture. Thrombus usually non-occlusive
Fibrocalcific plaque	Collagen-rich plaque with large areas of calcification. Necrotic core if present is small. Significant stenosis	Thrombus absent. May be clinically overt. Possibly the end stage of atheroma rupture/erosion and healing with calcification

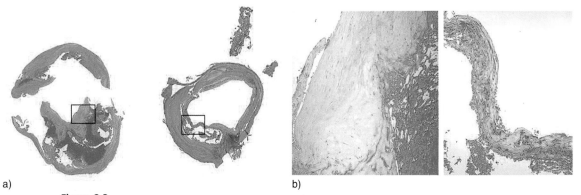

a)   b)

Figure 2.3
Microphotographs of fibrous cap atheromas. The boxed areas in (a) are magnified in (b). The fibrous cap in the left panels measures 350 µm and is free of inflammatory cells. This is, therefore, a thick fibrous cap atheroma. In contrast, the cap in the right panel measures <150 µm and is infiltrated by macrophages and lymphocytes (thin fibrous cap atheroma)

diabetes, hypertension, cigarette smoking, and a family history, independent of traits for hyperlipidaemia. The most important recent advance in our understanding of the pathogenesis is the growing evidence that inflammation and disordered immunity plays an important role in the development of lesions. Endothelial cells in early atherosclerotic lesions express selective adhesion molecules that bind certain classes of leukocytes. Hyperlipidaemia and haemodynamic stress may be a stimulus for this[4,5] and could explain why particular sites in the vascular tree are prone to the development of plaques. It is possible that other agents such as microorganisms (see below), products in cigarette smoke and abnormally glycosylated proteins may also induce endothelial dysfunction. Adherent leukocytes migrate into the intima where they express, or induce, other leukocytes or mesenchymal cells to express proinflammatory cytokines and chemokines. These have an important role in the perpetuation of the inflammatory process and the development of the plaque. Low-density lipoproteins (LDL) accumulate in the subendothelium but toxic oxygen species produced by activated intraplaque macrophages transform them into oxidized LDL. This modified LDL has a number of effects that together act to perpetuate the inflammatory process. Macrophages that express the scavenger receptor are able to ingest the modified LDL to become foam cells, key constituents of the atheromatous plaque. Despite much research in this area, the mechanism by which lipids become localized to the subendothelium is not known. It appears, however, that lipid accumulation precedes increases in the number of smooth muscle cells and macrophages within intimal masses.[6] SMCs are thought to have multiple roles in atherosclerotic lesions. Under the influence of inflammatory mediators, they migrate from the media into the intima where they proliferate and acquire a secretory phenotype, producing extracellular matrix molecules in an attempt to repair the damage induced by the inflammatory process. This results in the formation of the fibrous cap.

The role of infection and disordered immunity in the pathogenesis of atherosclerosis is one of the most active areas of recent research. There is strong epidemiological evidence of an association between extent of coronary artery atherosclerosis and infection by certain intracellular pathogens such as cytomegalovirus, herpes simplex virus (HSV-1), hepatitis A virus (HAV), *Helicobacter pylori*, *Chlamydia pneumoniae* and *Porphyromonas gingivalis*.[7–11] Several studies suggest that the presence of multiple pathogens (total pathogen burden) may be a stronger marker of risk than any individual infection alone.[12–13] It has been proposed that infections contribute to atherogenesis by inducing endothelial dysfunction and/or a proinflammatory effect on the vessel wall that is initiated at a local or systemic level. However, despite this strong epidemiological evidence it is not known whether this is a causal association or the result of a secondary variable, such as smoking. A causal role is supported by investigations that have demonstrated the ability of infectious agents to evoke cellular and molecular changes comparable to those seen in atherogenesis.[14–17] Studies that have demonstrated that lymphocytes derived from atheromatous plaques proliferate after exposure to bacterial antigens are of particular interest.[18]

DIFFERENT UNDERLYING PATHOLOGY OF DIFFERENT CLINICAL SYNDROMES

It is difficult for pathologists to explain why some patients with coronary narrowing have stable angina whereas others with a similar pattern of disease are symptom free. This is an area of research that has been largely ignored, as most recent studies have concentrated on the changes in patients with acute coronary syndromes or established myocardial infarction (Table 2.2).

REDUCTION IN BLOOD FLOW THROUGH THE ARTERIES

In the coronary arteries, enlarging atherosclerotic plaques may significantly reduce the size of the lumen leading to diminished coronary perfusion. If there is more than 75% reduction in luminal cross-sectional area, even moderate increases in myocardial demand cannot be met, resulting in myocardial ischaemia and the clinical syndrome of stable angina. However, not all enlarging atherosclerotic plaques are associated with development of luminal stenosis. The cross-sectional area of the coronary artery may increase to accommodate the plaque without any reduction in the cross-sectional area of the lumen.[19,20] This process is called 'positive remodelling', and is more often seen in eccentric plaques. The term 'negative remodelling' is applied when the development of a

Table 2.2: Pathology of stable angina and the acute coronary syndromes

	Coronary artery pathology	Clinocopathological comment
Stable angina	Atherosclerotic lesion with smooth outlines and minimal inflammation causing >75% reduction in luminal cross-sectional area Most significant lesions are concentric	Slowly enlarging lesions, not associated with plaque rupture, plaque erosion or development of acute thrombi Few recent studies of the pathology of stable angina
Unstable angina	Irregular atherosclerotic lesion complicated by plaque rupture or plaque erosion usually with development of acute thrombi	Acute, and probably progressive, reduction in luminal cross-sectional area It is presumed that anti-thrombotic therapy retards further thrombus formation
Acute myocardial infarct	Atherosclerotic lesions complicated by plaque rupture or erosion with development of acute thrombi or, rarely, intraplaque haemorrhage resulting in occlusion of coronary artery	Acute occlusion of coronary artery Underlying culprit atherosclerotic lesions may have caused only limited stenosis before rupture Thrombi partially, but not completely, lysed by thrombolytic therapy
Sudden death	Atherosclerotic lesion causing >75% reduction in luminal cross-sectonal area (<1 mm diameter at post-mortem) Acute thrombi identified in ~50% of cases	Healed or acute myocardial infarct in a proportion of cases In absence of significant atherosclerosis the many other causes of sudden death must be excluded

plaque is associated with an overall reduction in the cross-sectional area of the artery, over and above that caused by the lesion itself (Fig. 2.4). Negative remodelling is more often associated with concentric plaques. The development of a coronary stenosis is, therefore, dependent on the balance between plaque growth and the process of remodelling.

THROMBUS FORMATION

Acute coronary thrombosis can be precipitated by plaque rupture, plaque erosion or, occasionally, the rupture of a heavily calcified atheromatous mass.[3] In all cases, thrombogenic substances become exposed to the luminal blood, leading to platelet accumulation and activation. The coagulation cascade is activated, resulting in thrombin formation and fibrin deposition. Thrombin induces further platelet recruitment. Microscopically the thrombus consists of alternating pale layers of platelets and fibrin with red blood cells. When Zahn described these laminations in Geneva in the 19th century, he could have had no idea of the importance that they would assume 100 years

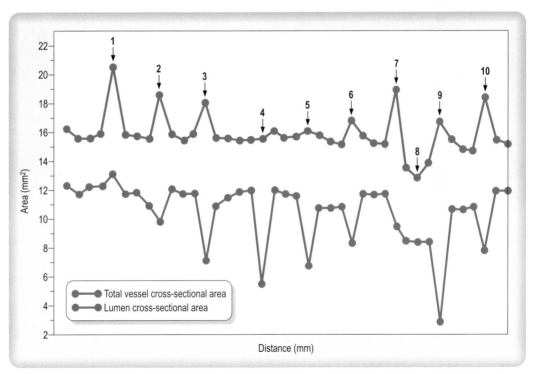

Figure 2.4
In this experiment, the cross-sectional area of the wall of a coronary artery (upper line) and the corresponding area of the lumen (lower line) was calculated from histological sections taken at regular intervals throughout its length. The numbers refer to individual atheromatous lesions. Note that some plaques cause a considerable increase in the size of the vessel wall but do not reduce the size of the lumen (e.g. lesions 1 and 7). This is positive remodelling. In contrast, other plaques cause less enlargement of the vessel wall but significant reduction in the size of the lumen (e.g. lesions 4 and 9). This is negative remodelling. With permission from Varnava A. Coronary artery remodelling. Heart 1998; 79: 109–110

later. Thrombolytic therapy causes breakdown of the fibrinous component of a thrombus but has no significant effect on the clumped masses of platelets.

Plaque rupture

Acutely ruptured plaques are characterized by an interrupted fibrous cap and a luminal thrombus that lies in continuity with the necrotic core (Fig. 2.5). Tissue factor, which is overexpressed by lipid-laden macrophages in the core of atherosclerotic lesions, appears to be responsible for the thrombogenicity of ruptured plaques. Partial luminal occlusion

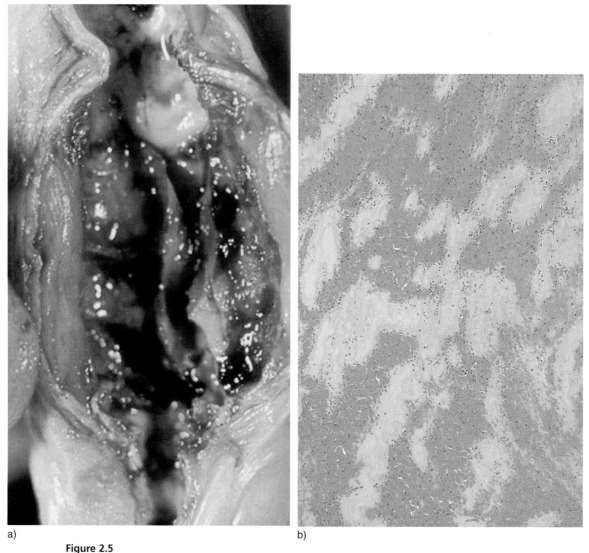

a)   b)

Figure 2.5
(a) Coronary artery thrombosis due to plaque rupture. A mass of thrombus occludes the lumen. Yellow material is plaque lipid. The microphotograph (b) is thrombus. Note the alternating layers of platelet masses (light pink) and fibrin with enmeshed red cells (dark red)

by a thrombus is associated with the development of unstable angina, while complete occlusion is associated with development of myocardial infarction or sudden death. There is also good evidence that plaque rupture can occur silently without causing symptoms and that repeated episodes of rupture followed by healing may be an important mechanism of increased luminal narrowing.[21] The fibrous cap appears to have a fundamental role in maintaining plaque integrity. Evidence indicates that the plaques most vulnerable to rupture are those with large lipid cores and thin fibrous caps containing large numbers of inflammatory cells (macrophages and T-cells) and relatively few SMCs.[22] In plaques with large lipid cores, haemodynamic stresses across the arterial wall during systole become concentrated on the fibrous cap, rendering it more vulnerable to disruption.[23,24] Plaques with large numbers of inflammatory cells are vulnerable for several reasons. Certain T-cell-derived signals incite intraplaque macrophages to secrete metalloproteinases that degrade the fibrous cap.[25,26] T-cells and macrophages can also release mediators that may inhibit SMC proliferation and collagen synthesis, and even induce them to undergo apoptosis.[27,28] Plaque composition may be more important than degree of stenosis in determining development of the acute coronary syndromes and, indeed, plaque rupture is often evident at sites of only modest luminal narrowing. One recent study indicates that plaques associated with positive remodelling are more vulnerable to rupture, which is possibly related to their higher lipid content and macrophage count.[29]

Van der Wal and colleagues (1998) demonstrated that culprit lesions of patients with unstable angina and myocardial infarction show increased numbers of IL-2R-positive T-cells, indicating that recent activation of the immune response within vulnerable plaques may play a key role in acute destablization of plaques and the development of the acute coronary syndromes.[30] This is supported by several population-based studies, which have shown that serum markers of inflammation in patients with unstable angina are raised when compared to patients with stable angina and controls.[31,32] A link between raised serum inflammatory markers and future cardiovascular events has also been demonstrated, supporting the notion that the inflammation is the cause rather than the effect of plaque rupture.[33]

Plaque erosion

This important mechanism of inducing thrombus formation has been discovered relatively recently. Plaque erosions are characterized by absence of endothelium and non-continuity between the thrombus and the core. In one study, the hearts of 685 patients with acute myocardial infarction were examined, and plaque erosion was found to underly one-quarter of the 291 thrombi identified.[34] There is a significantly higher prevalence of plaque erosion in women and individuals less than 50 years of age.[35,36] Eroded plaques are more commonly eccentric, usually have an abundance of smooth muscle cells and proteoglycans, and compared with ruptured plaques contain relatively little lipid and few inflammatory cells. However, as with plaque rupture, inflammation may be important in the pathogenesis of plaque erosion and repeated sub-clinical episodes of erosion may contribute to plaque growth.[37]

References

1. Stary HC, Chandler AB, Glagov S et al. 1994 A definition of initial, fatty streak, and intermediate lesions of atherosclerosis: a report from the Committee on Vascular Lesions of the Council on Atherosclerosis, American Heart Association. Arterioscler Thromb Vasc Biol 14: 840–856

2. Stary HC, Chandler AB, Dinsmore RE et al. 1995 A definition of advanced types of atherosclerotic lesions and a histological classification of atherosclerosis: a report from the Committee on Vascular Lesions of the Council on Atherosclerosis, American Heart Association. Arterioscler Thromb Vasc Biol 15: 1512–1531

3. Virmani R, Kolodgie FD, Burke AP et al. 2000 Lessons from sudden coronary death: A comprehensive morphological classification scheme for atherosclerotic lesions. Arterioscler Thromb Vasc Biol 20: 1262–1275

4. Kim DN, Schmee J, Lee KT et al. 1985 Atherosclerotic lesions in the coronary arteries of hyperlipidaemic swine, part 1: cell increases, divisions, losses and cells of origin in first 90 days on diet. Atherosclerosis 56: 169–188

5. Li H, Cybulsky MI, Gimbrone MA Jr et al. 1993 An athergenic diet rapidly induces VCAM-1, a cytokine regulatable mononuclear leukocyte adhesion molecule, in rabbit endothelium. Arterioscler Thromb Vasc Biol 13: 197–204

6. Nagel T, Resnick N, Atkinson WJ et al. 1994 Shear stress selectively upregulates intercellular adhesion molecule-1 expression in cultured human vascular endothelial cells. J Clin Invest 94: 885–891

7. Siscovick DS, Schwartz SM, Corey L et al. 2000 Chlamydia pneumoniae, herpes simplex virus type 1, and cytomegalovirus and incident myocardial infarction and coronary heart disease death in older adults: the cardiovascular health study. Circulation 102: 2335–2340

8. Zhu J, Quyyumi AA, Norman JE et al. 2000 The possible role of hepatitis A virus in the pathogenesis of atherosclerosis. J Infect Dis 182: 1583–1587

9. Pasceri V, Cammarota G, Patti G et al. 1998 Association of virulent Helicobacter pylori strains with ischaemic heart disease. Circulation 97: 1675–1679

10. Saikku P, Leinonen M, Mattila K et al. 1988 Serological evidence of an association of novel Chlamydia, TWAR, with chronic coronary heart disease and acute myocardial infarction. Lancet 2: 983–986

11. Li L, Messas E, Batista EL Jr et al. 2001 Porphyromonas gingivalis infection accelerates the progression of atherosclerosis in a heterozygous apolipoprotein E-deficient murine model. Circulation 103: 45–51

12. Zhu J, Nieto FJ, Horne BD et al. 2001 Prospective study of pathogen burden and risk of myocardial infarction or death. Circulation 103: 45–51

13. Epsinola-Klein C, Rupprecht HJ, Blankenberg S et al. 2002 Impact of infectious burden on extent and long-term prognosis of atherosclerosis. Circulation 105: 15–21

14. Vercellotti GM 1998 Effects of viral activation of the vessel wall on inflammation and thrombosis. Blood Coagul Fibrinolysis 9: S3–S6

15. Kalayoglu MV, Byrne GI 1998 Induction of macrophage foam cell formation by Chlamydia pneumoniae. J Infect Dis 177: 725–729

16. Zhou YF, Guetta E, Yu ZX et al. 1996 Human cytomegalovirus increases modified low density lipoprotein uptake and scavenger receptor mRNA expression in vascular smooth muscle cells. J Clin Invest 98: 2129–2138

17. Hajjar DP, Pomerantz KB, Falcone DJ et al. 1987 Herpes simplex virus infection in human arterial cells: implications in atherosclerosis. J Clin Invest 80: 1317–1321

18. Mosorin M, Surcel HM, Laurila A et al. 2000 Detection of Chlamydia pneumoniae-reactive T-lymphocytes in human atherosclerotic plaques of carotid artery. Arterioscler Thromb Vasc Biol 20: 1061–1067

19. Glagov S, Welsenberd E, Zarins CV et al. 1987 Compensatory enlargement of human atherosclerotic arteries. N Engl J Med 316: 1371–1375

20. Varnava A 1998 Coronary artery remodelling. Heart 79: 109–110

21. Burke AP, Kolodgie FD, Farb A et al. 2001 Healed plaque ruptures and sudden coronary death. Evidence that subclinical rupture has a role in plaque progression. Circulation 103: 934–940

22. Davies MJ, Richardson PD, Woolf, N et al. 1993 Risk of thrombosis in human atherosclerotic plaques: role of extracellualr lipid, macrophage, and smooth muscle cell content. Br Heart J 69: 377–381

23. Richardson PD, Davis MJ, Born GV 1989 Influence of plaque configuration and stress distribution on fissuring of coronary atherosclerotic plaques. Lancet 2: 941–944

24. Cheng GC, Loree HM, Kamm RD et al. 1993 Distribution of circumferential stress in ruptured and stable atherosclerotic lesions: a structural analysis with histopathological correlation. Circulation 87: 1179–1187

25. Galis ZS, Sukhova GK, Lark MK et al. 1994 Increased expression of matrix metalloproteinases and matrix degrading activity in vulnerable regions of human atherosclerotic plaques. J Clin Invest 94: 2493–2503

26. Nikkari ST, O'Brien KD, Ferguson M et al. 1995 Interstitial collagenase (MMP-1) expression in human carotid atherosclerosis. Circulation 92: 1393–1398

27. Amento EP, Ehsani N, Palmer H et al. 1991 Cytokines and growth factors positively and negatively regulate interstitial collagen gene expression in human vascular smooth muscle cells. Arteriosclerosis and Thrombosis 11: 1223–1230

28. Geng Y-J, Wu Q, Muszynski M et al. 1996 Apoptosis of vascular smooth muscle cells induced by in vitro stimulation with interferon-gamma, tumour necrosis factor-alpha, and interleukin-1-beta. Arterioscler Thromb Vasc Biol 16: 19–27

29. Varnava AM, Mills PG, Davies MJ 2002 Relationship between coronary artery remodelling and plaque vulnerability. Circulation 105: 939–943

30. van der Wal AC, Piek JJ, de Boer OJ et al. 1998 Recent activation of the plaque immune response in coronary lesions underlying acute coronary syndromes. Heart 80: 14–18

31. Berk BC, Weintraub WS, Alexander RW 1990 Elevation of C-reactive protein in 'active' coronary artery disease. Am J Cardiol 65: 168–72

32. Luizzo G, Biasucci LM, Gallimore JR et al. 1994 The prognostic value of C-reactive protein and serum amyloid A protein in severe unstable angina. N Engl J Med 331: 417–424

33. Kannel WB, Wolf PA, Castelli WP, D'Agostino RB 1987 Fibrinogen and risk of cardiovascular disease: the Framington study. JAMA 258: 1183–1186

34. Arbustini E, Dal Bello B, Morbini P et al. 1999 Plaque erosion is a major substrate for coronary thrombosis in acute myocardial infarction. Heart 82: 269–272

35. Farb A, Burke AP, Tang AL et al. 1996 Coronary plaque erosion without rupture into a lipid core. A frequent cause of coronary thrombosis in sudden coronary death. Circulation 93: 1354–1363

36. Burke AP, Farb A, Malcolm GT et al. 1998 Effect of risk factors on the mechanism of acute thrombosis and sudden coronary death in women. Circulation 97: 2110–2116

37. Henriques de Gouveia R, van der Wal AC, van der Loos CM, Becker AE 2002 Sudden unexpected death in young adults. Discrepancies between initiation of acute plaque complications and the onset of acute coronary death. Eur Heart J 23: 1433–1440

Cardiovascular risk factors

3

K. F. Fox

INTRODUCTION

It has been known for some time that coronary heart disease (CHD) is not evenly distributed between and within populations. Many of the **cardiovascular risk factors** that explain this inhomogeneity have also been long recognized. But our ability to intervene to reduce cardiovascular risk is a relatively recent development. Today, primary and secondary prevention of cardiovascular disease forms an equal partnership with symptom control in the practice of cardiology.

RISK FACTORS

Criteria have been established to determine the validity of risk factors. The association between the 'risk factor' and the disease should be strong, graded, independent, consistent, reversible and plausible. A number of cardiovascular risk factors fulfill all or nearly all of these criteria.

Table 3.1 lists the key risk factors that impact upon an individual's likelihood of developing CHD. The simultaneous occurrence of several well-recognized risk factors – abdominal obesity, elevated triglycerides, low high-density lipoprotein (HDL) cholesterol, small dense low-density lipoprotein (LDL) particles, hypertension and insulin resistance – form the 'metabolic syndrome' (also called the insulin-resistance syndrome or syndrome X, this is distinct from the 'syndrome X', which relates to chest pain with normal coronary arteries), which is a particularly atherogenic state.

MULTIFACTORIAL RISK

Epidemiological studies have clearly demonstrated that the risk of a person developing CHD is related to the total burden of risk factors. Thus, a heavy smoker with a low cholesterol and a low blood pressure may be at much lower risk than a moderate smoker with borderline hypertension and a slightly above average cholesterol. Determining priorities for primary prevention decisions is, therefore, based on the overall risk of CHD rather than individual risk factors, i.e. their multifactorial risk.

Table 3.1: Risk factors for the development of coronary heart disease

	Comments
Non-modifiable risk factors	
Age	Strong evidence for increased risk with age
Gender	Strong evidence for reduced risk in pre-menopausal women
Ethnicity	Differences are only partially explained by established risk factors
Family history	Differences are only partially explained by established risk factors
'Modifiable' risk factors	
Diet	'Mediterranean' diet with high intake of fruit and vegetables is protective, saturated fat adverse
Body mass index (BMI)	Increased BMI correlates with CHD risk but waist–hip ratio may be more closely related (centripetal obesity)
Exercise	Increased levels of aerobic exercise are protective
Lifestyle	Evidence for increased risk for 'Type A' personality and lack of control at work
Tobacco consumption	No randomized controlled trials (RCTs) exist, but overwhelming evidence supports a causal association with cigarette consumption and the efficacy of smoking cessation
Alcohol consumption	Low consumption (1–2 units/day) may be protective but excessive consumption is adverse
Hypertension	Essentially linear correlation of CHD risk with blood pressure with RCT evidence for treatment
Hyperlipidaemia	Strong correlation (total cholesterol:HDL cholesterol ratio is most predictive) with RCT evidence for treatment. Small LDL particles and oxidized LDL are particularly atherogenic While raised triglyceride levels are associated with increased CHD events, the relationship and benefits of treatment independent of cholesterol reduction are still unproven
Diabetes mellitus	Fasting glucose is essentially linearly correlated with CHD risk
Additional factors associated with increased risk of CHD	
Lipoprotein (Lpa)	Correlated with CHD risk but in general, non-modifiable in an individual
Homocysteine /folate/ vitamin E and other antioxidants	The exact relationships are debated Raised homocysteine is associated with increased CHD events but its independence from the association with low folate levels is uncertain Oxidized LDL is atherogenic but treatment trials with vitamin E have been disappointing Dietary increase in folate, fruit and vegetables is effective
Fibrinogen (coagulation and thrombolytic factors)	Pro-coagulant states and increased fibrinogen in particular are associated with increased CHD events
C-reactive protein (CRP) (inflammatory mediators)	CRP levels correlate with CHD events supporting the inflammatory/infective theories of atherosclerosis but at present not useful clinically

Using data from the Framingham study (a 50-year longitudinal study of cardiovascular disease amongst the population of Framingham, west of Boston), tables, calculation packages and charts have been prepared to estimate an individual's CHD risk using their age, gender, smoking status, blood pressure and cholesterol. The tables published by the Joint British Societies (British Cardiac Society, British Hyperlipidaemia Association, British Hypertension Society and British Diabetic Association) are shown in Figures 3.1a and 3.1b. These tables illustrate the importance of multifactorial risk and can be used to explore the impact of one risk factor (e.g. smoking status) depending on the level of other risk factors. Notes on use of the tables are given in Box 3.1.

PRIMARY PREVENTION

While individuals with the greatest burden of risk factors are at greatest risk of CHD events, most events occur in individuals at moderate risk because there are so many more such individuals. This is because major risk factors, such as cholesterol, are normally distributed in the population.

Primary prevention can, therefore, be approached in one of two ways:
1. *The population approach* – a modest reduction in the mean cholesterol of the population will significantly reduce the number of CHD events, but for any individual the absolute risk reduction is modest. It will be appreciated, however, that offering statins to the majority of the population is financially untenable.
2. *The high-risk individual approach* – by targeting individuals at highest risk, the majority of the population (and, therefore, the majority of events) will not be affected, but for the individuals involved, the absolute risk reduction may be substantial. Pharmacological therapy is an appropriate tool for these patients.

The National Service Framework for Coronary Heart Disease (NSF for CHD) advocates both approaches. Public health strategies such as healthy-eating campaigns are advocated, but targeting high-risk individuals for more intensive risk-factor reduction is also part of the strategy.

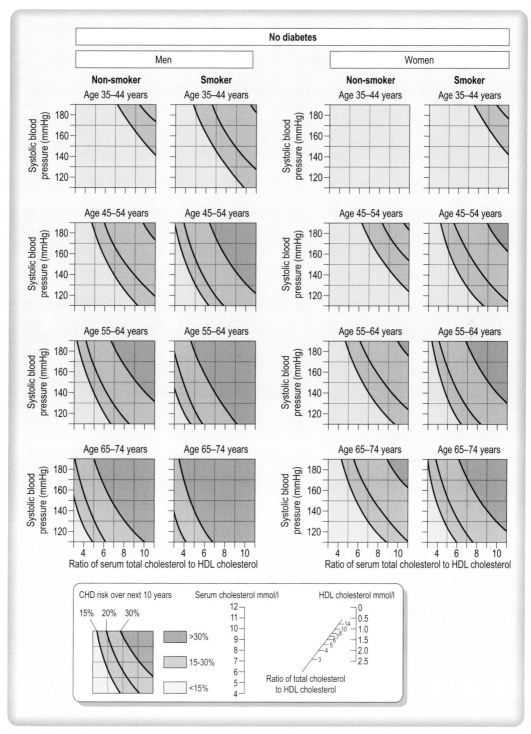

Figure 3.1a
Coronary risk prediction chart
Reproduced (and modified) with permission from Heart 1998; 80: S1–S29 © The University of Manchester

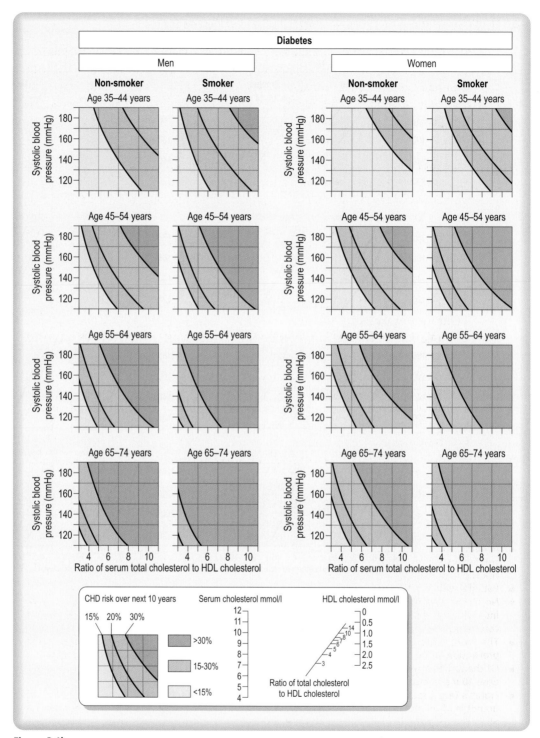

Figure 3.1b
Coronary risk prediction chart
Reproduced (and modified) with permission from Heart 1998; 80: S1–S29 © The University of Manchester

PATIENTS TARGETED FOR PRIMARY PREVENTION

Scientific evidence from randomized controlled trials (RCTs) supports pharmacological and other interventions in patients whose 10-year risk of a CHD event is around 15%. Economic and logistical considerations mean that this is not currently possible in the UK. For example, this would mean targeting 28% of English men aged 30–74. The Joint British Societies Guidelines and the NSF, therefore, propose targeting patients with a 10-year risk of a CHD event of >30% in the first instance.

Such individuals may be detected by planned screening or by opportunistic screening. Screening first-degree relatives of patients with premature CHD (men <55 years and women <65 years) is also an effective method of identifying patients at high risk for primary prevention.

Identified individuals should be offered interventions to address *all* modifiable risk factors (see Box 3.2 for additional patient-management notes):

- Lifestyle advice
- Dietary advice (Mediterranean diet rich in fruit and vegetables and low in red meat, saturated fats and salt)
- Moderation of alcohol consumption (<21 units/week for men and <14 units/week for women)
- Smoking cessation advice and support
- Encouragement to undertake aerobic exercise
- Advice to reduce weight where appropriate (BMI >30 kg/m^2 equates to obesity)
- Optimal glycaemic control
- Non-pharmacological and pharmacological intervention to achieve a blood pressure below 140/85 mmHg for non-diabetics and 130/80 mmHg for diabetics

---

Box 3.2: Notes on patient management in primary prevention

- Patients whose blood pressure warrants treatment in isolation (e.g. BP >160/100) should also have their other risk factors addressed whatever their risk, even in the unlikely event that their calculated 10-year CHD event risk is below 30%
- Patients with familial hypercholesterolaemia should always receive lipid-lowering therapy
- No specific targets or treatment levels are set for triglycerides (the relationship of triglycerides with CHD risk, independent of cholesterol, is complex, and the trials of independent therapy for triglycerides are less convincing than for cholesterol lowering)
- The current recommendations put an upper age limit of 70 years for screening for targeted primary prevention, although older patients would seem to have much to gain based on the trial data
- Of the statins available in the UK, only simvastatin (minimum dose 20 mg nocte) and pravastatin (minimum dose 40 mg nocte) have shown mortality reduction in large randomized controlled trials
- Fibrates (e.g. bezafibrate 400 mg od) are appropriate second-line agents where statins are not tolerated or do not lead to adequate lipid control, or where hypertriglyceridaemia predominates (triglycerides >5.0 mmol/l); however, when used in combination with statins, the possibility of myositis should be checked by monitoring of creatine kinase
- Consider the possibility of secondary hyperlipidaemia (e.g. renal dysfunction, hypothyroidism, excessive alcohol consumption, liver disease)
- For selection of anti-hypertensive medication see Chapter 15

- Non-pharmacological and pharmacological interventions (primarily statins) to achieve a total cholesterol <5.0 mmol/l and an LDL cholesterol <3.0 mmol/l. Revised guidelines from the Joint British Societies will revise these levels downwards to <4.0 mmol/l and 2.0 mmol/l, respectively
- Aspirin for patients with hypertension (once controlled) or those over 50 years of age or males at high risk.

SECONDARY PREVENTION

In managing patients with CHD, preventing events should run parallel to symptom control.

Patients with any manifestations of atherosclerotic disease should be offered secondary prevention, i.e. those with peripheral vascular disease and carotid arterial disease.

ANGINA, PERIPHERAL VASCULAR DISEASE AND CAROTID ARTERIAL DISEASE

There is little difference in the recommendations for secondary prevention for other manifestations of atherosclerotic disease compared to patients with CHD. Patients whose first manifestation of arterial disease is outside the heart are at high risk of CHD events. There are particular recommendations for post-MI patients (see below).

Principle interventions and targets:

- Antiplatelet therapy (aspirin 75 mg od or clopidogrel 75 mg od if intolerant). For patients with recurrent strokes there is evidence for a combination of aspirin and dipyridamole.
- Statin therapy (target: total cholesterol <5.0 mmol/l and LDL <3.0 mmol/l).
- BP <140/85 mmHg (and 130/80 mmHg in diabetics).
- Optimal glycaemic control in diabetics.
- Smoking cessation.
- Lifestyle and dietary modification (including alcohol consumption), exercise and weight reduction.

Statin therapy

Current guidelines recommend statin therapy in those with a total cholesterol level of 5.0 mmol/l and an LDL cholesterol level of 3.0 mmol/l (after a trial of dietary therapy). However, the recently reported Heart Protection Study (HPS) showed efficacy of simvastatin 40 mg nocte in patients with atherosclerotic disease and cholesterols >3.5 mmol/l (i.e. virtually all patients) and supports statin therapy for all patients with atherosclerotic disease.

Combining the guidelines and the HPS results, all patients with atherosclerotic disease should be treated with simvastatin 40 mg nocte. Starting simvastatin at 20 mg nocte for a few days may reduce the risk of gastrointestinal disturbance. If the target for cholesterol (total cholesterol <5.0 mmol/l, LDL cholesterol <3.0 mmol/l) is not achieved by 40 mg of simvastatin, an increased or alternative therapy is indicated. If the level is near target, increasing the dose of simvastatin to 80 mg may be effective; however, if there is a significant distance between the patient's cholesterol and the target, atorvastatin at a dose of 20–80 mg od has a more potent cholesterol-lowering effect.

Previously, trials of dietary therapy before pharmacological therapy and difficulties in interpreting cholesterol levels in the peri-infarct setting meant that there were arguments for the delay of statin therapy (as in the National Institute for Clinical Excellence (NICE) guidelines). However, the HPS data supporting the 'the earlier the better' view for statins and data showing current undertreatment of patients, all support starting statins as soon as the diagnosis of atherosclerotic disease is made.

SECONDARY PREVENTION MEASURES IN PATIENTS FOLLOWING MI

NICE have issued guidelines on 'prophylaxis for patients who have experienced a myocardial infarction' (Table 3.2) based on an extensive document from the North of

Table 3.2: Summary of the NICE guidelines for prophylaxis for patients who have experienced a myocardial infarction

	Drug treatment	Non-drug treatment
Prior myocardial infarction (no heart failure)	Early initiation (in hospital) of beta blocker + anti-platelet drug (aspirin) + ACE-inhibitor If not initiated in hospital, primary care should initiate ASAP Patients not taking a statin should be assessed and have treatment initiated 12 weeks after index myocardial infarction (MI)	Rehabilitation: – patients should be offered enrolment in a rehabilitation programme that has a prominent exercise component within it – be guided by functional ability and patient preference Diet: – not possible to recommend specific dietary manipulation due to nature of available evidence
Prior myocardial infarction (with heart failure)	Early initiation (in hospital) of an anti-platelet drug (aspirin) plus an ACE-inhibitor If not initiated in hospital, primary care should initiate ASAP Initiate spironolactone at any point in patients with moderate or severe heart failure (New York Heart Association (NYHA III or IV)) Initiate beta blockers at any point Start with low-dose and slowly increase, e.g. at fortnightly intervals, over a period of up to 12 weeks	
Prior myocardial infarction (with diabetes)	There is evidence that intensive insulin therapy initiated soon after admission for acute MI reduces mortality To achieve the benefits demonstrated in the single trial in this area involves four-daily insulin injections continuing for at least 3 months	

Box 3.3: Secondary prevention following myocardial infarction

- Beta blockers should not be initiated while patients have pulmonary oedema but should be deferred until the oedema has cleared. Beta blocker trials have used a number of different agents; atenolol (25–100 mg/day) is a popular but not exclusive choice in the UK. The RCTs showing the benefit of beta blockers in heart failure used carvedilol (starting dose 3.125 mg twice per day and target dose 25–50 mg twice per day), bisoprolol, and metoprolol CR (the latter is not licenced in the UK).
- Statin therapy should be offered to all in the light of the Heart Protection Study (discussed above).
- Ramipril, enalapril, captopril and lisinopril have all been shown in RCTs to benefit patients with heart failure but the Heart Outcomes Prevention Evaluation Study probably places ramipril (target dose 10 mg od) and perindopril (target dose 8 mg) as shown in the EUROPA trial, be used in any patient with CAD whether or not they have symptoms of heart failure or an impaired ejection fraction.
- Spironolactone has been shown in a single RCT (the randomized Aldactone evaluation study (RALES) to improve outcomes in patients with moderate or severe heart failure but it must be used in low doses (25–50 mg od) and monitoring of potassium and renal function undertaken (at least weekly initially). The recent EPHESUS study has shown the mortality benefits of eplerenone (selective aldosterone antagonist) in patients post-MI with evidence of heart failure.
- The Diabetes Mellitus, Insulin, Glucose Infusion in Acute Myocardial Infarction (DIGAMI) Study Group demonstrated the efficacy of intensive insulin therapy. Patients with diabetes (including newly diagnosed) should be commenced on intensive insulin therapy when hospitalized with an acute MI, which may require an initial 'sliding scale' of insulin. The DIGAMI trial maintained this intensive therapy for at least 3 months. Whether less intensive therapy works as well is unclear but optimal glycaemic control should be the aim.
- The target for blood pressure is <140/85 mmHg in non-diabetics and <130/80 mmHg in diabetics, just as for primary prevention, and may require additional antihypertensive therapy in addition to beta blockers and ACE inhibitors.
- Smoking cessation, lifestyle intervention, dietary advice, weight control and exercise are essential elements of a comprehensive multi-disciplinary programme of cardiac prevention and rehabilitation, which should be offered to all patients. Pro-active recruitment is needed and clinical support for risk-factor modification through integrated initiation and up-titration of drugs adds to the value of these programmes.
- In patients intolerant of aspirin, clopidogrel (75 mg od) is an appropriate alternative, although long-term safety data are awaited.
- Anticoagulants should be considered for patients with large anterior infarctions, left ventricular aneurysms, or paroxysmal tachyarrhythmias (in addition to aspirin unless absolute or relative contraindications exist in which case a balance must be struck).

England Guidelines Group. Notes on secondary prevention measures for patients following myocardial infarction are given in Box 3.3.

SUMMARY

The identification and treatment of cardiovascular risk factors is an integral part of modern cardiac practice. Patients at high risk of CHD events (>30% over 10 years) and those with clinical atherosclerotic disease should be offered interventions:

- Reduce BP <140/85 mmHg (130/80 mmHg in diabetics)
- Lipid-lowering therapy (statins) aiming for a total cholesterol <5.0 mmol/l, LDL cholesterol <3.0 mmol/l
- Anti-platelet therapy (aspirin)
- Optimal glycaemic control in diabetics
- Smoking cessation

- Lifestyle and dietary modification (including alcohol consumption), exercise and weight reduction.

Further reading

Braunwald E, Zipes D, Libby P (eds) 2001 Heart disease – a textbook of cardiovascular medicine, 6th edn. W.B. Saunders, Philadelphia

Heart Protection Study Collaborative Group 2002 MRC / BHF Heart Protection Study of cholesterol lowering with simvastatin in 20 536 high-risk individuals: a randomised placebo-controlled trial. Lancet 360: 7–22

Malmberg K 1997 Prospective randomised study of intensive insulin treatment on long term survival after myocardial infarction in patients with diabetes mellitus. DIGAMI (Diabetes Mellitus, Insulin, Glucose Infusion in Acute Myocardial Infarction) Study Group. BMJ 314: 1512–1515

National Institute for Clinical Excellence 2001 Prophylaxis for patients who have experienced a myocardial infarction. NICE, London (www.nice.org.uk)

North of England Evidence-based Guidelines Development Project 2000 Prophylaxis for patients who have experienced a myocardial infarction: drug treatment, cardiac rehabilitation and dietary manipulation. NICE, London (www.nice.org.uk)

Pitt B, Remme W, Zanned F et al. 2003 Eplerenone, a selective aldosterone blocker, in patients with left ventricular dysfunction after myocardial infarction. N Engl J Med 348: 1309–1321

Pitt B, Zannad F, Remme WJ, Cody R, Castaigne A, Pertz A, Palenski J, Wiles J 1999 The effect of spironolactone on morbidity and mortality on patients with severe heart failure. N Engl J Med 341: 709–717

The European trial on reduction of cardiac events with perindopril in stable coronary artery disease investigators. Efficacy of perindopril in reduction of cardiovascular events among patients with stable coronary artery disease; randomized double-blind, placebo-controlled multicentre trial (The EUROPA study) Lancet 2003 782–788

The Heart Outcomes Prevention Evaluation Study Investigators 2000 Effects of an angiotensin-converting-enzyme inhibitor, ramipril, on cardiovascular events in high risk patients. N Engl J Med 342: 145–153

The National Service Framework for Coronary Heart Disease 2000 HMSO, London

Wood DA, Durrington P, Poulter N, McInnes G, Rees A, Wray R on behalf of the British Cardiac Society, British Hyperlipidaemia Association, British Hypertension Society, British Diabetic Association 1998 Joint British recommendations on prevention of coronary heart disease in clinical practice. Heart 80 (Suppl 2): S1–S26

FREQUENTLY ASKED QUESTIONS

1. *Can patients use nicotine replacement therapy (NRT) following MI or unstable angina?* Continued smoking represents a major risk factor for further infarction and ischaemia. NRT use does improve smoking cessation rates. However, there is a (theoretical) danger that the nicotine content of NRT may precipitate ischaemia or infarction. Clear trial evidence to answer this question is unlikely and, therefore, a sensible approach is not to use NRT during the first 24–72 hours after MI or while patients are experiencing ongoing unstable symptoms. But after this time, if one feels that the chances of smoking cessation will be enhanced by the use of NRT, then use would seem reasonable.

2. *Do the recommendations apply equally in the elderly and very elderly?* The risk assessment tables and recommendations for primary prevention in the NSF for CHD address individuals up to 75 years of age. While this may appear ageist, the evidence for primary prevention in older patients is less clear and when combined with cost and ethical issues this appears a reasonable compromise. The elderly are generally under-represented in secondary prevention trials. However, there is little evidence of an

attenuation of benefit amongst older patients. Indeed, their higher absolute risk generally makes the benefit greater. Above the age of 85 years, data become very scanty and concerns regarding adverse effects increase. Inevitably decisions must be individualized. A sound approach is to initially consider treating patients the same, independent of age, and then to adapt the therapeutic strategy to take into consideration issues of polypharmacy, co-morbidity, and cognitive and physical frailty such that most patients in their late 70s would be offered the full range of therapies but these would be used sparingly in those over 90.

SELF-ASSESSMENT

Questions

a. A 54-year-old man with type 2 diabetes comes into your clinic asking if he should be taking one of those 'cholesterol-lowering wonder drugs'. He is well, has a total cholesterol of 5.2 mmol/l, an HDL cholesterol of 1.0 mmol/l, a blood pressure (after 5 minutes supine) of 155/80 mmHg and continues to smoke. Should he be given a prescription?
   He then explains that the reason for his concern follows a visit to his younger brother who is in hospital following a heart attack. Does this alter the decision?

b. In clinic a 73-year-old man presents 6 months after his first myocardial infarction. He is generally well but complaining of gastric upset from the aspirin despite proton pump inhibitors. He has stopped smoking but his total cholesterol is 5.5 mmol/l, despite 80 mg of simvastatin. He also takes ramipril 10 mg od. His blood pressure is 138/78 mmHg. He is not diabetic. How should his treatment be altered?

Answers

a. His initial calculated 10-year CHD risk is just under 30%. At this point he should be advised to stop smoking, improve his diet and lifestyle. Applying the 30% cut-off rule would not fulfill the criteria for statin therapy. He should, therefore, be offered a review and reassessment in a year's time.
   However, once the family history becomes apparent, this multiplies his risk by approximately 1.5 putting him above the 30% 10-year risk. In addition to smoking cessation advice and help, and optimization of his diabetes control, he should also be offered lifestyle measures and pharmacological therapy as needed (e.g. simvastatin or pravastatin) to bring his total cholesterol to <5.0 mmol/l (LDL cholesterol <3.0 mmol/l) and his blood pressure to <130/80 mmHg with an ACE inhibitor as a reasonable first choice.

b. In view of the persistent gastric symptoms it is reasonable to switch him to clopidogrel 75 mg od.
   His cholesterol is not controlled. It should be <5.0 mmol/l. Either switch to atorvastatin 20 mg (increasing to 80 mg od as needed) or add a fibrate (e.g. Bezalip Mono 400 mg od) monitoring creatine kinase closely because of the risk of myositis. He should be commenced on a beta blocker aiming for a resting pulse around 55–65 beats per minute).

Specialized cardiac investigations

T. Salukhe and D. Francis

INTRODUCTION

It is beyond the scope of this book to provide an extensive background to the appropriate use and interpretation of the resting electrocardiogram (ECG) and conventional exercise testing. Familiarity with these techniques is assumed, although specific texts dedicated to these techniques are cited at the end of the chapter.

CARDIOPULMONARY EXERCISE TESTING (DIAGNOSTIC EXERCISE PHYSIOLOGY)

PROBLEMS OF CLASSIC ASSESSMENT OF HEART FAILURE

Chronic heart failure (CHF) is a disease of disordered cardiopulmonary responses to exercise: patients in New York Heart Association (NYHA) Classes II and III, for example, have no symptoms in the absence of exercise. The classic convention of defining CHF in terms of symptoms, clinical signs, and findings on investigation has certain limitations (Box 4.1).

CARDIOPULMONARY EXERCISE TESTING EQUIPMENT

In essence, cardiopulmonary exercise testing (diagnostic exercise physiology) involves the measurement of respiratory oxygen uptake (VO_2), carbon dioxide production (VCO_2) and

---

Box 4.1: Limitations of classic heart failure assessment

- Although the principal symptoms of breathlessness and fatigue may be pronounced on exercise, these symptoms may overlap with those of patients with respiratory disease, and can even be reported by normal subjects.
- Signs of fluid retention do not always persist with optimal medical treatment and when they are found they do not necessarily signify cardiac failure.
- While imaging investigations may identify abnormalities in cardiac function at rest, there are difficulties in obtaining an objective, unifying measurement that may be useful across all forms of heart failure.
- None of the above observations can identify that exercise capacity is, indeed, limited by cardiovascular, rather than respiratory, musculoskeletal, or motivational causes.

ventilation (VE). VO_2 and VCO_2 may be measured breath-by-breath using a flowmeter close to the subject's mouth, in combination with a rapid on-line gas analyser. Alternatively, data can be obtained with less temporal resolution, but with less complex calibration, using inert gas dilution techniques, where the subject's expired air is mixed with a known flow rate of helium or argon and the resulting concentrations are assayed by mass spectrometer.

During the exercise test, VO_2 and VCO_2 can be observed by the supervising staff. At rest, VCO_2 is significantly less than VO_2, i.e. the respiratory exchange ratio (R), defined as VCO_2/VO_2, is less than 1.00. As exercise progresses, VO_2 and VCO_2 both rise in proportion at first, but eventually VO_2 begins to form a plateau. Thus, VCO_2 'overtakes' VO_2 and R exceeds 1.00.

The levelling off of VO_2 results from an inability of the cardiopulmonary system to transport more oxygen. Aside from transient fluxes into and out of compartments, VO_2 is the product of cardiac output and the arteriovenous difference in oxygen content. In heart failure, cardiac output cannot rise to the dramatic extent (typically tenfold) achievable in healthy subjects, and so VO_2 reaches a peak at an abnormally low level. VCO_2 does not form such a peak, because CO_2 transport is not limited by the saturation kinetics of oxygen transport.

If lung disease or lack of motivation cause cessation of exercise, the VO_2 will not have flattened off and, therefore, R will not have risen fully. Typically, a rise of at least 0.20 to a level of at least 1.00 (or 1.05) is prespecified to be satisfactory evidence of achievement of anaerobic metabolism.

VALUE OF DIAGNOSTIC EXERCISE PHYSIOLOGY

Diagnostic exercise physiology offers several valuable pieces of information to the clinician.
1. Peak oxygen uptake (VO_2) is particularly reproducible among the available measures of exercise capacity.
2. Peak VO_2 predicts mortality in CHF better than any resting measurement. This is recognized in guidelines for the management of severe CHF: a peak VO_2 below 14 ml/kg/min implies prognosis poor enough to warrant transplantation.
3. It can identify the cause of impaired exercise capacity specifically, whether it is caused by limitation of exercise aerobic response (characteristic of heart failure) or failure to utilize aerobic capacity fully (indicating that cardiac output is not the rate-limiting step.
4. The clinician can observe the behaviour of oxygen saturation on exercise. CHF on its own does not cause desaturation on exercise. In one series of 37 patients with CHF, the only three showing desaturation on exercise were found to have alternative diagnoses: patent foramen ovale with right-to-left shunt during exercise, pulmonary embolic disease, and clinically unsuspected obstructive airways disease.
5. The ventilatory response to exercise (slope of the ratio of expired ventilation to VCO_2) can be measured. This is abnormally augmented in many patients with CHF, closely related to symptoms of breathlessness, and carries additional prognostic significance that has recently been suggested to be even more powerful than that of peak VO_2.

6. Lastly, alongside these data, all the information obtained from a conventional exercise test is also available, including exercise-induced arrhythmias, ST segment changes, and chronotropic incompetence. These abnormalities may merit specific treatment.

CLINICAL APPLICATION IN HEART DISEASE

In CHF progressive shifts occur at a neuro-chemical, hormonal and molecular level in a compensatory manner in an effort to improve ventricular performance. The end results of these mechanisms include increased sympathetic tonicity, increased catecholamine levels, beta-receptor down-regulation and baroreflex modification. The varied mosaic of haemodynamic consequences is reflected in the wide range of exercise capacity in subjects with similarly impaired left ventricles. Indeed, the severity of exercise limitation in many heart failure patients is due to abnormalities in skeletal muscle metabolism. Such abnormalities arise from disuse de-conditioning and chronically impaired oxygen delivery (DO_2) in heart failure. Reduced DO_2, peak VO_2 and raised lactate levels all contribute to exercise related symptoms in CHF.

In stable heart failure, peak VO_2 is useful for stratifying patient risk, survival and the incidence of adverse cardiac events including death and need for transplantation. Peak VO_2 levels of greater than 20 ml O_2 kg^{-1}/min^{-1} and an anaerobic threshold (AT) greater than 14 ml O_2 kg^{-1}/min^{-1} are associated with a good long-term prognosis. Patients unable to achieve a VO_2 of 10 ml O_2 kg^{-1}/min^{-1} or an AT of 8 ml O_2 kg^{-1}/min^{-1} are usually unable to achieve a cardiac output of greater than 4 l/min^{-1} and have a poor prognosis. Failure of VO_2 to decrease 30 seconds after the termination of exercise is also a poor prognostic marker.

Recent work has suggested that the dynamics of ventilation may provide even more reproducible and prognostically helpful information than from peak VO_2 alone, by modelling the relationship between ventilation and gas transfer linearly (VE/VCO$_2$ slope) or non-linearly (oxygen uptake efficiency slope).

AMBULATORY ELECTROCARDIOGRAPHY

Prolonged ECG recording during normal activity is an indispensable tool in the documentation and qualification of cardiac arrhythmias, and their temporal relationship to the patients' symptoms; it is also useful in the evaluation of anti-arrhythmic therapy. Sophisticated software now allows for the analysis of other useful variables:

- R–R interval and heart rate variability
- QRS-T morphology and late potentials
- QT variability
- T-wave alternans.

Different modalities of ambulatory ECG (AECG) recording and their appropriate clinical application will be discussed in this chapter.

RECORDING MODALITIES

There are two broad categories of AECG recorders, namely, continuous Holter type recorders, which monitor over 24–48 hours and intermittent recorders, which can be kept by the patient for weeks or months and used to investigate events that occur less frequently.

Continuous recorders

For the investigation of arrhythmia, 24-hour recorders are often used as first line. Twenty-five to 50% of patients will experience symptoms during the time of recording, and arrhythmia is a cause in 2–15%, although this yield is increased slightly with longer or repeated recordings. When treating arrhythmia with drugs, it is seldom necessary to confirm the resolution of arrhythmia with repeat AECG. Although, when the efficacy of treatment or cause of continuing symptoms despite drug therapy is truly in question then repeat AECG may become appropriate. However, to exclude spontaneous variability over treatment effect, a 65% reduction in arrhythmia frequency after therapy is required.

Tape-free digital recorders can record electrical signals at a rate of 1000 signals per second; this allows for rapid acquisition of data, avoids the errors and biases of analogue-to-digital conversion, and also allows for a high resolution of ECG signal reproduction to perform tasks such as signal averaging and real-time QRS-T analysis. These devices are limited by their digital storage capacity and in the case of real-time on-line analysis, the dependence of software for the identification of abnormalities.

An additional and less widespread use of AECG is to assess myocardial ischaemia by looking for ST depression during daily activity and sleep. When investigating myocardial ischaemia, the variability in the frequency and magnitude of ST-segment depression is also marked. It is essential, therefore, to encourage patients to pursue their usual activities during time of recording.

Intermittent recorders

Three main types of patient-activated intermittent recorder are used to assess arrhythmias that occur too infrequently to be caught on conventional Holter monitoring:

1. The event recorder is a credit-card-sized device that the patient carries in a pocket or purse and applies to the chest when symptoms occur (naturally the onset of any arrhythmias will not be captured).
2. The external loop recorder, which resembles a simple three-lead light-weight Holter device with a small memory that records the ECG in a closed loop and only stores that latest few minutes of ECG data at any one time. When symptomatic the patient must activate the device to permanently store the last few minutes of ECG.
3. The implantable loop recorders are finger-sized devices implanted subcutaneously much like a pacemaker generator. After a symptomatic episode, the patient signals the loop recorder, using a magnetic key, to store the prior segment (typically 30–40 min) of loop recording for later transmission to the cardiology centre. These are particularly valuable for patients with unexplained, frequent syncope.

Although these recorders are very helpful for infrequent symptoms, it should be remembered that they all require patient activation and, therefore, cannot be applied to all patients.

INDICATIONS AND GUIDELINES FOR THE USE OF AECG

The logical application of AECG recording modalities depends largely on the quality and frequency of the patient's symptoms, their risk profile and ability to use devices appropriately. Specific indications are not discussed here but are summarized in the American College of Cardiology and American Heart Association guidelines in table form (Table 4.1).

Table 4.1: American College of Cardiology and American Heart Association guidelines

Indication	Class I	Class IIa	Class IIb	Class III
Assess symptoms possibly related to rhythm disturbances	Syncope, near syncope or episodic dizziness with no obvious cause Unexplained recurrent palpitations		Unexplained episodic shortness of breath, chest pain or fatigue Neurological events when transient atrial fibrillation or flutter is suspected Symptoms such as syncope, episodic dizziness or palpitations in which a cause other than arrhythmia is suspected but symptoms persist despite treatment of this other cause	
Arrhythmia detection to assess risk for future cardiac events in patients without symptoms from arrhythmia	None		Post-MI with left ventricular (LV) dysfunction (ejection fraction <40%) CHF Idiopathic hypertrophic cardiomyopathy	Myocardial contusion Systemic hypertension with LV hypertrophy Post-MI with normal LV function Pre-operative evaluation of patients for non-cardiac surgery Sleep apnoea Valvular heart disease
Measurement of HRV to assess risk for future cardiac events in patients without symptoms from arrhythmia			Post-MI with LV dysfunction (ejection fraction <40%) CHF Idiopathic hypertrophic cardiomyopathy	Post-MI patients with normal LV function Diabetic patients to evaluate diabetic neuropathy Patients with rhythm disturbances that preclude HRV analysis (i.e. atrial fibrillation)

Table 4.1: (Cont'd)

Indication	Class I	Class IIa	Class IIb	Class III
Assessment of antiarrhythmic therapy	To assess anti-arrhythmic drug response in individuals in whom baseline frequency of arrhythmia has been characterized as reproducible and of sufficient frequency to permit analysis	To detect proarrhythmogenic responses to antiarrhythmic therapy in patients at high risk	To assess rate control during atrial fibrillation To document recurrence of asymptomatic nonsustained arrhythmias during therapy during an outpatient setting	None
To assess pacemaker and ICD function	Evaluation of frequent symptoms and palpitation, syncope, or near syncope to assess device function to exclude myopotential inhibition and pacemaker-mediated tachycardia and to assist in the programming of enhanced features such as mode switching and rate responsivity Evaluation of suspected component failure when device interrogation is not definitive To assess the response to adjuvant drug therapy in patients receiving frequent ICD therapy		Evaluation of the immediate post-operative pacemaker function after the pacemaker or ICD implantation as an alternative to telemetry Evaluation of rate of SVT in patients with ICD	Assessment of ICD/pacemaker malfunction when device interrogation, ECG, or other available data are sufficient to establish underlying cause or diagnosis Routine follow-up in asymptomatic patients

ICD = implantable cardioverter defibrillator
HRV = heat rate variability
LV = left ventricle
SVT = supraventricular tachycardia

Class I: Conditions for which there is evidence and/or general agreement that a given procedure or treatment is useful and effective; Class II: Conditions where there is conflicting evidence or divergence of opinion on the usefulness or efficacy of treatment; Class IIa: Weight of evidence/opinion in favour of usefulness/efficacy; Class IIb: Usefulness/efficacy less well established by evidence/opinion; Class III: Conditions for which there is evidence and/or general agreement that a given procedure or treatment is not useful or is in some cases harmful

ADDITIONAL PARAMETERS ASSESSABLE WITH AECG

Heart rate variability

Frequency domain analysis of R–R variability is an accepted representation of the weight of sympathetic and parasympathetic tone on the heart. A normal physiological balance of sympathetic and parasympathetic activity manifests in high- (0.15–0.40 Hz) and low- (0.04–0.15 Hz) frequency components in R–R variability. Parasympathetic tone manifests in high-frequency (HF) spectral analysis, while low frequency (LF) reflects both sympathetic and parasympathetic tone. The LF:HF ratio is considered a measure of sympathovagal balance and reflects sympathetic modulation. Although a reduced variability is a marker of increased risk, this is most likely due to several different influences and simply reflects a reduction in periodicity or shift in autonomic tone. R–R variability is as accurate a predictor of all-cause mortality as left ventricular ejection fraction and non-sustained ventricular tachyarrhythmia (VT) in patients after myocardial infarction, and can be used in conjunction with other measures of risk to enhance predictive accuracy.

QT dispersion

Two hallmarks of re-entrant tachycardias are heterogeneity in refractoriness and conduction velocity. In its simplest form, QT dispersion can be assessed by measuring the difference between the shortest and longest QT interval in the surface leads, which is adjusted for heart rate. Several algorithms using different techniques for assessing QT dispersion are available. Abnormally high QT dispersion is associated with risk of arrhythmic death in a variety of disorders, although this is not a consistent finding. QT dispersion has been correlated with efficacy and pro-arrhythmic potential of drug therapy, however, its clinical value is yet to be established.

T-wave alternans

Variation in morphology and amplitude of the T wave and ST segment from beat to beat is associated with the development of ventricular tachyarrhythmias in myocardial ischaemia, long QT syndrome and patients with VTs. The mechanism behind T-wave alternation is not entirely clear, but it is, nevertheless, a marker of an electrically unstable myocardium prone to VT or ventricular fibrillation (VF) and may be useful to risk stratify patients.

Further reading

Crawford MH, Bernstein SJ, Deaedwania PC et al. ACC/AHA Guidelines for Ambulatory Electrocardiography: Executive Summary and Recommendations. A Report of the American College of Cardiology/American Heart Association Task Force on Practice Guidelines (Committee to Revise the Guidelines for Ambulatory Electrocardiography) Developed in Collaboration with the North American Society for Pacing and Electrophysiology. Circulation 1999; 100: 886–893.

Gibbons RJ, Balady GJ, Bricker JT et al. ACC/AHA 2002 Guideline update for Exercise Testing. A report of the American College of Cardiology/American Heart Association Task Force on Practice Guidelines (Committee on Exercise Testing). American College of Cardiology website available at: www.acc.org/clinical/guidelines/exercise/dirIndex.htm

Echocardiography

5

Rajan Sharma and S. J. Brecker

INTRODUCTION

This chapter aims to cover the use of echocardiography in the management of clinical disease processes. The detailed principles of ultrasound are not covered but it is hoped the reader will gain information that will allow better understanding of the reasons for requesting an echocardiogram and how the results should be interpreted in a clinical context. The assessment of valvular disease is not included in this section as it is dealt with in Chapter 11. Tissue Doppler imaging and stress echocardiography are included, but other newer modes of imaging, such as strain rate, myocardial contrast echocardiography, colour kinesis, 3-D echocardiography, intravascular ultrasound and hand-held echocardiography devices, are not mentioned. These topics are beyond the scope of this chapter, but more importantly, their routine use in clinical practice, at the time of writing, is still not defined.

Most large hospitals will perform thousands of transthoracic echocardiographs (TTEs) each year. The most common referral reasons are shown in Figure 5.1. Because it is

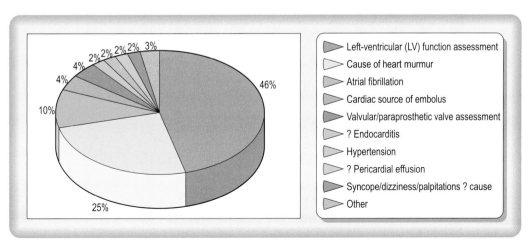

Figure 5.1
Common referral reasons for a transthoracic echocardiograph

relatively cheap and non-invasive, this figure will continue to rise. Access for general practitioners also continues to rise with the introduction of 'open-access' echocardiography clinics across the UK. At present, the vast majority of these scans are performed and reported by trained sonographers rather than doctors. Transoesophageal echocardiographs (TOEs) continue to be performed by cardiologists and, more recently, anaesthetists.

The role of echocardiography in common referral conditions is discussed below.

ASSESSMENT OF LEFT-VENTRICULAR FUNCTION

As Figure 5.1 shows, this is the commonest reason for requesting a transthoracic echocardiogram. An accurate assessment is, therefore, essential as it provides the requesting physician not only with a potential cause for symptoms, but also important prognostic information. Figure 5.2 outlines an approach to the echocardiograph assessment required. When assessing systolic function it is important to note that the conventional parasternal long axis M-mode measurements of the basal septum and posterior wall are only accurate if there are no regional differences in phase or amplitude of motion. The systolic and diastolic volumes (and hence ejection fraction) are estimated from linear dimensions using formulae assuming modified spherical geometry. In patients with bundle branch block or regional-wall motion abnormalities this technique is, therefore, inaccurate and another method of ejection fraction estimation must be used (see Figs 5.2 & 5.3).

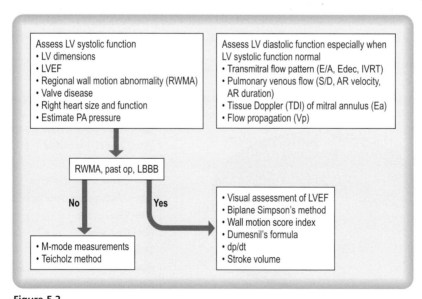

Figure 5.2
Patients referred for echocardiogram assessment of left-ventricular function
LV, left ventricular; LVEF, left ventricular ejection fraction; RWMA, regional wall motion abnormality; past op, previous cardiac operation; LBBB, left bundle branch block; Edec, early deceleration time; IVRT, isovolumic relaxation time

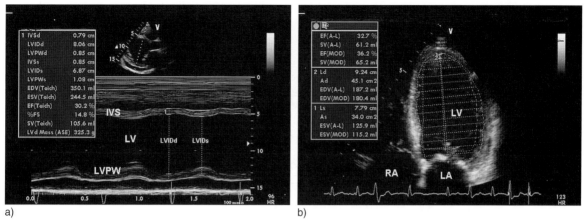

a)   b)

Figure 5.3
Systolic function estimation in a patient with dilated cardiomyopathy. (a) Assessment is made from linear M-mode measurements in parasternal long axis view. (b) Ejection fraction is calculated by Simpson's method. This technique requires planimetry of the endocardial border in systole and diastole, and assumes ventricular volume is the sum of the volumes of adjacent sets of discs of varying depth and cross-sectional area

The assessment of diastolic dysfunction is becoming increasingly important as we recognize that this is a potential cause for both symptoms and long-term morbidity. Pulsed Doppler of mitral valve flow is the most commonly used method of assessing diastolic function. In the presence of sinus rhythm 2 waves, 'E' and 'A' are produced, reflecting early filling of the left ventricle in diastole and atrial contraction respectively. Figure 5.4 shows the normal and abnormal filling patterns that can be produced. However, the normal and abnormal patterns are physiological descriptions and patients may move between them depending on the state of their disease, loading conditions, or treatment. It is, therefore, possible for a 'pseudonormal' transmitral Doppler pattern to occur in a patient with significant diastolic dysfunction depending on the loading conditions and treatment at the time. Other modes of assessment must always, therefore, be made before one can confidently exclude diastolic dysfunction in this situation (see Fig. 5.2).

FURTHER ROLE OF TRANSTHORACIC ECHOCARDIOGRAPHY

ATRIAL FIBRILLATION

TTE is useful to determine aetiology, guide therapeutic choice of cardioversion or rate control, and in helping to assess thromboembolic risk. In many cases, TTEs in patients with atrial fibrillation (AF) demonstrate an abnormality that affects clinical practice.

EVALUATION OF A HEART MURMUR

Studies suggest half of all TTEs performed to investigate a murmur will demonstrate an abnormality. This is most likely in patients over 60 where 55% of echocardiographs will

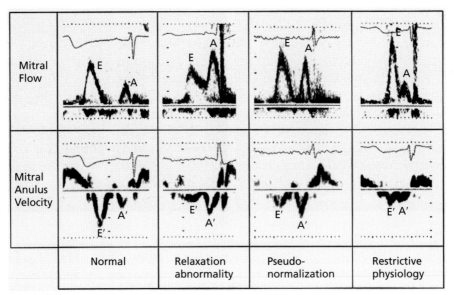

Figure 5.4
Four conventional patterns of pulsed Doppler mitral-flow velocity and tissue Doppler mitral annular velocity. Note: in the pseudonormal pattern, normal mitral inflow Doppler signal is matched by an abnormal relaxation pattern of mitral anulus velocity

be abnormal. On the other hand, in healthy young women with a murmur, the TTE is abnormal in only 5–10% cases.

HYPERTENSION

The presence of left-ventricular hypertrophy is an independent marker of cardiovascular risk in hypertension. It is for this reason that World Health Organization guidelines recommend echocardiography in these patients for risk stratification and to guide treatment.

PERICARDIAL EFFUSION

TTE is crucial in the assessment of suspected pericardial effusion for confirming diagnosis, assessing the presence of tamponade and guiding safe drainage. Indeed, suspected cardiac tamponade is one of the few reasons for requesting an emergency TTE (see Ch. 20).

SYNCOPE

In patients with a normal examination, electrocardiogram (ECG) and chest X-ray (CXR), an echocardiogram rarely shows a structural cardiac abnormality as a cause of syncope. However, an echocardiograph is considered mandatory if there is any suspicion of underlying structural heart disease.

ELDERLY

The role of echocardiography in evaluating elderly patients with suspected cardiac disease is often a cause of contention between geriatricians and other health-care professionals who believe the results will not affect management. However, 50% of patients over 80 years with suspected heart failure do, in fact, have normal systolic function. Indeed, diastolic dysfunction is a commoner cause of breathlessness in these patients. Sixty per cent of octogenarians with a heart murmur will have a cause detected by TTE. While many of these patients may not be suitable for surgery, the results do have long-term prognostic implications for the patient and family and direct the referring physician to prescribing and avoiding certain drugs. Echocardiography, therefore, has an important role to play in the management of elderly patients.

ECHOCARDIOGRAPHY IN MYOCARDIAL INFARCTION

Echocardiography plays an increasingly critical role in the management of patients with acute myocardial infarction (MI). The main uses are given below.

DIAGNOSIS OF ACUTE MYOCARDIAL INFARCTION

In patients with a good history but equivocal ECG, the presence of a regional-wall motion abnormality has a 50% positive predictive value for MI. Other causes of this include myocardial ischaemia, myocarditis and old scar tissue. The presence of normal wall thickness and reflectivity suggests an acute event. Importantly, the absence of regional wall motion abnormality in these patients suggests a very good prognosis. TTE, therefore, provides useful additional information in the diagnosis and risk stratification of patients presenting to the emergency department with chest pain and an equivocal ECG.

ASSESSMENT OF LEFT-VENTRICULAR FUNCTION

This remains one the most important prognostic markers post-MI and should be assessed in all such patients before discharge. The number of dysfunctional segments on echocardiograph gives a better assessment of infarct size than the ECG or biochemical markers of cardiac necrosis.

ASSESSMENT OF COMPLICATIONS

An emergency TTE should be sought if a patient develops shock after MI. As well as allowing assessment of left-ventricular function and filling pressure, several important mechanical causes can be diagnosed. These include ventricular septal rupture, mitral regurgitation due to papillary muscle rupture or ischaemia, ventricular-free wall rupture with pseudoaneurysm formation and right-ventricular infarction (complicates 30% inferior MIs). These conditions are associated with extremely high mortality unless treated early, so once the diagnosis is made early liaison with the local or regional cardiac

45

team is essential. In the absence of MI, the TTE may also give clues to other causes of shock and chest pain, such as aortic dissection or pulmonary embolus. Other mechanical complications of MI, such as LV aneurysm and thrombus formation, can also be easily detected by TTE.

LONG-TERM RISK STRATIFICATION

Pre-discharge dobutamine stress echocardiography or, more recently, myocardial contrast echocardiography allows detection of myocardial viability and ischaemia. These patients benefit most from early angiography and revascularization.

TRANSOESOPHAGEAL ECHOCARDIOGRAPHY (TOE)

Miniaturized electronic phased array transducer technology incorporated in a gastroscope-like instrument formed the basis of TOE in clinical cardiology. Over the last 15 years the use of this technique has grown enormously. A TOE is always indicated if the TTE fails to provide conclusive information, especially if the subject has poor acoustic windows. Because of the proximity of the oesophagus and the heart, TOE is especially useful in assessing the interatrial septum, the left atrial appendage and aortic pathology. The improved signal to noise ratio combined with the high resolution from high-frequency transducers and the lack of problems related to acoustic penetration also make TOE the technique of choice for investigation of mechanical valves. Box 5.1 shows the clinical conditions in which TOE is superior to TTE. However, TOE is more invasive than TTE and provides less quantitative information so careful consideration is advisable before making a request. In the assessment of aortic valve disease and left-ventricular function, TOE often adds little and even provides less information than a good quality TTE.

Typically the patient is nil by mouth for 4 hours and written consent obtained. Dentures are removed. Relative contraindications, such as a recent upper gastrointestinal bleed or dysphagia, are investigated beforehand. The procedure can be performed with or without sedation. Continuous pulse oximetry is advised as well as suction if required. Blood pressure before, during and after the procedure should be obtained. As well as the operator, a trained nurse and cardiac technician should also be present.

Box 5.1: Common indications for a transoesophageal echocardiogram

- Poor views from transthoracic echocardiogram
- Determining cardiac source of embolus
- Infective endocarditis
- Prosthetic valve evaluation
- Intraoperative application
- Catheter-based interventions
- Adult congenital heart disease (especially atrial septal defects)
- Mitral-valve disease requiring intervention

DETERMINING A CARDIAC SOURCE OF EMBOLUS

Up to 20% of all ischaemic strokes are caused by cardiogenic embolism (see Ch. 22). TOE has a much higher sensitivity than TTE as it allows better delineation of the atria (especially the left atrial appendage), the interatrial septum and the aortic arch. The exception is left-ventricular thrombus, which is usually better seen with TTE, although its presence can often be predicted clinically. Indeed, studies have shown that in the absence of clinical, ECG or laboratory evidence of heart disease, TTE is unlikely to yield findings that alter clinical management.

The aims of echocardiography are given below.

DETECTION OF A POSSIBLE DIRECT SOURCE OF EMBOLUS

Thrombus

This may be from the left atrial appendage, especially if the patient has atrial fibrillation, or ventricular in origin (see Fig. 5.5), if the patient has poor left-ventricular function (up to 20% may have apical thrombus) or a recent anterior MI (where thrombus may develop acutely in up to 40% cases).

Vegetation

The risk of embolism in all cases of bacterial endocarditis is 15–20% before the initiation of appropriate antibiotic therapy. The risk is especially high for vegetations greater than 1 cm and those attached to the anterior mitral valve leaflet.

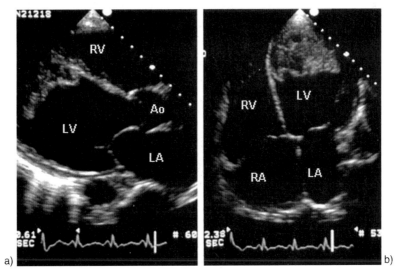

Figure 5.5
Left-ventricular apical thrombus in a patient seen on an echocardiogram performed 48 hours after an anterior myocardial infarction. (a) Parasternal long axis view. (b) Apical four chamber view

Myxoma

Left-atrial myxoma is found in 1% of all strokes in patients under 50 years.

DETECTION OF A POSSIBLE SUBSTRATE FOR EMBOLISM FORMATION

Patent foramen ovale

In a young patient with otherwise unexplained stroke the presence of a patent foramen ovale (PFO) (see Fig. 5.6) with right-to-left shunting, demonstrated with peripheral contrast injection and valsalva release, suggests a potential source of paradoxical embolism. In particular, the presence of a PFO with atrial septal aneurysm (Fig. 5.6) or with a major pulmonary embolus is associated with a high risk of embolic complications. In these circumstances percutaneous closure is recommended.

Aortic atheroma

Plaques of the aorta occur in about 25% of patients with previous embolic events. The risk of a second embolic event is high – 12% have recurrent stroke within 1 year. Plaque thickness (>4 mm) and superimposed mobile thrombi are independent risk factors for embolic events.

Low-flow state in the left atrium

This is identified by a large left atrium, spontaneous echocardiograph contrast (seen as a 'smoky' appearance) and decreased flow within a large left atrial appendage. Such low flow states are associated with increased thromboembolic risk and high recurrence rates of atrial fibrillation after a successful cardioversion.

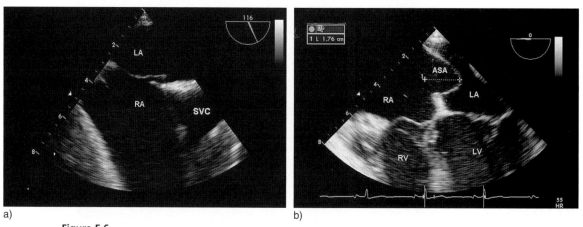

a)   b)

Figure 5.6
(a) Tranoesophageal echocardiograph (TOE) showing a patent foramen ovale. (b) TOE of an atrial septal aneurysm (ASA) bowing into the left atrium (LA). The presence of both in patients with previous embolic events necessitates percutaneous closure

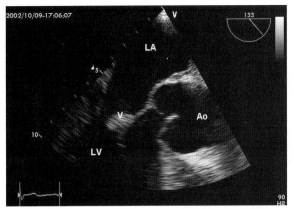

Figure 5.7
Transoesophageal echocardiograph showing a vegetation (V) on the anterior leaflet of the mitral valve. Note the relationship of this leaflet to the aortic valve, explaining why infection on one valve often spreads to the other

DIAGNOSIS OF INFECTIVE ENDOCARDITIS

The combination of echocardiographic findings with clinical parameters according to the Duke criteria has greatly improved the diagnostic accuracy of this potentially fatal disease. The hallmark echocardiograph feature is the presence of a vegetation (see Fig. 5.7), which is an oscillating mass moving independently of the structure to which it is attached. However, there are many causes of echocardiograph masses and their presence should always be interpreted in the clinical context.

TOE has a higher sensitivity (>90%) for detecting vegetations compared to TTE (<70%), especially smaller vegetations (<5 mm). TOE also facilitates the detection of left-ventricular outflow-tract complications (fistula, perforation), especially abscess formation, and prosthetic valve vegetations with a sensitivity of >80% versus 30% by TTE. Because of this, TOE is the primary diagnostic method of choice in patients with intermediate or high clinical suspicion of endocarditis. However, the technique is not 100% sensitive and in the case of mitral-valve root abscesses has a sensitivity of only 50%. Therefore, in cases with a high clinical index of suspicion, a normal TOE does not exclude infective endocarditis. In these situations close liaison with the microbiologist, referring physician and cardiologist is essential and a repeat TOE is usually recommended in 5–7 days.

INTRAOPERATIVE TOE

This is a continually growing application of TOE that is increasingly being performed by anaesthetists as well as cardiologists. The recognized uses are given below.

RECONSTRUCTIVE MITRAL-VALVE SURGERY

This remains the main use of intraoperative TOE in the UK. In cases of mitral regurgitation, precise information can be obtained concerning the mechanism (e.g. annular dilatation or the number of scallops involved in valve prolapse) as well as the severity, which allows the surgeon to decide whether valve repair or replacement is the best option. Intraoperative TOE allows immediate assessment of success of repair by detecting any residual mitral regurgitation, restriction of the repaired leaflet causing mitral stenosis, or development of systolic anterior motion of the mitral valve, which may produce an outflow tract gradient.

INTRA-AORTIC BALLOON PUMP INSERTION

Optimal placement of the balloon in the descending aorta.

INTRACARDIAC AIR VISUALIZATION

This can be visualized early and de-airing continued until TOE can no longer detect microbubbles, which may be responsible for most of the neuro-psychological syndromes often seen after open-heart surgery.

LEFT-VENTRICULAR FUNCTION

TOE allows global and regional assessment of left-ventricular function and is of particular importance in 'off-pump' surgery. It can identify regional-wall motion abnormalities as possible markers of hypoperfusion before and immediately after bypass.

POST-OPERATIVE HYPOTENSION

In patients with low cardiac output and hypotension in the intensive therapy unit, TOE assessment of the left ventricle rapidly allows discrimination between depressed myocardial function, hypovolaemia or cardiac tamponade.

AORTIC ATHEROMA

The presence of atheroma in the aortic arch and ascending aorta significantly increases the risk of stroke during cardiopulmonary bypass surgery. Detection by TOE is far more sensitive than simple palpation during surgery and alerts the surgeon with regard to cross clamping of the aorta.

REMOVAL OF INTRACARDIAC MASSES

This is particularly important with atrial myxomas where, as well as identifying the attachment point, TOE also guides the surgeon to the safest area for atrial cannulation.

ECHOCARDIOGRAPHY DURING CATHETER-BASED INTERVENTIONS

The combined use of echocardiography with fluoroscopy in catheter-based interventions continues to rise. Recognized applications are given here.

ATRIAL SEPTAL DEFECT CLOSURE

TTE often provides the diagnosis, allows assessment of right-heart size and function, together with calculation of the shunt ratio and pulmonary artery pressure. However, TOE assessment is crucial in selecting those defects suitable for percutaneous device closure. These assessments are difficult and should, ideally, be performed by those with experience of device closure. TOE defines the exact morphology, size and site of the defect, assessment of the pulmonary venous drainage, and identifies whether a suitable rim of tissue exists around the defect, over which the closure device can be safely deployed without compromising important nearby structures. During the procedure, TOE permits correct sizing and safe deployment of the device.

BALLOON MITRAL VALVULOPLASTY

TOE allows selection of those patients with severe mitral stenosis who are suitable for balloon valvuloplasty. Criteria for this include minimal calcification of the mitral leaflets and sub-valvar apparatus, no left-atrial appendage thrombus, and minimal mitral regurgitation. Post procedure, a TTE allows assessment of success (by calculating the mitral valve area) and excludes complications such as cardiac tamponade and significant mitral regurgitation.

ALCOHOL SEPTAL ABLATION IN HYPERTROPHIC CARDIOMYOPATHY

Myocardial contrast TTE with selective intracoronary injections enables the most appropriate septal perforator of the left anterior descending artery to be identified for alcohol ablation.

STENTING OF THE THORACIC AORTA

Assists in the guiding of stent placement for Type B dissection and for aortic coarctation.

RADIOFREQUENCY ABLATION

TOE helps with correct catheter positioning.

CONGENITAL HEART DISEASE

Applications include balloon positioning during aortic/pulmonary valvuloplasty, balloon dilatation of venous pathways post Mustard or Senning operation, and ventricular septal defect closure.

DOBUTAMINE STRESS ECHOCARDIOGRAPHY

Since its introduction over 10 years ago, stress echocardiography has become an established method for the diagnosis of coronary artery disease. Although dobutamine is the most commonly used stress agent, the procedure can be performed with exercise (usually bicycle), dipyridamole or pacing. The procedure compares favourably with other non-invasive procedures in detecting coronary artery disease with sensitivity, specificity and accuracy of 85–90%. The sensitivity is not reduced in the presence of left bundle branch block (LBBB) or atrial fibrillation. The procedure takes between 40 and 60 min and requires two trained staff.

Dobutamine is given by continuous infusion with incremental dose increases until target heart rate is achieved. Those unable to achieve target heart rate in this way are given atropine boluses. A baseline echocardiogram with two parasternal and three apical views is taken and the myocardial walls divided into 18 segments. The images are taken at low and peak-dose dobutamine, and recovery. All images are stored in digital format for off-line analysis. The development of new regional-wall motion abnormalities signifies ischaemia in that territory.

The procedure is safe with serious arrhythmias occurring in less than 1 in 2000. The most common side-effects are headache, nausea, chills, anxiety and hypotension. As with nuclear imaging, the development of chest pain or ECG changes during the test is not sensitive for ischaemia if there are no regional-wall abnormalities.

Absolute contraindications are rare and include poorly controlled hypertension or atrial fibrillation, known ventricular arrhythmias and hypokalaemia.

USES OF STRESS ECHOCARDIOGRAPHY

- Detection of coronary artery disease in patients with an equivocal exercise test result or in those unable to exercise or achieve a target heart rate.
- Provides prognostic information in those patients with proven coronary artery disease at angiography and identifies those who will benefit from revascularization.
- After MI to detect those with significant ischaemia or viability who require angiography and appropriate revascularization.
- To assess viability in those patients with poor left-ventricular function and coronary disease.
- To assess anaesthetic risk in patients awaiting non-cardiac major surgery.
- In valvular disease to assess dynamic gradients in mitral and aortic stenosis, and particularly to predict functional recovery in patients with severe aortic stenosis and poor left-ventricular function.
- To assess dynamic outflow tract obstruction in hypertrophic cardiomyopathy. In this situation bicycle or treadmill exercise is recommended as the stress agent rather than dobutamine.

LIMITATIONS

The main limitations of stress echocardiography are poor endocardial border definition and subjective interpretation of regional-wall abnormalities. However, use of second harmonic imaging and intravenous contrast agents has significantly improved endocardial definition in poor echocardiograph subjects. Tissue Doppler imaging with digital storage and off-line processing has allowed the procedure to become quantitative.

At present the procedure is rarely performed in district general hospitals and this is largely because of old equipment without the necessary software for image processing and off-line analysis, and the lack of training of staff.

TISSUE DOPPLER IMAGING

Doppler assessment of myocardial motion was first proposed in 1989, but even today it is little used in the day-to-day assessment of patients. The principles are the the same as for colour-flow mapping, except high-amplitude low-velocity filters are used to detect myocardial motion in preference to blood flow. For good 2-D tissue Doppler imaging, an echocardiograph machine with high frame rates and the ability to acquire digital images for off-line processing is required (Fig. 5.8).

Images are processed in spectral pulsed wave, colour M-mode and colour 2-D mode. Accurate quantification of regional myocardial motion in both systole and diastole, from multiple sites, can be acquired in seconds.

Lack of widespread clinical application is largely because of lack of training and old machines with inadequate frame rates.

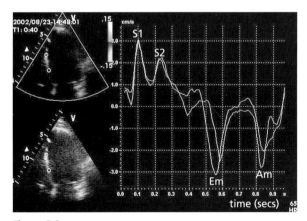

Figure 5.8
Tissue Doppler apical four chamber view showing myocardial velocity samples from the basal and mid septum. This typical pattern shows two systolic and two diastolic peaks
SI, isovolumetric contraction; S2, peak systolic velocity; Ea, peak early myocardial relaxation velocity; Am, late diastolic relaxation velocity

POTENTIAL CLINICAL APPLICATIONS

Systolic function

The technique allows assessment of longitudinal as well as transverse function and a more detailed analysis of left-ventricular function both globally and at segmental level.

Diastolic function

Accurate assessment of diastolic dysfunction can be obtained, even in conditions with raised pre-load that produce 'pseudo normalization' of standard Doppler mitral inflow velocities. Assessment is also useful in atrial fibrillation where, again, standard mitral inflow velocities cannot be used.

Differentiation of hypertrophic cardiomyopathy from physiological hypertrophy

Myocardial velocity gradients differ between these two groups who often have similar transmitral filling patterns from standard Doppler assessment.

Stress echocardiograph

This allows for the technique to be more quantitative.

Distinguish beween restriction and constriction

Segmental 'E' waves are large in constrictive pericarditis, but small in restrictive cardiomyopathy.

Assess filling pressures

This is performed by measuring mitral annular velocity and can avoid the use of invasive haemodynamic monitoring in critically ill patients.

Myocardial contrast echocardiograph

Power Doppler imaging combined with left-heart contrast agents allows assessment of microvascular integrity. At present, this technique is used as a research tool but holds great promise for assessment of microvascular perfusion and viability.

Biventricular pacing

This allows localization of the most appropriate cardiac vein to pace and optimization of pacemaker programming after implantation.

Further reading

American College of Cardiology/American Heart Association Task Force on Practice Guidelines 2002 ACC/AHA guidelines for the peri operative cardiovascular evaluation of non cardiac surgery. Circulation 105(10): 1257–1267

Cheitlin MD, Armstrong WF, Aurigemma GP et al. ACC/AHA/ASE 2003 Guideline update for the clinical application of echocardiography. Circulation 108: 1146–1162

Erbel R, Engberding R, Daniel W, Roelandt J, Visser C, Rennollet H et al. 1989 Echocardiography in the diagnosis of aortic dissection. Lancet 1: 457–461

Gasch WH 1994 Diagnosis and treatment of heart failure based on left ventricular systolic and diastolic dysfunction. JAMA 271: 1276–1280

Goldhaber SZ 2002 Echocardiography in the management of pulmonary embolism. Ann Intern Med 136(9): 691–700

Pearson AC, Labovitz AJ, Tatineni S, Gomez CR 1991 Superiority of transoesophageal echocardiography in detecting a cardiac source of embolism in patients with cerebral ischaemia of uncertain aetiology. J Am Coll Cardiol 17: 66–72

Pellikka PA, Roger VL, Oh JK, Miller FA, Seward JB, Tajik AJ 1995 Stress echocardiography. Part 2. Dobutamine stress echocardiography: techniques, implementation, clinical applications and correlations. Mayo Clinic Proc 70: 16–27

Price DJA, Wallbridge DR, Stewart MJ 2000 Tissue Doppler imaging: current and potential clinical applications. Heart 84(Suppl 2): 11–18

Schiller NB, Shah PM, Crawford M et al. 1989 Recommendations for quantitation of the left ventricle by two dimensional echocardiography. Am Soc Echocardiogr 2: 358–367

Shively BK, Gurule FT, Roldan CA, Leggett JN, Schiller NB. 1991 Diagnostic value of transoesophageal echocardiography compared to transthoracic echocardiography in infective endocarditis. J Am Coll Cardiol 18: 391–397

SELF-ASSESSMENT

Questions

What is the role of echocardiography in:

a. Aortic dissection
b. Congenital heart disease
c. Management of pulmonary embolism
d. Pre-operative cardiovascular evaluation for non-cardiac surgery
e. Pre-operative assessment of left-ventricular function
f. Pre-operative murmur evaluation
g. Pre-operative assessment of coronary artery disease.

Answers

a. The role of TOE in aortic dissection is covered in detail in Chapter 17.

b. Transthoracic echocardiography (TTE) gives the correct diagnosis in 90% of paediatric but only about 60% of adult congenital heart lesions. Transoesophageal echocardiography (TOE) is required for the correct diagnosis in the remaining cases, although magnetic resonance imaging (MRI), where available, is an excellent alternative.

c. TTE is not recommended for the diagnosis of acute pulmonary embolism as sensitivity and specificity are low. Thrombus is rarely seen. However, when the diagnosis is established it does identify those patients with poor prognosis who will benefit from thombolysis or embolectomy. Echocardiographic poor prognostic features in pulmonary embolus include:

- RV dilatation (RVEDD >30 mm, RVEDD/LVEDD >1), and hypokinesis (EDD = End diastolic diameter)
- raised PA pressure
- paradoxical motion of interventricular septum
- presence of a patent foramen ovale
- presence of free-floating thrombus in the right heart (rarely seen)
- low cardiac index.

Serial imaging of right-ventricular size and function and pulmonary artery pressure helps allow monitoring of the response to treatment and particularly identifies those who fail to respond to thrombolysis. Such patients should be considered for embolectomy. Patients with normal echocardiogram and normal systemic pressure have an extremely good prognosis and do not require thrombolysis or embolectomy.

TOE is reserved for critically ill patients and some case series report sensitivities and specificities as high as 85% for the diagnosis of proximal pulmonary emboli (Fig. 5.9). However, while the pulmonary arteries can be seen up to lobar level, the mid portion of the left main pulmonary artery is hidden by the left main bronchus.

d. Pre-operative echocardiography requests form an increasing workload for all cardiac departments. The American College of Cardiology/American Heart Association (ACC/AHA) guidelines article shown in the Further reading section is strongly recommended reading. High-risk non-cardiac surgery includes vascular procedures, emergency surgery and prolonged procedures involving large fluid shifts. Intrathoracic,

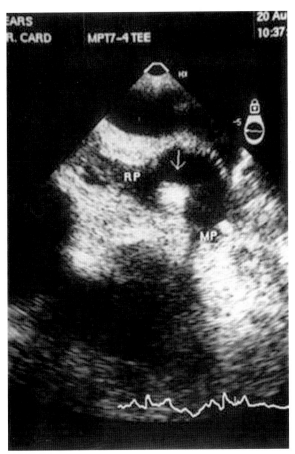

Figure 5.9
Transoesophageal echocardiograph showing thrombus (arrowed) in the main pulmonary artery (MP) in a patient presenting with shock and hypoxia requiring emergency ventilation RP, right pulmonary artery

intraperitoneal, orthopaedic and prostate surgery are considered intermediate risk, cataract and breast surgery low risk. Generally, cardiac evaluation is required for high- and intermediate-risk surgery only. (See also Ch. 25.)

e. A pre-operative TTE is advised for all patients with known or suspected heart failure with deteriorating symptoms, and for those with stable heart failure and no cardiac evaluation for 2 years. Screening all patients pre-operatively is not recommended.

f. A TTE is mandatory pre-operatively if a new murmur is detected and is not considered to be innocent. In patients with previous mild or moderate valvular disease, a TTE should be performed if no evaluation has occurred in the previous 2 years.

g. Stress echocardiography is one of the recommended non-invasive methods for this purpose. Patients who should be referred prior to high-risk surgery include those with proven stable coronary artery disease, those with suggestive symptoms and those with a high probability of coronary disease. Patients with unstable symptoms should, ideally, have angiography. Non-invasive assessment is not recommended in low-risk asymptomatic patients with isolated ventricular ectopics, bundle branch block or with evidence of pre-excitation.

Nuclear imaging

Chee Yee Loong and C. Anagnostopoulos

BASIC PRINCIPLES

All nuclear imaging techniques involve the internal administration of a radioisotope, which emits gamma photons by radioactive decay, followed by the imaging of radioactivity within an organ of interest using a gamma camera. The gamma camera has a scintillation detector, which interacts with the emitted photon to generate a light signal that is converted into an electrical signal enhanced by photomultipliers. In the 1970s, planar imaging was employed; modern gamma cameras comprise of one or more rotating detector(s) that permit single-photon emission computed tomographic (SPECT) imaging. Tomographic imaging provides a true 3-D display of the distribution of radioactivity, with resultant improved image contrast and the potential for quantification. The spatial resolution of modern gamma cameras ranges between 6 and 10 mm.

RADIONUCLIDE MYOCARDIAL PERFUSION IMAGING

Radionuclide myocardial perfusion imaging (MPI) is used to detect haemodynamically significant coronary artery disease (CAD). It involves the intravenous administration of a perfusion tracer, such as thallium-201, technetium-99m-labeled sestamibi or technetium-99m-labeled tetrofosmin, to evaluate regional coronary flow after stress and at rest. Stress may be performed by dynamic exercise or with pharmacological agents (adenosine, dipyridamole or dobutamine). Comparison of the stress and rest images permits comment on the presence, or otherwise, of inducible ischaemia and/or infarction, and hence on the likely presence, or absence, of flow-limiting coronary lesions (Fig. 6.1). The incorporation of ECG-gating provides additional information regarding regional and global left-ventricular function, as well as enhancing image interpretation. The recent application of non-uniform attenuation correction by transmission imaging may further improve diagnostic accuracy.

MPI is the only non-invasive and widely available method of assessing myocardial perfusion. The indications for MPI are summarized in Box 6.1.

Many studies have assessed the diagnostic accuracy of the technique for the detection of CAD, mostly by comparison to the coronary arteriogram as gold standard. Published

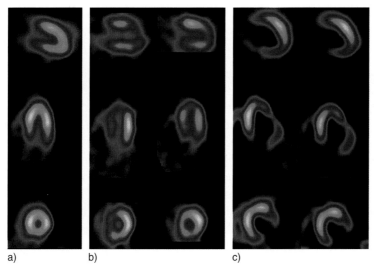

a)　　　　　　b)　　　　　　　　　c)

Figure 6.1
Examples of radionuclide myocardial perfusion scans (thallium-201). (a) Normal myocardial perfusion scan, showing homogeneous uptake of radiotracer throughout the left-ventricular myocardium (vertical long axis, horizontal long axis and short axis views respectively). (b) Inducible ischaemia in the left anterior descending (LAD) artery territory. The images after stress (left panel) show a moderate reduction in tracer uptake at the apex, apical anterior wall and septum; at rest (right panel), the images are normal. These scintigraphic findings are consistent with a proximal LAD lesion. (c) Fixed full-thickness myocardial infarction (MI) in the left circumflex (LCx) territory. The images after stress and at rest show absent tracer uptake at the inferolateral wall

---

Box 6.1: Indications for performing myocardial perfusion imaging

To assess the presence and degree of coronary obstruction in patients with suspected coronary artery disease (CAD)

To aid the management of patients with known CAD:

– to determine the likelihood of future coronary events, for instance, after myocardial infarction or related to proposed non-cardiac surgery
– to guide strategies of myocardial revascularization by determining the haemodynamic significance of coronary lesions
– to assess the adequacy of percutaneous and surgical revascularization

To assess myocardial viability and hibernation, particularly with reference to planned myocardial revascularization

Special indications:

– to assess the haemodynamic significance of known or suspected anomalous coronary arteries and muscle bridging
– to assess the haemodynamic significance of coronary aneurysms in Kawasaki's disease
– to assess the presence of microvascular disease, for instance, in diabetes mellitus, left-ventricular hypertrophy and syndrome X

---

figures for sensitivity and specificity vary according to certain factors, such as the population studied (sex, presenting symptoms, medication, presence of previous infarction, etc.), the imaging technique used (planar or SPECT, qualitative or quantitative analysis), and the experience of the centre. Using modern techniques with SPECT imaging, good accuracy can be achieved with a sensitivity of 91% and a specificity of 89%. This is significantly better than exercise electrocardiography, for which a large meta-analysis has shown a sensitivity of 68% and a specificity of 77%.

Beyond diagnosis, MPI contributes to the management of known or suspected CAD by assessing the likelihood of a future coronary event such as MI or coronary death. This can guide the need for invasive investigation and revascularization, and is also useful for risk stratification after acute MI or in patients undergoing non-cardiac surgery. MPI with vasodilator stress can be safely performed in stabilized patients as early as 4 days after acute MI. MPI is more powerful as an indicator of prognosis than clinical assessment, exercise electrocardiography and coronary angiography, and it provides incremental prognostic value even once the other tests have been performed. The key variables that predict future events are the extent and depth of the inducible ischaemia. Other features of increased risk are increased lung uptake of tracer on stress images (which indicates raised pulmonary capillary pressure either at rest or in response to stress) and ventricular dilatation that is greater in stress images than at rest. A normal perfusion scan indicates a likelihood of future coronary events of less than 1% per year, a rate that is lower than that in an asymptomatic population. Thus, whether CAD is present or not, further investigation can be avoided.

MPI can be valuable both before and after myocardial revascularization, either by angioplasty or bypass surgery. MPI is often the most reliable and objective way of demonstrating myocardial ischaemia, thus ensuring that revascularization is targeted at the culprit lesion(s). It is an excellent tool for predicting restenosis and clinical events after angioplasty, and this can be especially helpful in patients with recurrent but atypical symptoms.

ECG-gated tomographic MPI also permits the detection of myocardial hibernation within one imaging modality. Hibernating myocardium has the potential to recover function after revascularization, and, hence, it is important to detect this condition in patients with chronic ischaemic left-ventricular dysfunction. All three commonly used perfusion tracers are also good markers of viability, and ECG-gating permits the evaluation of regional function. Hibernating myocardial segments classically fulfill three scintigraphic criteria:

1. Viability: resting tracer uptake >50% of maximal
2. Dysfunction: akinesis (or severe hypokinesis) on ECG-gating
3. Ischaemia: improvement in tracer uptake from stress to rest images.

Studies have shown that there is good agreement between ECG-gated tomographic MPI and positron emission tomography (PET) using fluorine-18 fluorodeoxyglucose (a marker of glucose uptake), as well as with dobutamine stress echocardiography, for the detection of hibernating myocardium.

RADIONUCLIDE VENTRICULOGRAPHY

Radionuclide ventriculography is used for the assessment of ventricular function. In equilibrium radionuclide ventriculography (ERNV), red cells labelled with technetium-

99m are allowed to equilibrate in the blood pool and the heart is then imaged under the gamma camera. The waxing and waning of radioactivity within the ventricular chambers during diastole and systole, respectively, permits construction of a dynamic ventriculogram. Left-ventricular function can be evaluated quantitatively (by calculation of the ejection fraction) or qualitatively (by observation of wall movement). Global left-ventricular impairment is characteristic of cardiomyopathy, while regional defects are seen usually following MI. Stress radionuclide ventriculography using exercise or peripheral cold stimulation (cold pressor test) is used for detection of myocardial ischaemia – provocation of reversible regional-wall motion abnormalities is strongly suggestive of CAD. First-pass radionuclide ventriculography (FPRNV) is similar to ERNV except that a bolus of tracer is rapidly flushed through and its passage through the central circulation is imaged. FPRNV is often used to measure right-ventricular ejection fraction, as well as shunting in congenital heart disease.

INFARCT IMAGING

Infarct imaging (or hot-spot scintigraphy) permits the diagnosis of recent MI, but in practice it is rarely used. Technetium-99m-labelled pyrophosphate and indium-III-labelled anti-myosin antibody are taken up by recently infarcted myocardium, producing a localized 'hot spot' of radioactivity on the scintigram. Diagnostic sensitivity is greatest during the first week following infarction.

POSITRON EMISSION TOMOGRAPHY

PET uses positron-emitting radiopharmaceuticals and emission computed axial tomography to produce images of coronary flow and cardiac metabolism. The instrumentation consists of detector systems working in coincidence to register the paired annihilation 511-keV photons emitted by the tracer. PET devices record multiple slices of the heart simultaneously (usually between 3 and 18 slices). Stress and rest perfusion studies are performed using nitrogen-13 ammonia, oxygen-15 water or rubidium-82. Metabolic studies of the heart can be carried out using carbon-11 palmitate or fluorine-18 fluorodeoxyglucose. PET is a highly sensitive imaging modality, and is able to provide absolute quantification of myocardial perfusion and metabolism. The main drawback to this technique is cost. It requires expensive detectors and a cyclotron site for the production of most of the radiopharmaceuticals.

Further reading

Bateman TM 1997 Clinical relevance of a normal myocardial perfusion scintigraphic study. J Nucl Cardiol 4: 172–173

Beller GA, Zaret BL 2000 Contribution of nuclear cardiology to diagnosis and prognosis of patients with coronary artery disease. Circulation 101: 1465–1478

de Bono D 1999 Investigation and management of stable angina: revised guidelines 1998. Heart 81: 546–555

National Institute for Clinical Excellence 2003 Myocardial perfusion scintigraphy for the diagnosis and management of angina and myocardial infarction (no. 73). National Institute of Clinical Excellence, London, www.nice.org.uk/TA073guidance

Pennell DJ, Prvulovich E 1995 Clinicians guide to nuclear medicine: nuclear cardiology. British Nuclear Medicine Society, London

Schwaiger M, Melin J 1999 Cardiological applications of nuclear medicine. Lancet 354: 661–666

Underwood SR, Anagnostopoulos C 2001 Nuclear cardiology. In: Grainger RG, Allison DJ, Adam A, Dixon AK (eds). Diagnostic radiology, 4th edn. Churchill Livingstone, London, pp. 721–739

SELF-ASSESSMENT

Questions

a. When would one use technetium-99m-labelled tracers preferentially over thallium-201 in myocardial perfusion imaging?

b. What can nuclear imaging provide that conventional exercise electrocardiography cannot?

Answers

a. All three commercially available radiopharmaceuticals are excellent tracers of coronary blood flow. Thallium-201 has better myocardial uptake characteristics and, in theory, provides defects with greater contrast, but sestamibi and tetrofosmin are superior in terms of physical characteristics. The higher energy of technetium-99m means that there is less susceptibility to attenuation and scatter. Hence, technetium-99m-labelled tracers should be preferentially used over thallium-201 in patients where attenuation and scatter are likely to degrade image quality, such as obese patients and women, as well as when ECG-gating is required (e.g. hibernation studies).

b. Both exercise electrocardiography (ECG) and radionuclide myocardial perfusion imaging (MPI) are non-invasive tests for detecting coronary artery disease (CAD). Exercise ECG is cheap and widely available, but suffers from a suboptimal diagnostic accuracy, particularly in women. In addition, it is of limited diagnostic value in patients who are unable to exercise to an adequate workload and in those with resting ECG abnormalities; in patients with left bundle branch block (LBBB), exercise ECG has no diagnostic value for CAD. Radionuclide MPI, although more expensive than exercise ECG, is highly cost effective. It is useful in patients who are unable to exercise, since it can be combined with pharmacological stress. It has a better diagnostic accuracy, particularly in women, and has diagnostic value in patients with LBBB and other resting ECG abnormalities. Finally, it is superior to exercise ECG in detecting the extent of CAD, as well as in localizing the coronary stenosis.

Magnetic resonance imaging and computed tomography

7

A. Elkington

CARDIOVASCULAR MAGNETIC RESONANCE

Cardiovascular magnetic resonance (CMR) is a rapidly developing technique, with increasing availability and indications. CMR does not expose the patient to ionizing radiation making it a safe modality for clinical trials and serial patient studies. Approximately 1% of patients are unable to undergo a CMR study due to claustrophobia.

CARDIAC MASS AND VOLUMES

CMR is the gold standard for measuring cardiac volumes, function and mass. The high reproducibility of CMR allows smaller sample sizes when assessing changes in left-ventricular volumes in response to treatment. Figure 7.1 shows a typical example of a four-chamber, two-chamber and short-axis (SA) stack study in a normal subject, from which cardiac volumes are calculated.

COMPLEX ANATOMY

CMR is not limited by imaging planes, allowing complete assessment of complex anatomy, for example in patients with congenital heart disease. Volumes of shunts and the pressure gradient across valves can be quantitatively measured. CMR is particularly good for visualizing the central pulmonary arteries, thoracic aorta and defining complex anomalies involving the great vessels and ventricles.

CONTRAST-ENHANCED MAGNETIC RESONANCE ANGIOGRAPHY

3-D contrast-enhanced magnetic resonance angiography (MRA) is a powerful tool for visualizing the aorta, carotids and renal arteries – allowing exclusion of such diseases as coarctation and renal artery stenosis. CMR has a specificity and sensitivity of nearly 100% in the diagnosis of aortic dissection (see Ch. 17). Figure 7.2 shows a surface-rendered, maximum-intensity projection contrast-enhanced MR angiogram of the thoracic aorta in a patient with a tight coarctation.

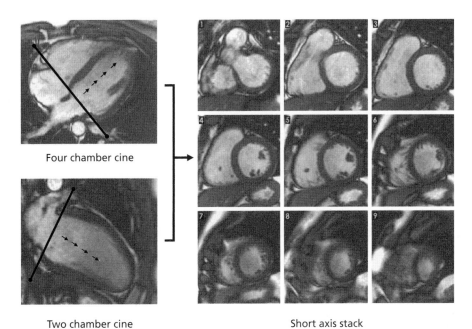

Four chamber cine

Two chamber cine

Short axis stack

Figure 7.1
How cardiac volumes and mass are calculated using CMR. From the four-chamber and two-chamber end-diastolic views, a series of contiguous basal to apex short axis slices are acquired, encompassing the entire left and right ventricles. The endocardial and epicardial borders are traced, from which ventricular volumes and mass are calculated

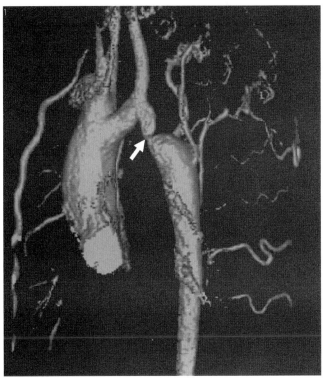

Figure 7.2
Surface rendered contrast-enhanced MR angiogram of the thoracic aorta. Arrow indicates tight coarctation

VIABILITY

CMR can detect myocardial infarction, following injection of a gadolinium chelate ('late enhancement'), with greater accuracy than single-photon emission computed tomography (SPECT) or positron emission tomography (PET). Recent studies have indicated that the extent of late enhancement can predict functional recovery of myocardium after revascularization. Figure 7.3 shows how late enhancement allows excellent demonstration of areas of infarction. Late enhancement techniques can also aid the diagnosis of cardiomyopathies, for example infiltrative cardiomyopathies or hypertrophic cardiomyopathy. Figure 7.4 shows a case of hypertrophic cardiomyopathy, with areas of late enhancement following injection of gadolinium.

CORONARY MAGNETIC RESONANCE ANGIOGRAPHY

Coronary MRA is clinically useful in diagnosing and excluding anomalous coronary arteries. However, coronary MRA has not yet become suitable for routine screening for coronary artery disease, although recent data suggest that it is able to exclude triple vessel and left main stem disease with a high degree of confidence.

PERFUSION CARDIOVASCULAR MAGNETIC RESONANCE

Perfusion CMR offers an attractive alternative to the current methods available for assessing myocardial perfusion. It is ionizing radiation free, has excellent spatial resolution and can be combined with other aspects of CMR. Studies indicate that

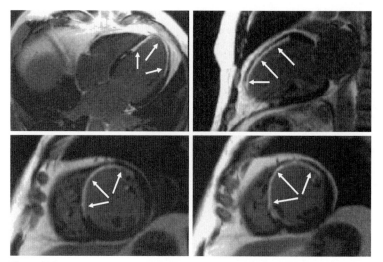

Figure 7.3
Late enhancement following gadolinium injection CMR study in the four-chamber, two-chamber and short-axis views, in a patient with near transmural anteroseptal myocardial infarction. Arrows indicate the areas of enhancement (white) indicative of infarction

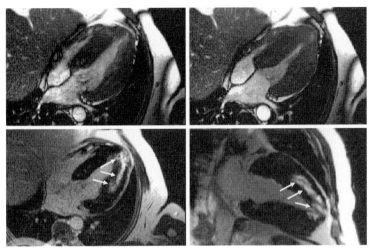

Figure 7.4
Top row shows end-diastolic and end-systolic four-chamber views by CMR in a patient with hypertrophic cardiomyopathy. Bottom row shows late enhancement images following gadolinium injection in the same patient. Arrows indicate areas of late enhancement, in a pattern typical of hypertrophic cardiomyopathy

perfusion CMR has similar sensitivity and specificity of SPECT for the detection of significant coronary disease. However, further development of the technique is needed before it is suitable for routine clinical use.

COMPUTED TOMOGRAPHY

Conventional computed tomography (CT) has been widely used in the diagnosis of pulmonary embolus, aortic dissection and pericardial disease. With the development of electron beam CT (EBCT) and multislice spiral CT the range of cardiac indications for referral has expanded.

PULMONARY EMBOLISM

CT is the gold standard for the diagnosis of pulmonary embolism and at some centres it is replacing X-ray angiography and nuclear perfusion imaging.

AORTIC DISSECTION AND ANEURYSM

CT has an accuracy of 95%, and is the equivalent of CMR and better than X-ray angiography in the diagnosis of aortic dissection. CT is an effective way of measuring the maximum diameter of an aneurysm and monitoring the diameter over time (see Ch. 17).

PERICARDIAL DISEASE

CT is particularly effective at detecting thickening of the pericardium, defined as greater than 4 mm, which is one of the main discriminatory factors between constrictive pericarditis and restrictive cardiomyopathy.

CORONARY CALCIFICATION

Coronary calcification usually indicates the presence of atherosclerosis. CT has been used in the past few years for the detection of calcification within the coronary arteries (Fig. 7.5). A calcium score is calculated from the total area of calcium multiplied by density weighting. In comparison to coronary angiography, coronary calcification has a high sensitivity for predicting significant coronary stenoses (approximately 90%), but only moderate specificity. The role of CT in detecting coronary calcification in asymptomatic individuals is controversial. CT-defined calcification was found to be about equivalent, but no better, than risk factors assessment in identifying patients who will suffer coronary events in a 3–4 year follow-up period.

COMPUTED TOMOGRAPHY CORONARY ANGIOGRAPHY

Contrast enhanced CT has been shown to be effective in visualizing the lumen of the major coronary arteries. Sensitivities of 74–92% and specificities of 79–94% for identifying haemodynamically significant coronary artery stenoses have been found.

PULMONARY VENOGRAPHY

An increasing indication is the assessment of patients' pulmonary veins pre- and post-pulmonary vein ablation for atrial fibrillation.

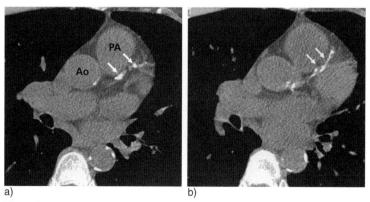

a)   b)

Figure 7.5
Two transverse cuts by CT. Arrows indicate areas of calcification in the left main stem and left anterior descending artery. Ao, aorta; PA, main pulmonary artery

INTRAVASCULAR ULTRASONOGRAPHY

Contrast angiography is limited in its ability to quantitate the extent and distribution of coronary atherosclerosis. Intravascular ultrasonography (IVUS) is a safe, accurate, reproducible technique for detecting vessel wall pathology. In particular, IVUS provides unique insights into the changes in vessel wall pathology during percutaneous coronary intervention (PCI). Current catheter-based IVUS systems are able to assess vessels down to a lumen diameter of 1 mm. However, the widespread use of IVUS has been limited due to its cost, technical difficulty, and lengthy set-up for occasional users.

Further reading

Higgins CB, De Roos A. Cardiovascular MRI and MRA. Lippincott Williams and Wilkins 2003.
Manning WJ, Pennell DJ. Cardiovascular Magnetic Resonance. Churchill Livingstone 2002.
Ohnesorge BM, Becker CR, Flohr TG, Reiser MF. Multi-slice CT in Cardiac Imaging. Springer 2002.

SELF-ASSESSMENT

Questions

a. What are the benefits of a coronary magnetic resonance (CMR) study as compared with other imaging techniques?
b. What are the contraindications to a CMR study?
c. What is the benefit of a computed tomography coronary calcification study?

Answers

a. The table below gives the relative strengths and weaknesses of a range of imaging techniques. Three pluses (+) indicates current gold standard, while minus (–) indicates modality is not suited for that field.

	X-ray angiography	CMR	CT	Echo	SPECT	PET
Function and mass	++	+++	+	++	+	+
Ischaemia	–	+	–	+	+++	+++
Viability	–	+++	–	+	+	+++
Great vessels	++	+++	+++	+	–	–
Coronaries	+++	+	+	–	–	–
Valves	+	++	–	+++	–	–
Morphology	+	+++	+	++	–	–
Pericardial disease	–	++	+++	++	–	–

CMR = cardiovascular magnetic resonance; CT = computed tomography; SPECT = single photon emission computed tomography; PET = positron emission tomography

b. Pacemaker, cerebral clips and ferromagnetic material in the eye (for example metal filings from lathe work) are contraindications. Note: prosthetic valves, coronary stents and hip replacements are not contraindications.
c. In asymptomatic individuals the evidence does not at present indicate improved prognostic evaluation over careful assessment on the basis of risk factors. In patients with suspected coronary artery disease, electron beam computed tomography (EBCT) coronary calcification assessment provides good sensitivity, but only moderate specificity for predicting significant coronary stenoses.

Cardiovascular disease markers

8

P. O. Collinson

INTRODUCTION

The atheromatous plaque defines the pathophysiology of cardiovascular disease (CVD). The concept of plaque development and progression is central to a rational understanding of the pathogenesis, pathology, diagnosis and management of coronary artery disease (CAD). Following initial formation, plaque development may progress with production of a stable or unstable lesion. An unstable plaque with erosion or rupture represents the final common pathway of all acute coronary syndromes (ACS). Cardiac biomarkers can be used to assess all stages of the evolution of this process but can conveniently be divided into those used to assess four processess: the risk of developing CVD, the risk of plaque rupture, the diagnosis and prognosis in ACS, and the assessment of myocardial function (Fig. 8.1).

BIOMARKERS OF PLAQUE DEVELOPMENT AND PROGRESSION

Plaque initiation occurs as a result of the interaction of genetic and environmental factors. Post-mortem studies have shown that the earliest atheromatous changes can be detected in children and young adults. Lipoproteins contribute to plaque development. Some lipoprotein fractions (such as oxidized low-density lipoproteins (LDL), small dense LDL and intermediate density lipoprotein) are particularly atherogenic. Direct measurement of apolipoprotein b and calculation of the non-high-density lipoprotein (HDL) cholesterol fraction are currently the best tools to assess the amount of the most atherogenic components. Lipoprotein interaction is reflected in the total cholesterol/HDL ratio. In addition to lipoproteins, there are other markers of the risk of plaque development and progression. Lipoprotein(a) (Lp(a)) is a complex lipoprotein with a central core of LDL covalently linked to a polypeptide chain of apolipoprotein(a). Apolipoprotein(a) shows sequence homology with plasminogen and has been proposed as a link between plaque rupture and thrombosis. Homocysteine is a risk marker for development and progression of CVD, although its precise role remains to be fully defined. Endothelial injury is the initial basis of plaque formation and it has been suggested that this may be due to a direct effect of homocysteine on endothelial cells. Measurement of Lp(a), homocysteine and

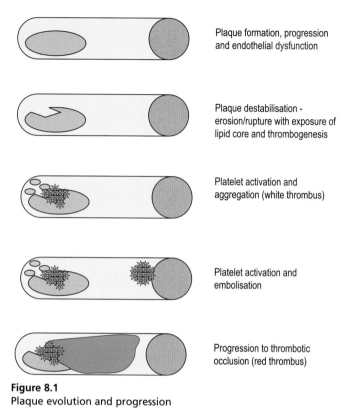

Plaque formation, progression and endothelial dysfunction

Plaque destabilisation - erosion/rupture with exposure of lipid core and thrombogenesis

Platelet activation and aggregation (white thrombus)

Platelet activation and embolisation

Progression to thrombotic occlusion (red thrombus)

Figure 8.1
Plaque evolution and progression

Box 8.1: Biomarkers for assessment of risk of cardiovascular disease

- Total cholesterol, LDL and HDL
- Total cholesterol/HDL ratio
- Apolipoproteins a and b
- Lp(a)
- Homocysteine

---

lipoproteins forms part of an optimal assessment in combination with the classical risk factors, however, these are not routinely measured in all UK hopitals at present (Box 8.1).

BIOMARKERS OF PLAQUE STABILITY

Atheromatous plaques contain a range of inflammatory cells. Studies have shown that there is expression of cytokines and interleukins within the plaque. Endothelial injury results in progressive recruitment of mononuclear cells within the atheromatous plaque and is part of the process of plaque development. Levels of interleukins such as IL-6 are increased in patients at risk of developing CVD and in patients with ACS. Interleukin levels rise and fall rapidly but result in the production of an acute phase response, with

---

Box 8.2: C reactive proteins for risk assessment

- Low risk <1 mg/l
- Intermediate risk 1–3 mg/l
- High risk >3 mg/l

---

elevation of acute phase reactants such as C-reactive protein (CRP) and serum amyloid A protein (SAA).

A large series of studies have shown that CRP can be related to risk of a subsequent cardiac event in patients both with and without pre-existing CVD. The CRP levels reported in these studies are low, in the range 0–3 mg/l. They can be measured using modern 'sensitive' CRP methods. Methods currently in routine use are for detection of infection and measure in the range 10–1000 mg/l so are unsuitable for this role. The clinical role of inflammatory markers is not yet fully defined. Interleukin-6 (IL-6) is probably a better marker in ACS than CRP but is less convenient for routine measurement. Whether measurement of either can contribute to the management of ACS is not yet known. The current role of CRP is as a risk predictor for primary prevention of CVD. Sensitive CRP can be shown to be an independent and additive risk factor to total cholesterol and LDL measurements. Aspirin treatment is associated with reduction in CRP and lower risk of cardiovascular events. Treatment with statins is also associated with reduction in CRP and a low CRP, plus a low LDL has been shown to indicate the lowest risk group (Box 8.2).

BIOMARKERS OF PLAQUE RUPTURE

Cardiovascular risk is related to the degree of atheromatous disease, 'plaque burden'. Plaque rupture is often multiple. A stable plaque is one with a thick overlying cap and minimal evidence of inflammatory activity. The inflammatory process within plaques results in plaque instability and a predisposition to plaque rupture. The traditional view of atheromatous disease is a progressive narrowing with flow limitation and symptom development. This is not the case. From 70 to 80% of plaques causing ACS are not flow limiting. Plaque rupture or erosion occurs with exposure of the plaque core containing thrombogenic plaque contents. This results in platelet aggregation with formation of 'white thrombus' and initiation of the clotting cascade. The risk of progression of disease will then be a balance between the tendency towards platelet aggregation and thrombosis and the anti-thrombotic activity of the blood. This is reflected in the relationship between elevations of thrombotic markers and risk of CVD events. The activation of the coagulation system can be assessed by functional tests that measure activity or by measuring concentrations of precursors or reaction products of activation. The half-life of both precursors and products adds to the complication of interpreting these measurements.

Markers of coagulation which are raised in acute coronary syndromes include prothrombin fragments F1 + 2 and Factor VIIa. Elevation of thrombin/antithrombin complex associated with and related to cardiac troponin elevation has also been described. Impaired thrombolysis with elevated plasminogen activator and plasminogen activator inhibitor-1 (PAI-1) has been described in ACS. This elevation is associated with increased risk of cardiac events. Elevated PAI-1 is associated with failure of or inadequate response to thrombolysis. However, routine use of these markers outside the research setting is not currently practical.

BIOMARKERS FOR DIAGNOSIS AND PROGNOSIS IN ACUTE CORONARY SYNDROMES

The initial platelet/fibrinogen/fibrin aggregates are unstable and fragments break off with downstream embolization and microinfarction by occlusion of small vessels. This produces minimal release of markers of myocyte necrosis. These lesions may then heal with no further evidence of significant cardiac damage. Lesion progression will result in full activation of the coagulation cascade and production of an occlusive fibrin thrombus, a 'red thrombus'. This will result in a large area of infarction corresponding to the territory supplied by the culprit lesion artery with a more substantial release of markers of myocyte necrosis (see Fig. 8.2).

Markers of myocyte necrosis can be divided into cytosolic proteins and structural proteins. Cytosolic proteins include enzymes, such as creatine kinase (CK) and lactate dehydrogenase and proteins, such as myoglobin. In routine clinical practice measurement of CK and its MB isoenzyme (CK-MB) are most often used. CK-MB is not cardiac specific. It is also found in skeletal muscle, 3–10% of total activity, compared to the 25–45% found in the myocardium, but there is much more skeletal than cardiac muscle.

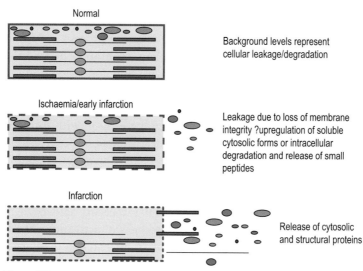

Figure 8.2
Schematic representation of release of cardiac biomarkers during ischaemia and infarction

CK and CK-MB levels rise 4-6 hours after acute myocardial infarction (AMI) and peak at 21–24 hours. Myoglobin offers an earlier marker. It can be detected 2 hours post AMI and peaks at 12 hours. It, therefore, has a short time window, so can miss late presentations.

Only two cardiac structural proteins are measured routinely: the cardiac troponins (cTn), cardiac troponin T (cTnT) and cardiac troponin I (cTnI). They are part of the troponin–tropomyosin complex that regulates muscular contraction. They are the products of individual genes and are found only in the myocardium. The major advantages of measurement of cTn measurement are the following:

- Cardiac specific – Elevations of CK and CK-MB due to skeletal muscle damage do not cause cTn elevation. If CK or CK-MB is elevated but cTn is not, the patient does not have AMI.
- Sensitive to cardiac damage missed by CK and CK-MB and can be used to predict outcome – A number of studies have shown that cTn elevations without elevated CK or CK-MB predict an increased risk of cardiac death or AMI.
- Can be used to plan management – The absence of cTn elevation 12 hours from symptoms excludes AMI. When combined with stress testing or perfusion imaging, patients can be accurately risk stratified. A negative cTn and a negative functional test defines a low risk group. Conversely, in patients with non-ST elevation MI/unstable angina, low-molecular-weight heparin, glycoprotein IIb/IIIa antagonists or revascularization show maximal benefit if cTn is elevated.
- Long time window – Detection of myocardial infarction up to 5–7 days post event is possible (Fig. 8.3). This also means that for infarct timing or detection of re-infarction a short time window marker is desirable. The combination of cTn plus myoglobin, CK or CK-MB can be used.

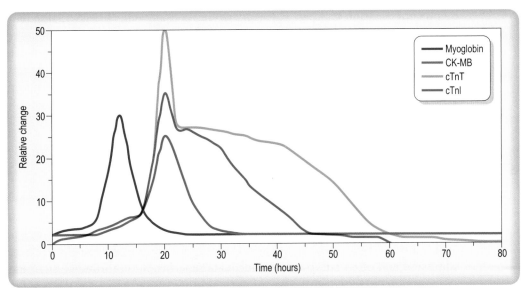

Figure 8.3
Release kinetics of conventional cytosolic biomarkers compared with cardiac troponin T and I

AMI has been redefined to include cTn as the 'gold standard' test; a typical rise and fall of troponin with at least one of the following:

1. ischaemic symptoms
2. new Q waves
3. ischaemic electrocardiograph changes
4. need for percutaneous coronary intervention (PCI)

or

5. pathological findings of an acute AMI.

This has been defined as the maximal concentration of cTnT or cTnI exceeding the 99th centile of the values for a reference control group.

Elevation of cTn means cardiac damage, but AMI is a **clinical** diagnosis. This is part of the AMI definition. A knife through the heart produces chest pain, it causes cTn elevation – but it is not an AMI! Elevation of cTn will occur in any clinical situations that cause cardiac damage. These can be divided into those primarily due to rupture of an atheromatous plaque, primary ischaemic cardiac injury (PICI); those secondary to ischaemic coronary disease, secondary ischaemic coronary injury (SICI); and those due to non-ischaemic coronary injury (NICI). Examples are summarized in Table 8.1.

STRATEGIES FOR TEST UTILIZATION

The ECG and clinical features or scoring systems such as the thrombolysis in myocardial ischaemia (TIMI) risk score are used to assign patients into risk categories. The TIMI risk score for unstable angina/non-ST elevation MI is a simple prognostication scheme that categorizes a patient's risk of death and ischaemic events and provides a basis for therapeutic decision making. This is based on the following characteristics: patient age, at least three risk factors for coronary artery disease, significant coronary stenosis, ST segment deviation, severe anginal symptoms (e.g. greater than or equal to two anginal events in the last 24 hours), use of aspirin in the last 7 days and elevated serum cardiac markers. A score of 0 to 7 can then be derived for prognostic purposes. Interpretation of cardiac biomarkers is then performed according to risk group. Specific scenarios are now discussed in turn.

ST ELEVATION MYOCARDIAL INFARCTION

In this group, management is aimed at opening the occluded artery. Cardiac biomarker measurements have no role if thrombolysis is the primary management pathway and a single cTn measurement at 12–24 hours from admission to confirm diagnosis and quantitate damage is sufficient. Approximately one-third of patients have elevated cTn on admission and often fail to achieve adequate reperfusion on thrombolysis. Patients from this group may be candidates for primary angioplasty since this has the best chance of achieving TIMI III flow overall.

Table 8.1: Classification of troponin release by pathophysiology

Primary ischaemic cardiac injury

Thrombotic coronary artery occlusion due to platelets/fibrin	ST elevation MI Non-ST elevation MI	

Secondary ischaemic cardiac injury

Coronary intervention	Primary PCI	Distal embolization from clot or atheroma Side branch occlusion
	Elective PCI	Distal embolization from atheroma or debris Side branch occlusion
	CABG	Global ischaemia from inadequate perfusion, inadequate myocardial cell protection or anoxia
Sympathomimetics	Cocaine Catecholamine storm Head injury, stroke, intracerebral bleed	
Pulmonary embolus	Presumed right heart strain or hypoxia	
Coronary artery spasm	Japan – up to 10% on admissions	
Coronary artery embolization	Clot Air CABG	
Coronary artery inflammation with microvascular occlusion	Vasculitides Connective-tissue disease SLE	
End-stage renal failure	More severe CAD but 50% have normal coronaries	
Rhythm disturbances	Prolonged tachyarrhythmia or bradyarrhythymia with IHD	
Acute heart failure	More commonly with concomitant IHD	
Direct coronary artery trauma	RTA	
Extreme endurance exercise	Extreme marathons Extreme training	Wall motion abnormalities cTn +ve deaths presumed due to extreme oxygen debt producing ischaemia

Non-ischaemic cardiac injury

Known causes of myocarditis	Infection	Bacterial Viral
	Inflammation Auto-Immune	Polymyositis Scleroderma Sarcoid
	Drugs	Alcohol Chemotherapy
Cardiac trauma	Direct	RTA Stabbing
	Cardiac surgery	
Metabolic/toxic	Renal failure Multiple organ failure	

RTA = road traffic accident
MI = myocardial infarction
PCI = percutaneous coronary intervention
CABG = coronary artery bypass grafting

SLE = systemic lupus erythematosus
CAD = coronary artery disease
IHD = ischaemic heart disease

HIGH-RISK ACUTE CORONARY SYNDROME

Management is based around risk stratification and appropriate revascularization (Fig. 8.4).

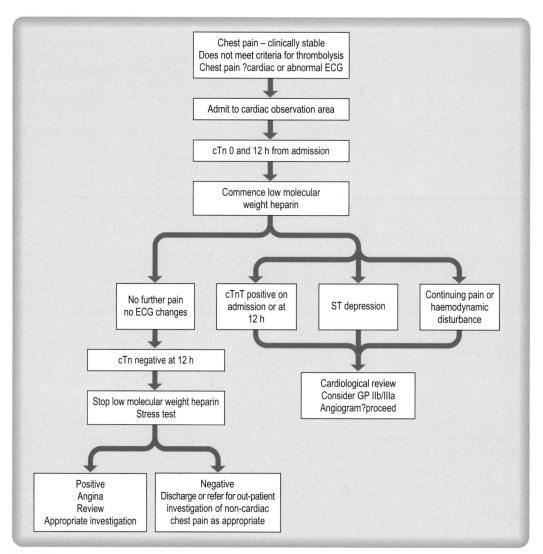

Figure 8.4
Strategy for management of high-risk acute coronary syndrome patients. All patients should initially receive aspirin. The adjunctive use of clopidogrel and beta blocker will depend on the individual presentation

LOW-RISK ACUTE CORONARY SYNDROME

A number of units have adopted a rapid rule out for this group based on a combination of patient selection followed by a rapid (4–6 hour) testing strategy. For this to succeed the patients must meet the following criteria:

- Have a normal ECG
- Have an atypical history for ACS with no obvious non-cardiac cause of chest pain
- Be clinically at low risk.

This group has a low incidence of AMI, typically 5%, and is at low risk of death. Biochemical testing at 4–6 hours will detect at least 90% of the AMI cases (Fig. 8.5).

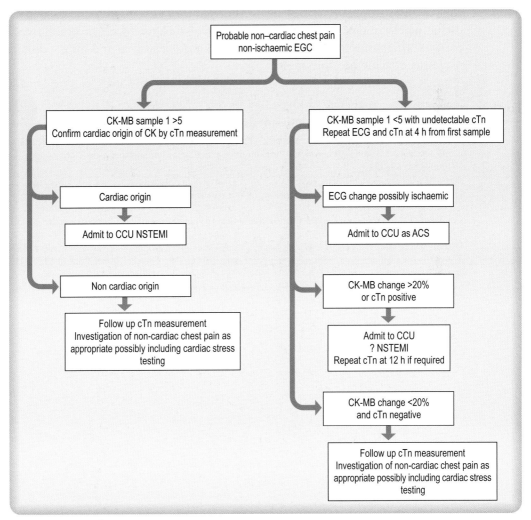

Figure 8.5
Example of a rule-out protocol for low-risk acute coronary syndrome patients
ACS = acute coronary syndrome; NSTEMI = non ST elevation myocardial infarction

After discharge, there should be follow-up cTn testing as an outpatient within 72 hours and appropriate further investigation including cardiac stress testing if appropriate.

BIOMARKERS OF MYOCARDIAL FUNCTION

Measurement of cTn can be used to assess the degree of damage, and conventional imaging and ejection fraction assessment when measured in the plateau phase of release, 12–24 hours after admission. A more direct measure of cardiac function is by measurement of natriuretic peptides. The most useful clinically is B-type natriuretic peptide (BNP). This is secreted as a prohormone, proBNP then cleaved to N-terminal proBNP (NTpBNP) and BNP. Measurement of both is routinely available using the same equipment as troponin measurement. Although they have been found to be particularly useful in detection of cardiac failure, they can also be used for risk stratification in patients with suspected non-ST elevation MI/unstable angina and for the differential diagnosis of acute breathlessness.

Further reading

Antman EM, Cohen M, Bernink PJ, McCabe CH, Horacek T, Papuchis G et al. 2000 The TIMI risk score for unstable angina/non-ST elevation MI: A method for prognostication and therapeutic decision making. JAMA 2000: **284**: 835–842

Bertrand ME, Simoons ML, Fox KA, Wallentin LC, Hamm CW, McFadden E et al. 2002 Management of acute coronary syndromes in patients presenting without persistent ST-segment elevation. Eur Heart J 2002; **23**: 1809–1840

Collinson PO, Chamberlain L 2001 Cardiac markers in the diagnosis of acute coronary syndromes. Curr Cardiol Rep 3: 280–288

Olatidoye AG, Wu AH, Feng YJ, Waters D 1998 Prognostic role of troponin T versus troponin I in unstable angina pectoris for cardiac events with meta-analysis comparing published studies. Am J Cardiol 81: 1405–1410

Wu AH, Apple FS, Gibler WB, Jesse RL, Warshaw MM, Valdes R, Jr. 1999 National Academy of Clinical Biochemistry Standards of Laboratory Practice: recommendations for the use of cardiac markers in coronary artery diseases. Clin Chem 45: 1104–1121

SELF-ASSESSMENT

Questions

a. What is the role of new markers such as C reactive protein (CRP) for risk assessment of suspected cardiovascular disease (CVD) patients?

b. Does the absence of troponin elevation in a chest pain patient exclude ischaemic heart disease (IHD)?

c. Should I measure cardiac troponin T or cardiac troponin I?

Answers

a. The current role of risk markers such as homocysteine, Lp(a) and sensitive CRP is to improve risk stratification in borderline cases or to target more aggressive treatment. If a patient is found to be at intermediate risk by conventional risk factors (including lipoprotein measurement), but with an elevated risk marker, intensive treatment of conventional risk factors, including the use of lipid lowering drugs, is indicated. There is currently no indication for use of such agents in patients where the CRP is elevated but the low-density lipoprotein (LDL) is below treatment guidelines. Trials are ongoing in this area. When utilizing CRP for primary prevention risk assessment, at least three measurements should be made, 2–3 weeks apart as elevations can occur due to intercurrent illness. The lowest value obtained should be used for risk stratification.

b. Although it excludes an active ruptured plaque, **no cTn elevation does not equal no IHD**. Measurements detect if there has been myocyte necrosis. The detection of a functional stenosis requires appropriate follow-up stress testing.

c. Studies have shown cTnT and cTnI measurements to be clinically equivalent in the majority of circumstances. There is only one method of measuring cTnT but a number of methods of measuring cTnI. The cTnI methods do not all give the same answer and some methods have better performance than others do. Be aware what the local laboratory measures and if it is recognized for risk stratification. Finally, if you want to measure cTn on the coronary care unit or in the emergency department, use a method that gives the same result as the lab – and measure the same troponin.

Management of chronic, stable, ischaemic heart disease

9

J. P. Carpenter and R. Mansfield

BURDEN OF DISEASE

A comprehensive overview is provided in Chapter 1.

PATHOPHYSIOLOGY OF MYOCARDIAL ISCHAEMIA

Angina is a manifestation of myocardial ischaemia resulting from an imbalance between myocardial oxygen demand and supply (Fig. 9.1). Therapeutic interventions aim to redress this imbalance. Myocardial ischaemia leads to impairment of left-ventricular function, which, in turn, causes a reduction in coronary blood flow and oxygen supply. This is further compounded by sympathetic drive and chatecholamine release, which, by inducing a tachycardia, results in increased myocardial oxygen demand. Coronary artery blood flow occurs primarily during diastole and as tachycardia decreases diastolic filling time there is a corresponding reduction in coronary perfusion. Chronic ischaemia may lead to a prolonged state of reversible left-ventricular dysfunction (hibernating myocardium).

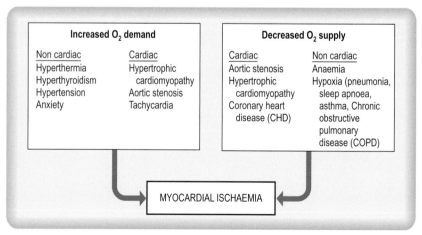

Figure 9.1
Factors affecting myocardial oxygen supply and demand

CLINICAL FEATURES

In the initial assessment and diagnosis of angina, the history is of paramount importance as there may be few clinical signs.

SYMPTOMS

Angina is frequently described as a retrosternal pain or discomfort. Typically exertional, it is aggravated by cold weather and may be precipitated by a heavy meal or emotional upset. Its character is usually that of a heaviness, gripping or pressure which may also be felt in the arms, neck, jaw, shoulder or back. It is relieved with rest or sublingual glyceryl trinitrate (GTN). Associated dyspnoea or lightheadedness is not uncommon.

The term atypical chest pain should be discouraged and a distinction made between atypical angina – myocardial ischaemia associated with atypical symptoms (for instance, burning retrosternal pain) – and chest pain due to some other cause (Box 9.1).

The Canadian Cardiovascular Society Classification (Box 9.2) of angina is widely used in symptom assessment.

Prinzmetal (variant) type angina develops spontaneously, is associated with ST elevation and is thought to be due to an increase in coronary tone (Box 9.3). Prinzmetal originally described focal coronary spasm at the site of atherosclerotic plaque, but in 10% of cases the coronary arteries are normal. Caution should be exercised in attributing symptoms to this in the presence of recognized risk factors for coronary heart disease (CHD) (see Ch. 3). Cigarette smoking is an important risk factor for Prinzmetal angina, possibly the result of endothelial dysfunction.

Box 9.1: Possible causes of non-ischaemic chest pain

Cardiovascular – aortic dissection, pericarditis

Respiratory – pulmonary embolus, pneumothorax, pneumonia, pleurisy

Gastrointestinal – oesophagitis, oesophageal spasm, oesophageal reflux, peptic ulceration, gall stones, pancreatitis

Chest wall – costochondritis, herpes zoster, muscular, cervical root pain

Other – hyperventilation, anxiety

Box 9.2: The Canadian Cardiovascular Society Classification of angina

Class I – ordinary physical exertion does not cause angina

Class II – angina occurs with walking or climbing stairs rapidly, emotional stress or walking more than 200 m on the level

Class III – marked limitation of ordinary physical activity

Class IV – angina with any physical activity, may be present at rest

> **Box 9.3: Angina in the absence of ischaemic heart disease**
>
> Coronary spasm
> Syndrome X
> Prinzmetals angina
> Aortic stenosis
> Hypertrophic cardiomyopathy
> Hypertension

EXAMINATION

Cardiovascular examination is often normal in patients with angina but physical signs specific to any underlying cause such as aortic valve disease may be present.

INVESTIGATIONS

Each year half a million patients consult their general practitioner with angina. Initial assessment and investigation can be conducted in the general practice (GP) surgery but referral to a chest pain clinic for exercise testing is appropriate for most patients (Fig. 9.2). The National Service Framework for CHD has set standards for the investigation and management of stable angina. Most NHS Trusts now have rapid access chest pain clinics supported by clear referral criteria for GPs and protocols for investigation, which lead to the rapid assessment and accurate diagnosis of people with suspected angina. Patients should be seen within 2 weeks of referral.

BLOOD TESTS

All patients should have blood taken to identify risk factors (hyperlipidaemia, diabetes) and precipitating conditions such as anaemia or thyroid dysfunction.

ELECTROCARDIOGRAPH

A 12-lead electrocardiograph (ECG) is frequently normal (50%) but may show evidence of prior myocardial infarction (MI). Other ECG abnormalities including atrial fibrillation and left-ventricular hypertrophy (LVH) may identify alternative mechanisms for angina.

EXERCISE TESTING

Exercise testing remains the mainstay of confirming the diagnosis and risk stratification in chronic stable angina and can be used to assess the efficacy of current therapy. Treadmill rather than bicycle ergometer is the preferred method of increasing the speed and gradient with time whilst monitoring the 12-lead ECG and haemodynamic response. The Bruce protocol is used most commonly.

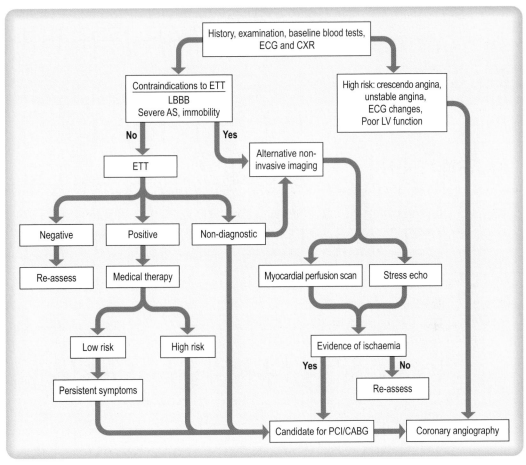

Figure 9.2
Flow chart for the investigation of patients with chronic stable ischaemic heart disease
PCI, percutaneous coronary intervention; LV, left ventricular; LBBB, left bundle branch block;
AS, aortic stenosis; ETT, exercise tolerance test; CABG, coronary artery bypass graft

Exercise electrocardiography has a sensitivity of around 65% and specificity of approximately 90%. The pre-test likelihood of CHD is important when referring patients for exercise testing. The predictive accuracy of diagnosing coronary artery disease depends partly on the prevalence in the target population (as stated by Bayesian theory). A man aged 65 years with typical angina has a 94% pre-test risk of having coronary artery disease and a positive exercise test is likely to be a true-positive result. A woman aged 35 years, however, with non-anginal chest pain has only a 0.8% risk of coronary disease and, for this reason, one must be cautious about undertaking exercise testing in such patients. False-positive results are common in middle-aged women. Horizontal or downsloping ST depression (>1 mm) during exercise or recovery signifies myocardial ischaemia and a positive test (Fig. 9.3). Upsloping ST depression is a normal finding on exercise. Other positive endpoints include a fall in blood pressure at peak exercise (>20 mmHg), ST elevation and typical angina. A positive test within the first two stages of the Bruce protocol should be investigated by angiography if appropriate.

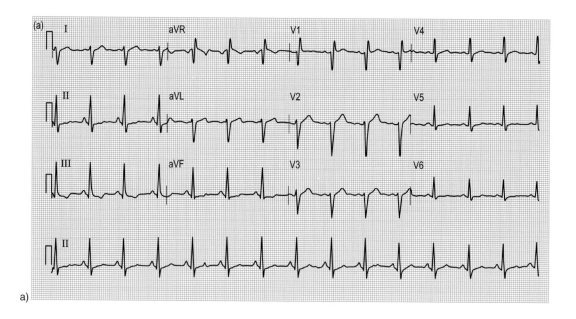

a)

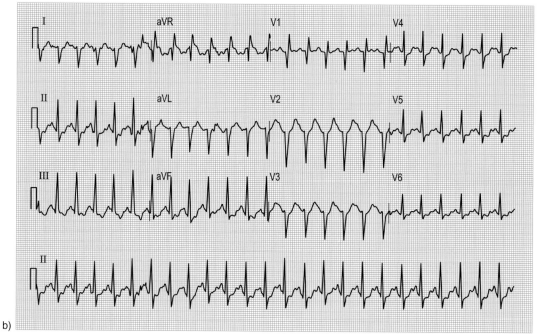

b)

Figure 9.3
Electrocardiograph tracings (a) at rest and (b) at peak exercise showing ST segment depression and a positive exercise test result

Box 9.4: Factors limiting the interpretation of the exercise electrocardiograph

Digoxin: causes ST depression in up to 40% of apparently healthy normal individuals

Beta-blockers: modulate the haemodynamic response to exercise and should be withdrawn for 48 hours before the test in certain situations

Antihypertensive agents and nitrates: alter the haemodynamic response to exercise

Left bundle branch block: precludes reliable analysis of the ST segment

Right bundle branch block: ST depression in V1–3 has no association with ischaemia, but is significant when in the inferior or lateral leads

LVH with repolarization abnormality: increased false-positive rate

If the patient reaches their target heart rate without symptoms, the blood pressure rises gradually at each stage and there are no significant ECG changes then this constitutes a negative test.

Contraindications to exercise testing are few and include uncontrolled hypertension and severe aortic stenosis but several factors may limit its value (Box 9.4).

MYOCARDIAL PERFUSION IMAGING

Nuclear techniques enable the assessment of myocardial perfusion and viability (see Ch. 6). They are indicated for both the diagnosis of CHD and to assess the functional significance of disease identified at angiography. Myocardial perfusion scintigraphy is an appropriate initial investigation for patients with an intermediate probability of CHD who will be unable to exercise adequately and those whose exercise ECG is uninterpretable due to resting ECG abnormalities such as left bundle branch block (LBBB). Myocardial stress can be dynamic (exercise testing) or pharmacological using either an infusion of adenosine (which causes coronary vasodilation) or dobutamine.

Radioactive tracers (thallium-201 or technetium (Tc-99) labelled analogues) are administered intravenously and are taken up by viable cardiac myocytes. A comparison is made between rest and stress. Normal myocardium shows a uniform uptake of tracer. A defect at rest and stress (fixed) implies infarction but a defect seen only on stress (reversible) indicates ischaemia (Fig. 9.4).

STRESS ECHOCARDIOGRAPHY

Myocardial contractility usually increases with stress. In the presence of reversible ischaemia, the myocardium may contract normally at rest, but following stress function deteriorates giving a wall motion abnormality seen on 2-D echo (see Chapter 5). Areas of myocardium that are akinetic at rest show a differing response to stress depending on

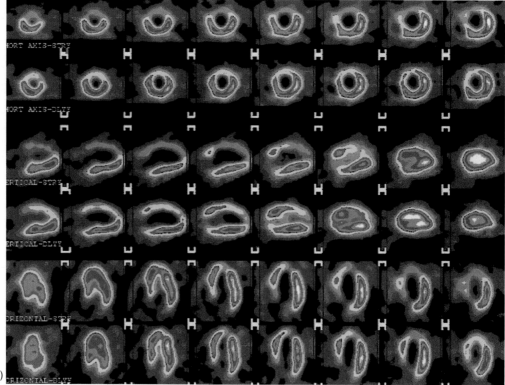

Figure 9.4
Myocardial perfusion images (a) acquired following adenosine stress in a 48-year-old lady correlate with the severe stenosis (b, p. 89) seen in the proximal left anterior descending (LAD) at angiography (arrow). (Courtesy of Dr Julie Fitzgerald)

whether or not they are viable. Viable myocardium will regain some, if not all, function, whereas infarcted areas will remain akinetic. This technique is heavily operator dependent but a useful adjunct in the non-invasive assessment of CHD.

COMPUTED TOMOGRAPHY AND CARDIAC MAGNETIC RESONANCE IMAGING

Refer to Chapter 7 for a complete coverage.

CORONARY ANGIOGRAPHY

Angiography remains the 'gold standard' for determining the presence, pattern and severity of CHD. Performed via the femoral artery, brachial or radial artery, it is readily

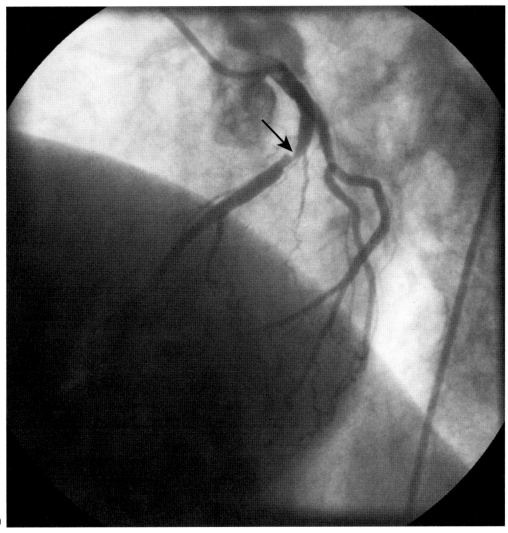

b)

Figure 9.4 (*Cont'd*)
Severe stenosis in the proximal LAD at angiography (arrow). (Courtesy of Dr Julie Fitzgerald. A schematic
of coronary anatomy is shown in Fig. 9.5)

available and safe with an overall mortality of less than 0.1% (Table 9.1). It should be
performed when symptoms are not adequately controlled with medical therapy, when a
definitive diagnosis is necessary or when non-invasive testing is suggestive of an impaired
prognosis (Box 9.5). Every centre performing angiography should have systems in place to
ensure that referral for invasive investigation is appropriate and that patients are adequately
prepared prior to the procedure. Patients with severe peripheral vascular disease,
symptomatic heart failure, advanced diabetes, valve replacement, other medical problems or
simply those who may present a technical challenge should be identified. In these situations
especially, it is important that both patient and operator are optimally prepared.

Table 9.1: Risk of coronary angiography

Death	0.07–0.12%
Stroke	0.14–0.25%
Myocardial infarction	0.1–0.16%
Arrhythmia	0.2–0.4%
Complicated arterial access	0.17–0.25%
Contrast allergy	0.1%

Box 9.5: Indications for coronary angiography

Stable angina if non-invasive testing indicates ischaemia at moderate or low work load

Post myocardial infarction if non-invasive testing indicates ischaemia at moderate or low work load

Persistent symptoms not adequately controlled by medical therapy

Post successfully resuscitated cardiac arrest

Post myocardial infarction or in context of stable angina if diagnosis is mandatory for occupation, e.g. HGV driver

Asymptomatic if non-invasive screening indicates any abnormality and diagnosis mandatory for occupation, e.g. pilot

Previous coronary artery bypass graft (CABG) or percutaneous coronary intervention (PCI) with early recurrent angina

Previous CABG or PCI if recurrent symptoms not controlled by medication

Prior to major non-cardiac surgery, if symptoms or non-invasive testing suggest presence of extensive CHD

Angiographic findings should *always* be interpreted in the light of the patient's symptoms and the results of other cardiac investigations such as exercise testing or perfusion scanning. Only then can an appropriate management strategy be implemented.

MANAGEMENT

Management of chronic stable angina depends on the extent of disease, left-ventricular systolic performance (both important indicators of prognosis) and the patient's age and symptoms. There are three broad treatment options: medical therapy (including risk factor modification), PCI (angioplasty) or CABG. The aims of treatment are to improve symptoms, limit progression of disease and reduce the risk of MI and mortality. In all patients with established CHD, secondary prevention is of paramount importance.

ANTIPLATELET AGENTS

Aspirin (75 mg) use is associated with a 33% reduction in major cardiovascular events. Clopidogrel is also of prognostic benefit and a safe alternative to aspirin. However, there

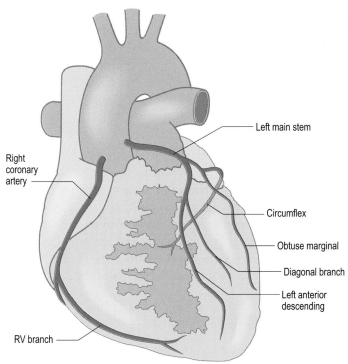

Figure 9.5
Left and right coronary arteries and branches

is no clear evidence that clopidogrel confers a significant benefit over aspirin alone. Studies combining the agents are ongoing.

LIPID-LOWERING AGENTS

The Scandinavian Simvastatin Survival Study (4S) showed conclusively that treatment of hypercholesterolaemia with statins in patients with coronary disease resulted in a dramatic reduction in MI, revascularization rate and risk of death. Initial dietary advice and subsequent use of a statin is recommended to lower the total cholesterol (see Chapter 3).

The recently published Heart Protection Study provides evidence that addition of simvastatin to existing treatments in high-risk individuals with CHD produces a substantial additional benefit in reducing the rates of MI, stroke, revascularization and death irrespective of the patient's initial cholesterol concentrations.

ACE INHIBITORS

The value of ACE inhibition post MI and in heart failure is unquestionable but there is now additional evidence of a prognostic benefit in stable angina. The HOPE study (in which 50% of patients had stable angina) was terminated early due to the consistent benefit of ramipril in lowering the rates of MI, stroke and cardiovascular death. A 20% relative risk reduction in cardiovascular death, myocardial infarction and cardiac arrest was seen in patients treated with an ACE inhibitor in the European Trial of Reduction of Cardiac Events with Perindopril in Stable Coronary Disease (EUROPA) study.

BETA-BLOCKERS

Beta-blockers should be considered first-line therapy in symptom control for stable angina. They act mainly on the β-1 receptors slowing the heart rate and decreasing myocardial contractility thereby reducing myocardial oxygen demand. Cardio-selective agents (atenolol and metoprolol) may be tolerated in mild airways disease and in patients with peripheral vascular disease. The non-selective agents with intrinsic sympathomimetic activity (pindolol) cause less of a reduction in heart rate and are rarely used in practice as a result. There are limited data on the prognostic benefit of beta-blockade, but it seems probable that these drugs have the potential to reduce the risk of MI.

CALCIUM CHANNEL ANTAGONISTS

Calcium channel antagonists induce coronary and peripheral vasodilatation. Reduction in afterload and smooth muscle relaxation contribute to a decline in myocardial oxygen demand. Verapamil and diltiazem are negatively inotropic and slow the heart rate. The dihydropyridine group (e.g. nifedipine and amlodipine) frequently cause reflex tachycardia and so these drugs should be used in combination with a beta-blocker to avoid such consequences. Short-acting, rapid-release preparations of the dihydropyridine group are not recommended. All calcium antagonists should be used with caution in heart failure. Calcium antagonists should be used if beta-blockers are contraindicated and are of particular value in vasospastic angina. Prognostic data are lacking.

NITRATES

All patients with angina should be prescribed sublingual nitrates. Nitrate therapy is very effective (by causing venodilatation and a reduction in afterload) but tolerance can develop and GTN syncope is not uncommon. Oral nitrate preparations should be prescribed with a nitrate-free period or as a long-acting preparation. They are of use in syndrome X and vasospasm. On the available evidence nitrates do not confer prognostic benefit.

NICORANDIL

The potassium channel opener nicorandil appears to have cardioprotective effects over and above its benefit in relieving angina. The IONA study demonstrated that stable angina patients treated with nicorandil had a significant reduction in major coronary events compared to placebo. It should be used as second- or third-line therapy for angina after instigation of therapy with beta-blockers, calcium channel blockers or oral nitrates. Patients on nicorandil do not seem to develop tolerance to its effects and, although it contains a nitrate moiety, which may induce tolerance, the potassium channel opening action is sustained.

ANTICOAGULANTS

Most of the data supporting anticoagulation are in secondary prevention following MI. In combination with antiplatelet therapy, warfarin provides a significant benefit over aspirin alone but only when the International Normalized Ratio (INR) is greater than 2.0. Extrapolation to patients with chronic stable angina may be possible but the observed increase in bleeding and the logistical problems in monitoring such therapy in the large population of patients with CHD could limit its widespread acceptance. The addition of the new oral direct thrombin inhibitor, ximelagatran, to aspirin post MI has been shown to be superior to aspirin alone in reducing all-cause death, non-fatal MI and severe recurrent ischaemia. There are no data for ximelagatran in chronic stable angina.

ANTI-OXIDANTS

There is no conclusive evidence that anti-oxidants such as vitamin E are of prognostic benefit.

OTHER AGENTS

There are a few other agents for the treatment of chronic stable angina, as yet unlicensed in the UK or still undergoing research trials.

Molsidomine has a nitrate-like moiety and acts in a similar way to nitrates. Trimetazidine is a metabolic agent, which acts by reducing fatty acid metabolism, increasing myocardial glucose oxidation and protecting myocytes against ischaemia. Ivabradine, an I_f channel inhibitor aimed at heart rate reduction is undergoing trials.

ROLE OF RATE CONTROL IN STABLE ANGINA

Tachycardia leads to increased myocardial oxygen demand and a reduced oxygen supply by shortening diastole and thus reducing the time available for coronary blood flow. It follows that if the heart rate is controlled, coronary perfusion increases thereby reducing myocardial oxygen demand resulting in a potent anti-ischaemic effect. Indeed, a linear relationship exists between increasing heart rate and cardiovascular mortality.

CHOICE OF DRUG THERAPY

Monotherapy should be pursued but if insufficient to improve symptoms then a second agent can be added. A usual combination is a beta-blocker and calcium antagonist. There is little evidence that adding a third agent is more effective than dual therapy and so if needed the patient should be re-assessed and considered for PCI or CABG.

PERCUTANEOUS CORONARY INTERVENTION

Percutaneous transluminal coronary angioplasty (PTCA) is highly effective in relieving angina and improving exercise tolerance. Over 30 000 PTCA or related procedures (now referred to generically as PCI) were carried out in the UK in 2000 and these numbers are likely to increase further (Fig. 9.6).

Endothelial loss and plaque dissection are ubiquitous features of PTCA and re-narrowing (restenosis) was initially seen in up to 40% of cases. Stents were developed to treat complex dissection and are associated with a reduction in the need for repeat target vessel revascularization and modest decrease in angiographic restenosis rates to around 20%. An early complication of stenting was acute thrombosis and it is current practice to give a minimum of a 28-day course of clopidogrel, *in addition* to aspirin to those patients in whom a stent is deployed, after which time re-endothelialization of the arterial wall (and stent struts) should be complete.

Drug-eluting stents (DES), coated with the anti-proliferative agents sirolimus or paclitaxel, have recently become available and are associated with a striking reduction in restenosis rates and are currently recommended for the treatment of long stenoses or lesions in small vessels. When DES are used a combination of aspirin and clopidogrel is continued for 6–9 months.

High-risk PCI cases (e.g. bifurcation lesions, multivessel disease and diabetics) often require adjunctive treatment with glycoprotein IIb/IIIa inhibitors. Of the available agents it is only abciximab (Reopro) that is licensed for this indication.

The procedural success of PCI is high (95%) and whilst it is highly effective in relieving symptoms there are no convincing data that PCI is superior to medical therapy in reducing the rate of MI or death. The risks of PCI are low (mortality <0.7%) and risk of urgent CABG is 0.4%. Such procedures no longer need to be carried out with the support of cardiac surgeons 'on site'.

Repeat angioplasty is the treatment of choice for in-stent restenosis but with an increased risk of recurrence. Brachytherapy, the use of ionizing radiation to ablate the cells in the arterial wall responsible for restenosis, is currently licensed for the treatments of in-stent restenosis but is not without its limitations. In-stent restenosis continues to present a challenge to clinicians and vascular biologists alike.

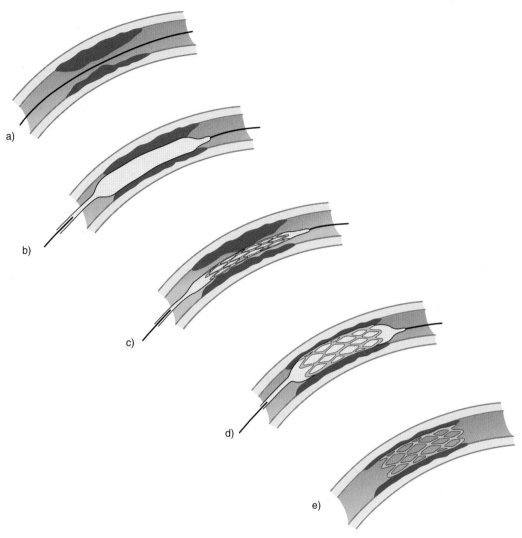

Figure 9.6
(a) Following the passage of a guide wire across the stenosis, (b) a balloon is positioned and inflated to pre-dilate the plaque. (c) A balloon-mounted stent is then placed within the stenosis. (d) High-pressure inflation of the balloon results in stent deployment. (e) The balloon is deflated and removed leaving the stent in-situ and the vessel patent

CORONARY ARTERY SURGERY

Surgical revascularization or CABG using venous or arterial conduits is highly effective in relieving angina. Importantly, CABG has also been shown to improve prognosis in patients with left main stem (LMS) disease, three-vessel disease (with or without left-ventricular systolic dysfunction) or two-vessel disease involving the proximal left-anterior descending artery (LAD). CABG does nothing to reduce the risk of myocardial infarction. 95

A single graft to one artery may improve symptoms but has no prognostic benefit. The trials demonstrating prognostic benefit for these patterns of disease were from an era predating the advent of such important medical therapies as ACE inhibitors and lipid lowering agents as well as the now widespread use of the internal mammary artery (IMA). The observed longevity of arterial conduits (10-year patency of IMA 90% vs saphenous vein graft 50%) has increased their use to include free radial artery grafts. Thirty-day operative mortality after bypass surgery is 1–3% rising to 7% for re-operation. Increasing age, renal disease, female sex and diabetes are all associated with increased in-hospital mortality. Diabetic patients do, however, have a significantly lower 5-year mortality with CABG than with PCI. Peri-operative complications include MI (5%) and stroke (2%). An additional concern following cardiopulmonary bypass is neuropsychometric damage but it is hoped that the increasing use of off-pump 'beating heart surgery' (up to 50% in some institutions) will lead to a significant reduction in this problem.

APPROPRIATE REFERRAL FOR PERCUTANEOUS CORONARY INTERVENTION OR CORONARY ARTERY BYPASS GRAFTING

The previous discussion highlights which patients are likely to benefit from PCI or CABG (Fig. 9.7) but as angioplasty techniques and, in particular, equipment have continued to develop, the distinction between these two treatment options for patients with two- or three-vessel disease has become less clear.

The Arterial Revascularisation Therapy Study (ARTS) and Stent or Surgery (SOS) study have investigated the role of PCI and stenting in multivessel disease in whom equivalent revascularization could be achieved with either PCI or CABG. Both trials demonstrated

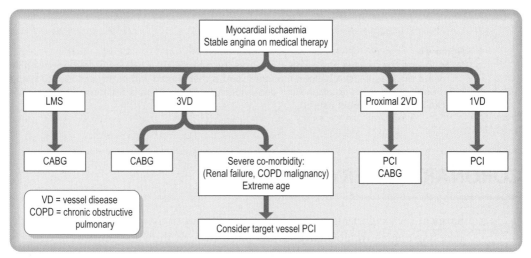

Figure 9.7
Flow chart of revascularization strategies in chronic stable angina
VD, Vessel disease; COPD, Chronic obstructive pulmonary disease; LMS, Left main stem

the additional need for repeat revascularization in the PCI group but offered the same degree of protection against death and myocardial infarction following PCI or CABG.

SPECIAL CIRCUMSTANCES

WOMEN

Coronary artery disease is often under-diagnosed in women. The prevalence is lower in premenopausal women than men of the same age and atypical symptoms are often dismissed. In addition, exercise testing is often falsely positive and women are less likely than men to be referred for coronary angiography. There is also a greater incidence of finding normal coronary arterial anatomy. Due to the lower sensitivity of exercise testing, perfusion scanning or stress echocardiography should be considered more often. If women have symptoms typical of angina and a positive exercise test, they should have angiography – they benefit in exactly the same way as men from drug therapy and revascularization. Interestingly, their morbidity following MI is increased .

DIABETIC PATIENTS

There is a high incidence of coronary artery disease in the diabetic population. Patients with diabetes may present late or with atypical symptoms in view of the autonomic neuropathy associated with the condition. Silent ischaemia and even infarction is common. Good glycaemic control is important in the management to prevent progression of disease (see p. 23).

Investigation and management should be performed as detailed above and patients referred for PCI or CABG as appropriate. Diabetics have a worse prognosis and outcome whatever treatment strategy is followed. Restenosis is more common following PCI and hence the need for repeated procedures. CABG provides a greater benefit in terms of mortality but carries a greater peri-operative risk than in non-diabetics.

ASIAN PATIENTS

Patients from Southern Asia are noted to have more severe coronary artery disease at an earlier age than Caucasian counterparts. There is a higher incidence of diabetes and insulin resistance as well as hypertension in this population. Symptoms of ischaemia are often atypical at presentation and, therefore, it is important to consider the diagnosis of ischaemic heart disease and have a lower threshold for investigation.

POST-CORONARY ARTERY BYPASS GRAFTING ANGINA

Some patients will have a recurrence of their symptoms after CABG. They should be carefully re-assessed as for *de-novo* angina. Medical therapy should be pursued to relieve symptoms. Angiography may be needed to assess both native arteries and graft function.

PCI is used increasingly now for venous and arterial graft disease and may eliminate the need for re-operation. Indeed, the presence of patent grafts may enable PCI of previously unsuitable lesions in the native circulation. Re-operation is a difficult area as a co-existent patent left internal mammary artery (LIMA) graft can be damaged on repeat sternotomy. The development and/or progression of graft or native arterial disease highlight the need for ongoing risk factor modification after surgery.

SYNDROME X

Syndrome X is defined as typical angina accompanied by objective evidence of myocardial ischaemia (e.g. positive exercise test) but with normal coronary arteries. The symptoms are less consistently associated with exercise and patients often experience longer periods of pain. The underlying pathophysiology is not clear, but probably relates to small vessel disease. The symptoms respond to nitrates, calcium antagonists and possibly oestrogen therapy and there is a good overall prognosis.

REFRACTORY ANGINA

There are an increasing number of patients with intractable angina in whom further medical, percutaneous or surgical intervention is not possible. These patients are often extremely limited by their symptoms and are difficult to treat. Multidisciplinary management involving a pain clinic is extremely useful. Possible interventions include simple oral analgesia (including opiates), stellate ganglion blocks, trial of neurostimulatory devices (both transcutaneous and implanted spinal cord stimulators) and even external counterpulsation devices.

Further reading

ACC/AHA/ACP 1999 ASIM Guidelines for the management of patients with chronic stable angina. A report of The American College of Cardiology/American Heart Association Task Force on Practice Guidelines. Journal of the American College of Cardiology 33 (7): 2092–2197

Dagenais GR, Yusuf S, Bourassa MG, Yi Q, Bosch J, Lonn EM, Kouz S, Grover J on behalf of the HOPE investigators 2001 Effect of ramipril on coronary events in high-risk patients. Results of the Heart Outcomes Prevention Evaluation Study. Circulation 104: 522–526

De Feyter PJ, Nieman K 2002 New coronary imaging techniques: what to expect? Heart 87: 195–197

Department of Health 2000 National Service Framework for Coronary Heart Disease. Department of Health, London

Morice MC, Serruys PW, Sousa JE et al. RAVEL Study Group 2002 Randomised study with the sirolimus-coated Bx velocity balloon-expandable stent in the treatment of patients with de novo native coronary artery lesions. N Engl J Med 346: 1770–177

MRC/BHF 2002 Heart Protection Study of cholesterol lowering with simvastatin in 20,536 high-risk individuals: a randomised placebo-controlled trial. Heart Protection Collaborative Group. Lancet 360: 7–22

Scandinavian Simvastatin Survival Study 1994 Randomised trial of cholesterol lowering in 4444 patients with coronary heart disease: the Scandinavian Simvastatin Survival Study (4S). Lancet 344: 1383–1389

Serruys PW, de Jaegere P, Kiemeneij F et al. 1994 A comparison of balloon-expandable stent implantation with balloon angioplasty in patients with coronary disease. The Benestent Study Group. N Eng J Med 331: 489–495

Serruys PW, Unger F, Sousa JE et al. 2001 Arterial Revascularisation Therapies Study Group. N Eng J Med 344: 1117–1124

Task Force of the European Society of Cardiology 1997 Management of stable angina pectoris. Recommendations of the Task Force of the European Society of Cardiology. European Heart Journal 18: 394–413

The EURopean trial On reduction of cardiac events with perindopril in stable coronary. Artery disease investigations. Efficacy of Perindopril in reduction of cardiovascular events among patients with stable coronary artery disease: randomised, double-blind, placebo-controlled, multicentre trial (the EUROPA study). Lancet 2003; 362: 782–788

Weissberg PL 2000 Atherogenesis: current understanding of the causes of atheroma. Heart 83: 247–252

Yusuf S, Zucker D, Peduzzi et al. 1994 Effect of coronary artery bypass graft surgery on survival: overview of 10 year results from randomised trials by the Coronary Artery Bypass Graft Surgery Trialists Collaboration. Lancet 344: 563–570

SELF-ASSESSMENT

Questions

1. A 48-year-old HGV driver attends his GP with a 4-week history of 'retrosternal burning' associated with dyspnoea whilst behind the wheel and after walking uphill. He is overweight, smokes 30 cigarettes a day and has a positive family history of coronary heart disease (CHD). His only medication is salbutamol for asthma. His GP suspects CHD as a cause for his symptoms and refers him to you in the local chest pain clinic. The results of his electrocardiograph (ECG) (normal) and blood tests (cholesterol 6.3 mmol/l) are attached to the referral.
   a. What further assessment is needed?
   b. What treatment would you initiate?
   c. He is referred on for a coronary angiogram. The left coronary artery is normal. What does this view (Fig. 9.8) of the right coronary artery show?
   d. What treatment would you now offer him?
   e. He subsequently undergoes successful PCI to the right coronary artery. What further follow-up should he be offered?
   f. What advice would you give him regards his employment?

2. A 42-year-old lady with chest pain after eating was referred for further investigation. She smoked 10 cigarettes a day and had a positive family history of CHD. Two years previously she had received treatment for oesophageal reflux. She had been commenced on aspirin and a beta-blocker by her GP.
   a. What investigation would you recommend?
   b. What advice would you give her regarding her medication prior to attending for her exercise ECG?

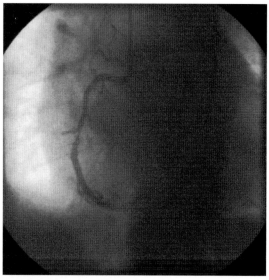

Figure 9.8
Angiogram of the right coronary artery

c. The exercise test was positive with 1 mm inferior (leads III and AVF) ST segment depression within 6 minutes of the Bruce protocol. What should be done next?
d. The angiogram demonstrated normal coronary arteries and normal left-ventricular systolic function. What are the possible explanations?
e. How would you approach this problem?
f. A diagnosis of syndrome X is subsequently made. What treatment would you recommend?

Answers

1. a. Presuming that his symptoms have been stable and you do not suspect unstable or crescendo angina then he should have an exercise tolerance test using the full Bruce protocol.
b. Irrespective of the exercise test result he should be treated with aspirin 75 mg od and commenced on a statin. Antianginal therapy, including a GTN spray, should also be commenced. In view of his history of asthma you may elect to use a calcium antagonist as a first-line agent, although he may, if his asthma is mild, tolerate a selective beta-blocker. An ACE inhibitor should also be considered.
He must be told to stop smoking and receive dietary advice.
It is also extremely important that he is told to stop driving his heavy goods vehicle and that he must notify the DVLA of this advice.
c. This angiogram of the right coronary artery shows a severe stenosis in the mid course of the vessel.
d. If he is symptom free on medical therapy then neither PCI nor CABG (he has single vessel disease) is indicated. If he continues to be symptomatic despite medical therapy then PCI would be an appropriate treatment option.
e. He must continue to address his lifestyle to reduce his risk factors. As he is symptom free he can discontinue the antianginal therapy but must continue the aspirin (and adjunctive anti-platelet therapy advised by the interventional cardiologist) and the statin.
A follow-up exercise test must be carried out at 6 weeks, and if satisfactory then he should be enrolled into a formal programme of cardiac rehabilitation.
f. In order to satisfy the DVLA criteria for return of his HGV licence he needs to complete 9 minutes of the full Bruce protocol exercise test without symptoms, hypotension, ventricular tachycardia or ECG changes of ischaemia (>2 mm horizontal or down sloping ST segment depression). Anti-anginal therapy (i.e. beta-blockers, calcium antagonists and nitrates) must be stopped 48 hours before the test. ACE inhibitors can be continued.

2. a. An exercise ECG may be appropriate but would depend on the pre-test probability of a positive test (Bayes theorem). As she gave a history of exertional angina an exercise ECG was performed.
b. As the purpose of the test is to establish a diagnosis of CHD the beta-blocker should be discontinued for 48 hours beforehand. Exercise testing is also carried out for prognostic reasons, i.e. following interventions such as percutaneous coronary intervention (PCI) and CABG, in which case it is not always necessary to discontinue such treatment prior to the test.

c. In view of the test result, risk factors and her young age she should be investigated by coronary angiography.

d. Classic angina, a positive exercise test and normal coronary arteries at angiography are features of syndrome X. Another possibility is that her symptoms are, once again, related to oesophageal reflux and that the exercise ECG is merely a false-positive test.

e. The relation of her symptoms to food may be important. Exclusion of ongoing gastrointestinal problems can be carried out safely and may be sensible in view of her prior history and the complexity of treating patients with syndrome X. Upper gastrointestinal endoscopy or oesophageal manometry may be appropriate. There is a role for myocardial perfusion scanning in assessing patients who may have syndrome X. Such imaging may help in this situation to determine if this is primarily a cardiac or gastrointestinal problem.

f. She should be reassured that the condition is benign. The aspirin does not need to be continued. The most frequently used agents in this condition are calcium antagonists, in particular diltiazem. Other options include oral nitrate preparations and the use of oestrogen therapy.

Management of acute coronary syndromes

10

S. J. Patel and J. Coutts

INTRODUCTION

Acute coronary syndromes (ACS) incorporate a spectrum of clinical presentations of coronary artery disease (CAD) including: unstable angina (UA), myocardial infarction (MI) without persistent electrocardiogram (ECG) ST elevation, i.e. non-ST elevation MI (NSTEMI), and acute ST elevation MI (STEMI). There are approximately 120 000 ACS admissions (excluding STEMI) per annum to hospitals in the UK. Despite the use of standard therapies, the rate of adverse events (recurrent UA, MI, death, cerebrovascular accident (CVA or stroke)) remains high (Fig. 10.1). Prompt diagnosis and management are, therefore, paramount in their successful management.

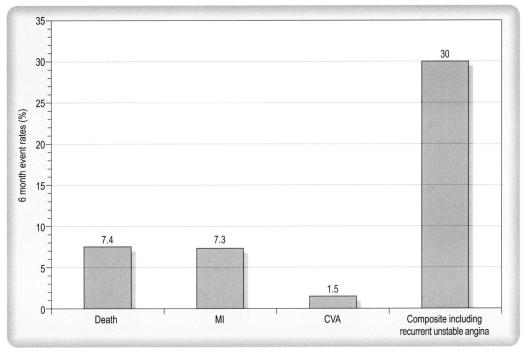

Figure 10.1
Major adverse cardiovascular event (MACE) rates at 6 months in patients presenting with acute coronary syndromes based on data from PRAIS-UK

The central pathophysiological mechanism in the development of an ACS is plaque disruption, superimposed platelet aggregation and subsequent thrombus formation (Fig. 10.2). The immediate consequence of thrombosis depends on its site and severity. The 'culprit' lesion responsible for the development of an ACS may not be severe with respect to pre-existing luminal obstruction; lesions with <50% obstruction have been shown to be responsible for the development of MI.

Asymptomatic plaque rupture is not uncommon as plaque healing may occur without significant occlusion. At the other extreme, complete occlusion of a large epicardial vessel may occur, and in the absence of adequate collateralization, transmural ischaemia may develop progressing to infarction in the absence of prompt reperfusion. On the ECG, this is typically associated with ST elevation and the development of Q waves, i.e. STEMI.

Between these two extremes is a spectrum of possibilities including partial occlusion of large epicardial vessels, distal embolization of thrombus, and occlusion of small vessels whereby damage may occur to the myocardium, but falls short of a 'full thickness' transmural infarct. The distinction between these clinical scenarios is important, as they require different management regimes; for example in the treatment of acute STEMI strategies promoting reperfusion with thrombolysis or percutaneous revascularization are indicated, whereas for UA or NSTEMI this is not always the case.

MANAGEMENT OF PATIENTS WITH SUSPECTED ACUTE CORONARY SYNDROME

The aims of managing patients presenting with a suspected ACS are to:

1. Confirm the diagnosis
2. Assess the degree of risk of adverse events such as MI and death
3. Restore coronary flow as appropriate
4. Treat associated complications
5. Minimize the risk of recurrence.

DIAGNOSIS

This is based upon clinical assessment, the ECG and biochemical markers of myocardial necrosis.

All patients presenting with symptoms consistent with an ACS should be referred for urgent assessment, for example to the A&E department. Presentation is typically with ischaemic chest discomfort at rest or on minimal exertion lasting for more than 10–15 minutes. This may occur without previous symptoms or as an abrupt worsening of pre-existing angina. Atypical presentations may occur, particularly in the elderly and diabetics; for instance, it is well recognized that STEMI may present as acute confusion in the elderly.

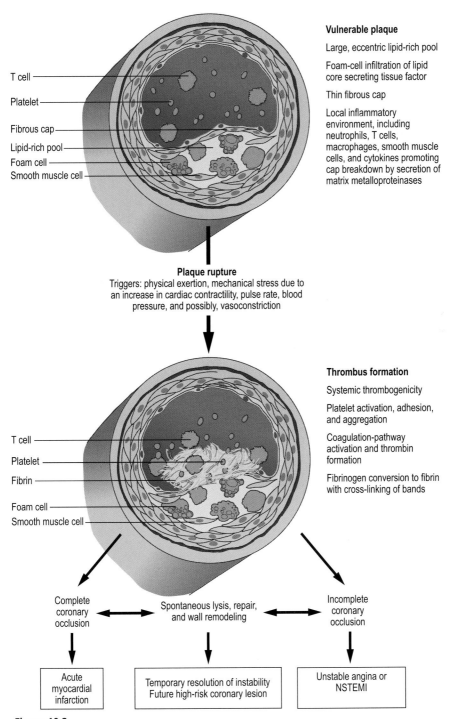

Vulnerable plaque

Large, eccentric lipid-rich pool

Foam-cell infiltration of lipid core secreting tissue factor

Thin fibrous cap

Local inflammatory environment, including neutrophils, T cells, macrophages, smooth muscle cells, and cytokines promoting cap breakdown by secretion of matrix metalloproteinases

T cell
Platelet
Fibrous cap
Lipid-rich pool
Foam cell
Smooth muscle cell

Plaque rupture
Triggers: physical exertion, mechanical stress due to an increase in cardiac contractility, pulse rate, blood pressure, and possibly, vasoconstriction

Thrombus formation

Systemic thrombogenicity

Platelet activation, adhesion, and aggregation

Coagulation-pathway activation and thrombin formation

Fibrinogen conversion to fibrin with cross-linking of bands

T cell
Platelet
Fibrin
Foam cell
Smooth muscle cell

Complete coronary occlusion ⟷ Spontaneous lysis, repair, and wall remodeling ⟷ Incomplete coronary occlusion

Acute myocardial infarction

Temporary resolution of instability Future high-risk coronary lesion

Unstable angina or NSTEMI

Figure 10.2
The pathophysiology of an acute coronary syndrome (Reproduced with kind permission from Yeghiazarians Y, New England Journal of Medicine 2000; 342: 101–114)

TREATMENT AND INVESTIGATION IN SUSPECTED ACUTE CORONARY SYNDROME (Fig. 10.3)

Analgesia should be provided. Ischaemic pain is associated with catecholamine release and consequently an increase in myocardial oxygen demand (MVO_2). Morphine/diamorphine, potent opioid analgesics with an anxiolytic effect, have beneficial haemodynamic effects (venodilatation, a mild reduction in heart rate through increased vagal tone and lowering of systolic blood pressure) and as such are recommended for those patients whose symptoms have not resolved with initial sublingual GTN use.

Provide supplemental *oxygen* to maintain arterial oxygen saturations above 90% where possible.

Treat associated haemodynamic instability, arrhythmias and pulmonary oedema (see below). Meanwhile *perform an ECG promptly*. The ECG should be repeated with a

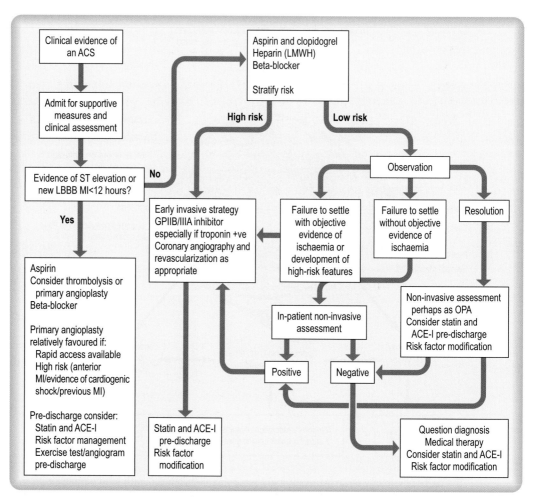

Figure 10.3
A flow chart for the management of patients presenting with a suspected acute coronary syndrome
ACEI, angiotensin converting enzyme inhibitor; LBBB, Left bundle branch block; ACS, Acute coronary syndrome; OPA, out-patients appointment; LMWH, Low molecular weight heparin

change in clinical status or if initially non-diagnostic. The ECG is the primary risk stratifying investigation. It may provide evidence of underlying coronary artery disease by one of the following: ST segment depression, T-wave inversion, transient ST elevation, pathological Q waves or left bundle branch block (LBBB). New persistent ST elevation or new LBBB in the context of cardiac ischaemic pain represents an acute MI; such patients should be considered for prompt reperfusion therapy.

ST elevation or new left bundle branch block shown on electrocardiogram

If the ECG shows ST elevation or new LBBB this is the best evidence that a major epicardial vessel is occluded. The patient is at high risk, and strategies should be considered to promote early reperfusion. It is not necessary to wait for biochemical markers. Time is of the essence – 'time is muscle' – and the condition should be regarded as a medical emergency.

Thrombolysis as a means of achieving reperfusion should be considered for all acute MI patients with acute STEMI or new LBBB. Streptokinase (SK), tissue plasminogen activator (tPA) and the newer plasminogen activators (reteplase-rPA, tenecteplase-TNK) have been shown to reduce mortality significantly (by ~20%), the degree of reduction being inversely related to the time from symptom onset to initiation of therapy.[1,2] For patients treated within the first hour of symptom onset, the so-called 'golden hour', mortality is reduced by more than 50%.[3] Pre-hospital fibrinolysis can also reduce mortality and should be considered when transport time to an acute hospital exceeds 60 minutes.[4] Improved vessel patency is associated with a better clinical outcome. Lytics, however, are limited in their ability to achieve vessel patency with patency rates of 30% for SK and 54% for tPA at 90 minutes.[5] Primary angioplasty appears to be superior in this respect achieving patency rates >90%.[6]

Aspirin (300 mg) is an effective thrombolytic. In the ISIS-2 study its benefits were found to be additive to those of streptokinase, and it is therefore given unless specifically contraindicated.[2] Heparin (see below) is given in conjunction with many thrombolysis regimes (e.g. with tPA and TNK). There is no convincing evidence of a benefit when given after SK.

Percutaneous revascularization in acute MI is an attractive option, as restoration of antegrade blood flow in the culprit coronary artery is of paramount importance. Primary angioplasty (1^0 PCI) is an alternative to thrombolysis and may be the only option promoting reperfusion in those where lysis is contraindicated. 1^0 PCI results in saving two additional lives per 100 patients treated compared with thrombolysis and is associated with a lower risk of stroke and re-infarction.[6,7] Analyses suggest that it may be as cost efficient if not cheaper than thrombolysis.

There is strong evidence supporting the view that 1^0 PCI is the treatment of choice for acute STEMI, providing it is available in an appropriate setting and a timely fashion. Trials are underway to investigate whether a combination of low-dose thrombolytic and antiplatelet agents (i.e. abciximab), with PCI – 'facilitated PCI' – will enhance macro- and micro-vascular reperfusion in the context of acute STEMI.

Abnormal electrocardiogram without ST elevation or left bundle branch block, but with T wave inversion or ST segment depression

This may be because the patient has an acute coronary event falling short of major epicardial vessel occlusion, i.e. UA or NSTEMI. The distinction is necessarily imperfect as, for instance, proximal occlusion of a dominant circumflex vessel may give rise to a full-thickness posterior infarction that may initially present only with anterior ST depression. It is also important to consider alternative diagnoses, such as a pulmonary embolism or left-ventricular hypertrophy.

The patient should be admitted and monitored, and ECGs must be repeated frequently, particularly with worsening of pain, since the development of ST elevation or new LBBB necessitates urgent revascularization (pharmacologically or mechanically).

Cardiac enzymes such as creatine kinase (CK or CK-MB) and other markers of myocyte necrosis such as troponin T or I may be elevated, which would support a diagnosis of an ACS (see Ch. 8). Elevation of biochemical markers is not instantaneous such that a negative troponin cannot be viewed as excluding myocardial damage unless the sample is drawn 12 hours after the onset of chest pain.

Trials involving the use of thrombolytics in such ACS patients (NSTEMI) have failed to demonstrate any benefit, with TIMI IIIB showing an adverse outcome.[8]

Aspirin (ASA) (Fig. 10.4) mediates its antiplatelet effect via inhibition of thromboxane A2 generation through cyclo-oxygenase. It is established as the first-line therapy in all patients with a confirmed ACS (STEMI and NSTEMI); if contraindicated, clopidogrel should be given.[9,10]

Clopidogrel (Fig. 10.4) is a thienopyridine derivative that inhibits ADP-dependent platelet activation. Based on the results of two recent studies, CURE and PCI-CURE, clopidogrel plays an important role in those patients with NSTEMI ACS being treated non-invasively and invasively, achieving 20% and 30% risk reductions in adverse event rates respectively; in the trials this benefit was maintained in the long-term at 9 and 12 months.[11,12] Although there was a significant increase in major bleeding events, there was no increase in life-threatening bleeds. Clopidogrel should, therefore, be used synergistically with ASA in hospitalized ACS patients, particularly those with high-risk features.

Heparin exerts its anticoagulant effect by accelerating the inhibitory action of antithrombin III on thrombin and factor Xa. Unfractionated heparin (UFH) has been shown to provide a significant, albeit short-term, benefit in the reduction of adverse events.[13] However, its bioavailability is poor and its anticoagulant effect is unpredictable. Although weight-adjusted regimes yield more predictable anticoagulation, a major limitation is the need for regular monitoring of the activated partial thromboplastin time (APTT). The low-molecular-weight heparins (LMWHs), enoxaparin and dalteparin, administered subcutaneously have decreased plasma protein and endothelial cell binding, a longer half-life and dose-independent clearance. This results in more predictable and sustained anticoagulation compared with intravenous (IV) UFH. Therefore, major

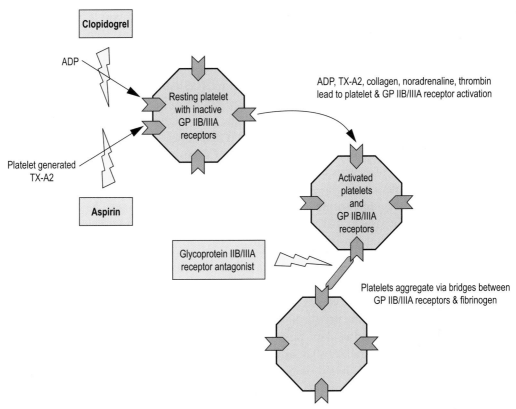

Figure 10.4
Modes of action for various anti-platelet agents
ADP, adenosine diphosphate; TX-A2, thromboxane A2

advantages of LMWHs include an easier route of administration and the freedom from routine laboratory monitoring. Large studies have shown that they are at least equivalent, and in the case of enoxaparin, superior, to UFH in the management of ACS patients.[14] LMWHs should be given for at least 48 hours and continued for several days in cases of recurrent ischaemia or when myocardial revascularization is delayed.[15]

Direct thrombin inhibitors, such as hirudin, have been evaluated in ACS trials. Benefits over UFH have been small and inconsistent. Hirudin agents have, therefore, not achieved widespread acceptance, probably because of, at best, the small benefit and a perceived increased bleeding risk. At present, hirudin is indicated only for those patients who have developed heparin-induced thrombocytopaenia. Reports on bivalirudin (a synthetic hirudin derivative) show initial promise but further trials are awaited.

The glycoprotein (GP IIB/IIIA) platelet surface receptor undergoes a conformational change in the face of platelet aggregation, increasing its affinity for binding to fibrinogen and other ligands. This is the final common pathway for platelet aggregation and, consequently, antagonism of the receptor using GP IIB/IIIA receptor antagonists (Fig. 10.4) results in potent inhibition of aggregation, the primary culprit in ACS. Antagonists include: abciximab (Reopro™), the F_{ab} fragment of the humanized murine antibody to the receptor; the smaller synthetic peptide eptifibatide (Integrilin™) and the non-peptide molecule tirofiban (Aggrastat™). Abciximab has been studied extensively in the context of percutaneous coronary intervention (PCI) where its administration to elective patients and those presenting with ACS has consistently shown a significant reduction in events.[16–18] However, its role in ACS patients where PCI is not considered to be the primary therapeutic strategy is questionable.[19] In this respect, eptifibatide and tirofiban may provide a reduction in events, particularly in those presenting with high-risk features such as ST depression and elevated troponins.[20,21] The recently published UK National Institute for Clinical Excellence (NICE) guidelines recommend the prompt initiation of small molecule agents as part of the primary treatment strategy and as a 'bridge' to PCI where possible – the 'upstream' strategy.[22] However, on the basis of a wealth of data including the findings of the TARGET trial, abciximab appears to be the more effective agent for the 'in the catheter-lab' strategy and, as such, it is currently the only GP IIB/IIIA inhibitor in the UK licensed for use in this setting.[23]

Nitrates primarily mediate their anti-ischaemic effect by a reduction in ventricular pre- and also after-load thereby decreasing MVO_2. Trial data in ACS patients assessing symptom relief or a reduction in events are limited. Although a meta-analysis of trials evaluating IV nitrates in AMI in the pre-thrombolytic era suggested a reduction in mortality, later trials to specifically address this issue failed to demonstrate such a benefit.[24] This may have been due to confounding variables such as the pre-hospital and hospital use of nitrates in the 'control' group. Nevertheless, based on pathophysiological principles and clinical experience, sublingual nitrates should be administered for the immediate relief of ischaemia, followed by an IV infusion if symptoms and/or signs of ischaemia persist.

With regard to percutaneous revascularization in ACS (UA and NSTEMI), much debate has arisen in the past about the conservative versus invasive management of ACS patients. VANQWISH suggested that a routine invasive strategy may be harmful, but the trial was limited by a high rate of crossover, a relatively low-risk study population and a high operative mortality rate in the coronary artery bypass graft surgery (CABG) invasive arm.[25] FRISC II has further clarified the issue.[26] FRISC II with TACTICS-TIMI 18, were conducted in an era of stenting, LMWH and GP IIB/IIIA inhibitors. They defined a more 'selective' approach to early revascularization, with the greatest reduction in adverse events being seen in those at highest risk, i.e. elevated troponins and/or ECG ST depression.[27] The results of the UK-based RITA-3 trial have recently been published. This trial was designed to test the hypothesis that early angiography with revascularization where clinically appropriate would be better than conservative management in patients presenting with unstable angina or NSTEMI.[28] The primary endpoint for this trial was a combination of death, non-fatal MI or refractory angina at 4 months. It is important to note that the use of anti-platelet therapy such as GP IIB/IIIA inhibitors and the nature and extent of revascularization (balloon angioplasty, stenting or CABG) was left to the discretion of the clinician. The results demonstrated a significant reduction in the primary combined endpoint in the invasive arm (9.6% vs. 14.5% in the conservative arm, $P<0.001$). This was predominantly due to halving the rate of refractory angina in the invasively treated arm (4.4% vs. 9.3%, $P<0.0001$). There was no difference in mortality or subsequent MI.

MANAGEMENT OTHER THAN ANTI-THROMBOTIC, ANTI-PLATELET AND REVASCULARIZATION THERAPY

The management of ACS patients has two principal aims, the relief of ischaemia and the prevention of serious events, i.e. death or MI. As already discussed above, this is best achieved by a combination of anti-ischaemic, anti-platelet and anti-thrombotic therapy, and, in some cases, by the use of invasive procedures, the intensity of treatment being tailored to the patient's individual risk. However, besides implementing strategies for reperfusion and treating flow-limiting stenoses, in all cases of coronary artery disease (STEMI, NSTEMI and angina) further pharmacological and lifestyle steps should be taken to reduce the ischaemic burden and minimize risk.

Modifiable risk factors should be assessed; in particular smoking, hypertension and diabetes. Rigorous control of blood glucose levels is associated with improved survival post-MI. In all diabetic patients, whether insulin-dependent or not, post-infarct insulin regimes should be considered.

Beta-blockers (BBs) are competitive antagonists of the β-adrenoceptor that reduce ischaemia by reducing MVO_2 and improving coronary flow. This is achieved by lowering heart rate, systolic blood pressure and myocardial contraction. BBs should be considered for all ACS patients particularly those presenting with acute STEMI, where they reduce the extent of infarction and incidence of associated complications, e.g. myocardial rupture.[29] Although there are only limited outcome data in ACS (UA/non-STEMI), a meta-analysis involving patients with threatened acute MI demonstrated a 13% risk reduction in progression to established acute MI. There is no convincing evidence that IV administration is better or worse than oral. Where there is a contraindication to BBs, a rate-limiting calcium channel blocker (CCB) such as diltiazem should be considered.

Angiotensin converting enzyme inhibitors (ACE-I) have been shown to reduce mortality in patients with acute MI or recent MI with LV systolic dysfunction.[30] They are also beneficial in high- and low-risk coronary artery disease patients with normal LV function.[31] They should, therefore, be considered for all patients with LV dysfunction, those presenting with acute MI, and ACS as well as all patients with stable coronary artery disease.

Statins mediate their effects not only through lipid lowering but also as a result of their pleiotrophic effects, i.e. enhancement of endothelial function, reduction in platelet activation, anti-inflammatory and anti-thrombotic effects. Such effects may account in part for the benefit seen with early statin initiation in ACS patients irrespective of the baseline lipid profile. In MIRACL, patients were randomized to either 80 mg atorvastatin or placebo within 96 hours of presentation; 4-month follow-up demonstrated a 16% risk reduction in adverse events, primarily as a result of reduction in recurrent symptomatic ischaemia.[32] The Heart Protection Study has demonstrated the benefit of statin therapy in high-risk patients with normal/low LDL levels.[33] Lipid reduction therapy is recognized as a means of reducing post-MI cardiovascular morbidity and mortality; landmark trials such as 4S have shown a 25–30% reduction in event rates.[34] Such therapy should, therefore, be considered early in the management of all ACS patients (irrespective of baseline lipid profile) and maintained indefinitely since withdrawal has been associated with an adverse outcome.[35]

Anticoagulation with warfarin after STEMI is associated with increased survival. In one large study, 1214 patients were randomized post-STEMI (mean 27 days) to warfarin or placebo for an average of 37 months. There was a significant 24% reduction in mortality ($P<0.05$). Studies comparing warfarin and aspirin with aspirin alone in patients with non-ST elevation ACS reveal a significant reduction in ischaemic events with the addition of warfarin. Despite evidence of benefits, warfarin has not come into widespread use probably because of the perceived bleeding risk, and the inconvenience and limitations that it imposes on the patient. The safety profile of warfarin in conjunction with newer anti-platelet agents (in particular clopidogrel) remains to be established. The authors do not routinely prescribe warfarin post-STEMI.

COMPLICATIONS OF ST ELEVATION MYOCARDIAL INFARCTION

The complications of STEMI relate primarily to the degree of myocardial damage. The most consistent marker of survival after a STEMI is left-ventricular ejection fraction. Damage to specific areas may be associated with specific complications, e.g. complete heart block after damage to the AV-node or mitral regurgitation after papillary muscle dysfunction. Strategies that reduce infarct size by promoting early reperfusion are, therefore, likely to reduce the risk of subsequent complications.

PUMP FAILURE

Left-ventricular impairment

A linear relationship between ventricular filling pressure and work output demonstrated in animal preparations and in the critically ill tacitly underlies the clinical management of patients with impaired left-ventricular function. The slope of this relationship varies with the degree of left-ventricular dysfunction. The management of fluid balance in these patients becomes a titration of filling pressure to a level achieving adequate cardiac output without inducing excessive pulmonary venous pressures.

The degree of left-ventricular impairment varies during the progress of the infarction, there being an initial 'honeymoon period', falling to a nadir in function at 12–48 hours and subsequently the possibility of a degree of improvement over the next few days. Improvement is critically dependant on the degree of salvage of myocardium, hence the vital role of reperfusion strategies.

In cases without major pump failure, haemodynamic parameters can be adjusted with non-invasive monitoring. Clinical assessment can be used to seek evidence of raised left-atrial pressure and adequate cardiac output, with fluid balance being adjusted accordingly whilst the effects of interventions are monitored.

Breathlessness secondary to raised left-atrial pressure or frank pulmonary oedema, in the absence of systemic hypotension, has traditionally been treated with diuretics. It is likely that the acute benefits from IV diuretics are as much related to their vasodilator properties as to diuresis. High circulating catecholamine levels in the immediate post-ACS period promote a high systemic vascular resistance, resulting in high left-atrial pressures through an increased left ventricular afterload. Vasodilator therapies, initially IV diamorphine and nitrates, followed by oral ACE inhibition, represent a more attractive and logical approach to the treatment of pulmonary oedema, with evidence of greater efficacy than a diuretic based strategy.

In cases of low cardiac output and/or systemic hypotension, the first issue is an assessment of left-ventricular filling pressure. In the absence of raised left-atrial pressure as assessed by the absence of pulmonary oedema clinically, radiographically or from assessment of gas transfer, a fluid challenge should be considered. Clinical improvement confirms the initial assessment. However, where filling pressures are felt to be high and systemic perfusion remains poor, or where interventions do not result in the expected clinical improvement, invasive monitoring is indicated.

Invasive monitoring

Indwelling arterial cannulation for direct pressure measurement, typically radially in patients receiving anticoagulants, allows accurate measurement of responses to therapy and arterial blood sampling. Right-atrial pressure measured via a central line (ideally internal jugular) can be a poor guide to left-atrial pressure, for example in cases of severe left-ventricular dysfunction, left-atrial pressure may be considerably higher than right-atrial pressure by an unknown quantity.

In practical terms, the key question asked of a monitoring system is the adequacy of left-ventricular filling pressure. Accurate measurement of cardiac output is interesting but the crude estimations available from non-invasive clinical assessment such as warmth of the peripheries, volume of the pulses, adequacy of urine output, lactate level, etc., are usually sufficient.

Traditionally the invasive tool of choice has been the balloon-tipped pulmonary artery catheter (PAC). Use of the PAC has associated risks, and data are lacking in STEMI to demonstrate a benefit. Indeed, there are some data to suggest a detriment in their use in the critically ill, although this is open to debate. The use of the PAC remains a matter of controversy. The authors feel that where clinical evidence is lacking, the benefits of measuring key physiological parameters as a guide to therapy probably outweigh the risks. Alternative tools to monitor fluid status and cardiac output include double indicator arterial dilution and the derivative PICO system. These provide, in addition to a thermodilution derived cardiac output, an estimation of total lung water, which can be an accurate guide to fluid balance.

Vasoactive agents

Where left-atrial filling pressures are deemed adequate or excessive, and cardiac output remains inadequate, i.e. cardiogenic shock, vasoactive agents are indicated. The choice of inotrope varies between different institutions and physicians, since there are no convincing trial data to promote any given strategy. Given the presumed greater myocardial efficiency in increasing flow rather than pressure, vasodilating inotropes such as dobutamine or milrinone are preferred. Vasoconstricting inotropes such as adrenaline may be used in combination with a vasodilator, such as intravenous nitrate. In all cases there is a price to pay, the increased inotropy being associated with tachycardia and increased myocardial oxygen demand and, consequently, the risk of developing tachyarrhythmias. Whilst vasodilatation is advocated, arterial blood pressure needs to be kept above a certain level in order to maintain adequate perfusion particularly in the coronary, cerebral and splanchnic beds. This level will vary from patient to patient and there is no substitute for repeated clinical assessment of myocardial and cerebral function, and urine output in determining the optimum level.

The calcium sensitizing agent, levosimendan, represents an interesting concept. The energetic cost of calcium fluxes across myocardial membranes, triggering the contractile apparatus, represents a significant proportion of myocardial energy balance. By sensitizing the contractile apparatus to calcium, the same work output can be achieved from a smaller calcium flux, promoting a higher level of myocardial efficiency. Levosimendan remains unlicensed in the UK, but anecdotal trial data show initial promise.

Intra-aortic balloon pumps

Intra-aortic balloon counter-pulsation devices (IABP) represent an attractive 'inotrope'. The sudden deflation of the balloon in the descending thoracic aorta during systole gives the benefits of profound vasodilatation to the failing left ventricle. Subsequent balloon inflation during diastole then results in an augmented proximal aortic pressure promoting coronary and cerebral blood flow. A typical balloon of 40 ml volume, operating at 80 beats per minute, results in a displacement of just over 3 l/min. Since there is reversal of flow in the descending thoracic aorta during balloon deflation, this does not equate to a similar increase in cardiac output; depending on the level of systemic tone, increases in the order of 1–1.5 l/min might be expected.

Intra-aortic balloon pumping is not, however, without problems. The device relies on an aortic valve of reasonable competence. Access is via a large (typically 8 or 9Fr) arterial sheath and local vascular complications are not uncommon as formal anticoagulation is required. The patient needs to lie relatively flat to avoid compression of the tubing, which may present its own difficulties in the non-ventilated patient with high left-atrial pressure. The complications tend to be time dependent, hence their use is primarily as a holding measure whilst awaiting a significant recovery in myocardial function, perhaps from an impending revascularization procedure (CABG or PCI).

Metabolic parameters

Whilst managing the patient with severe left-ventricular impairment, a global approach is required with optimization of all aspects of care, for example ensuring adequate nutrition, seeking and treating infections, and control of metabolic status. Tight control of blood sugar using insulin sliding scales is associated with an improved outcome in critically ill patients. Electrolytes and pH should be monitored and corrected accordingly.

Assisted ventilation

High left-atrial pressures, even in the absence of pulmonary oedema, are associated with a reduced lung compliance and hence an increased work of breathing. Patients may require assistance in maintaining adequate oxygenation and reducing this work. Continuous positive airway pressure (CPAP) circuits are effective and may, if used at a sufficiently early stage, obviate the need for endotracheal intubation. More complex non-invasive support modalities, e.g. biphasic positive airway pressure (BIPAP), are probably superior in reducing the work of breathing, but require more co-operation from the patient. Non-invasive ventilatory support systems are undoubtedly underused in coronary care units. In severe cases (i.e. respiratory failure), formal endotracheal intubation should be considered. This should be viewed as a 'holding measure', in a manner analogous to IABP usage, where there is an expectation of significant myocardial recovery.

Physiological right-ventricular failure

Inferior and infero-posterior STEMI may result in an effective failure of the right ventricle. This may present clinically as an apparently low cardiac output, with raised systemic venous pressures, in the context of low left-atrial pressures. If not apparent clinically, the syndrome may be confirmed with pulmonary artery (PA) catheterization. In contrast to left-ventricular impairment, systemic vasodilatation may be unhelpful, resulting in deteriorating cardiac output because of the low left-ventricular filling pressure. Maintenance of adequate systemic perfusion pressure is dependant on fluid loading, with or without inotropic support.

Arrhythmias

Rhythm disturbances in ACS are not uncommon. Heart block arising from damage to the conduction system may result in atrioventricular (AV) block and interventricular conduction deficits. Complete heart block occurs less frequently in patients with STEMI and often resolves spontaneously if reperfusion therapies are given early. Temporary pacing is strongly indicated if:

- there is persistent haemodynamic disturbance related to the bradycardia
- the ventricular escape rhythm is broad.

In the context of a narrow complex escape rhythm of a rate sufficient to provide adequate cardiac output, an expectant approach is reasonable but requires close monitoring, with recourse to urgent temporary pacing if required. If significant block persists after 5–7 days, there is a high likelihood of requiring permanent pacing.

In the authors' opinion, a perceived need for temporary pacing is rarely, if ever, a sufficient reason to delay/withhold thrombolysis. Thrombolysis may negate the need for pacing and temporary pharmacological measures (e.g. atropine) may be sufficient until reperfusion has occurred. Thrombolytic agents with a short half-life (e.g. tPA) are preferred if there is a high likelihood of needing central venous cannulation.

Tachyarrhythmias are not uncommon post-STEMI. Their management is discussed in Chapter 14.

Valve dysfunction

Valvular dysfunction in patients with ACS may be as a co-existent feature or as a result of myocardial damage. Inferior STEMI in particular may result in mitral regurgitation either as a result of papillary muscle dysfunction/rupture, or as a result of the immobility of the inferior wall and consequent splinting of the posterior leaflet in an open position.

Perforation

Rupture of the left-ventricular wall occurs most commonly within 24 hours or between 3 and 5 days post-infarction. Rupture of the free wall is generally fatal resulting in tamponade and cardiac arrest resistant to resuscitation, although there are reports of short-term survival due to 'walling off' of the defect with pericardium. The frequency of rupture is reduced in cases where appropriate thrombolysis has been given, and with the use of beta-blockade.

Ventricular septal defects

Rupture of the interventricular septum is associated with a high mortality. Left-to-right shunting results in right-ventricular volume overload. The patient may present with recurrent pain, and/or haemodynamic instability with tachycardia and hypotension. There is generally a harsh pan-systolic murmur with or without a thrill, often without evidence of significantly elevated left-atrial pressures. Diagnosis can be confirmed on echocardiography and/or pulmonary artery catheterization, both of which may be used to calculate the size of the shunt. Historically, management was initially conservative, supporting the circulation with vasodilating inotropes, or preferably an IABP, with the plan to repair the defect surgically 3–6 weeks post-infarct. However, initial mortality was high, and in the authors' experience, conservative management appears associated with clinical deterioration. Current guidelines promote immediate physical closure irrespective of clinical state. Closure can be achieved surgically, or more recently with the use of percutaneous devices, although in this context they remain experimental.

CONCLUSION

Successful management of an acute coronary syndrome requires careful assessment of risk/benefit at each stage, tailoring the therapeutic strategies employed to the individual patient. Various tools continue to be developed to help stratify risk, although clinical assessment and reassessment remain amongst the most useful.

References

1. The GISSI Trial Group 1986 Effectiveness of intravenous thrombolytic treatment in acute myocardial infarction. Gruppo Italiano per lo Studio della Streptochinasi nell'Infarto Miocardico (GISSI). Lancet 1(8478): 397–402

2. The ISIS-2 (Second International Study of Infarct Survival) Collaborative Group 1988 Randomised trial of intravenous streptokinase, oral aspirin, both, or neither among 17,187 cases of suspected acute myocardial infarction: ISIS-2. Lancet 2(8607): 349–360

3. The Fibrinolytic Therapy Trialists' (FTT) Collaborative Group 1994 Indications for fibrinolytic therapy in suspected acute myocardial infarction: collaborative overview of early mortality and major morbidity results from all randomised trials of more than 1000 patients. Lancet 343(8893): 311–322

4. The GREAT Group 1992 Feasibility, safety, and efficacy of domiciliary thrombolysis by general practitioners: Grampian region early anistreplase trial. BMJ 305(6853): 548–553

5. The GUSTO Angiographic Investigators 1993 The effects of tissue plasminogen activator, streptokinase, or both on coronary-artery patency, ventricular function, and survival after acute myocardial infarction. N Engl J Med 329(22): 1615–1622

6. Grines CL, Browne KF, Marco J et al. 1993 A comparison of immediate angioplasty with thrombolytic therapy for acute myocardial infarction. The Primary Angioplasty in Myocardial Infarction Study Group. N Engl J Med 328(10): 673–679

7. Zijlstra F, Hoorntje JC, de Boer MJ et al. 1999 Long-term benefit of primary angioplasty as compared with thrombolytic therapy for acute myocardial infarction. N Engl J Med 341(19): 1413–1419

8. The TIMI IIIB Investigators 1994 Effects of tissue plasminogen activator and a comparison of early invasive and conservative strategies in unstable angina and non-Q-wave myocardial infarction. Results of the TIMI IIIB Trial. Thrombolysis in Myocardial Ischemia. Circulation 89(4): 1545–1556

9. The Antiplatelet Trialists' Collaboration 1994 Collaborative overview of randomised trials of antiplatelet therapy–I: Prevention of death, myocardial infarction, and stroke by prolonged antiplatelet therapy in various categories of patients. BMJ 308(6921): 81–106

10. The CAPRIE Steering Committee 1996 A randomised, blinded, trial of clopidogrel versus aspirin in patients at risk of ischaemic events (CAPRIE). Lancet 348(9038): 1329–1339

11. Yusuf S, Zhao F, Mehta SR, Chrolavicius S, Tognoni G, Fox KK 2001 Effects of clopidogrel in addition to aspirin in patients with acute coronary syndromes without ST-segment elevation; the CURE Study. N Engl J Med 345(7): 494–502

12. Mehta SR, Yusuf S, Peters RJ et al. 2001 Effects of pretreatment with clopidogrel and aspirin followed by long-term therapy in patients undergoing percutaneous coronary intervention: the PCI-CURE study. Lancet 358(9281): 527–533

13. Theroux P, Ouimet H, McCans J et al. 1988 Aspirin, heparin, or both to treat acute unstable angina. N Engl J Med 319(17): 1105–1111

14. Cohen M, Demers C, Gurfinkel EP et al. 1997 A comparison of low-molecular-weight heparin with unfractionated heparin for unstable coronary artery disease. Efficacy and Safety of Subcutaneous Enoxaparin in Non-Q-Wave Coronary Events (ESSENCE) Study Group. N Engl J Med 337(7): 447–452

15. The Fragmin and Fast Revascularisation during InStability in Coronary artery disease Investigators 1999 Long-term low-molecular-mass heparin in unstable coronary-artery disease: FRISC II prospective randomised multicentre study. Lancet 354(9180): 701–707

16. The EPILOG Investigators 1997 Platelet glycoprotein IIb/IIIa receptor blockade and low-dose heparin during percutaneous coronary revascularization. The EPILOG Investigators. N Engl J Med 336(24): 1689–1696

17. The CAPTURE Investigators 1997 Randomised placebo-controlled trial of abciximab before and during coronary intervention in refractory unstable angina: the CAPTURE Study. Lancet 349(9063): 1429–1435

18. The EPISTENT Investigators 1998 Randomised placebo-controlled and balloon-angioplasty-controlled trial to assess safety of coronary stenting with use of platelet glycoprotein- IIb/IIIa blockade. The EPISTENT Investigators. Evaluation of Platelet IIb/IIIa Inhibitor for Stenting. Lancet 352(9122): 87–92

19. The GUSTO IV ACS Investigators, Simoons ML 2001 Effect of glycoprotein IIb/IIIa receptor blocker abciximab on outcome in patients with acute coronary syndromes without early coronary revascularisation: the GUSTO IV-ACS randomised trial. Lancet 357(9272): 1915–1924

20. The PURSUIT Trial Investigators 1998 Inhibition of platelet glycoprotein IIb/IIIa with eptifibatide in patients with acute coronary syndromes. The PURSUIT Trial Investigators. Platelet Glycoprotein IIb/IIIa in Unstable Angina: Receptor Suppression Using Integrilin Therapy. N Engl J Med 339(7): 436–443

21. The PRISM-PLUS Investigators 1998 Inhibition of the platelet glycoprotein IIb/IIIa receptor with tirofiban in unstable angina and non-Q-wave myocardial infarction. Platelet Receptor Inhibition in Ischemic Syndrome

Management in Patients Limited by Unstable Signs and Symptoms (PRISM-PLUS) Study Investigators. N Engl J Med 338(21): 1488–1497

22. National Institute for Clinical Excellence 2002 Final Appraisal Determination: The use of glycoprotein IIb/IIIa inhibitors in the treatment of acute coronary syndromes. Ref Type: Generic www.nice.org.uk

23. The TARGET Investigators, Topol EJ, Moliterno DJ, Herrmann HC et al. 2001 Comparison of two platelet glycoprotein IIb/IIIa inhibitors, tirofiban and abciximab, for the prevention of ischemic events with percutaneous coronary revascularization. N Engl J Med 344(25): 1888–1894

24. The ISIS-4 (Fourth International Study of Infarct Survival) Collaborative Group 1995 ISIS-4: a randomised factorial trial assessing early oral captopril, oral mononitrate, and intravenous magnesium sulphate in 58,050 patients with suspected acute myocardial infarction. Lancet 345(8951): 669–685

25. Boden WE, O'Rourke RA, Crawford MH et al. 1998 Outcomes in patients with acute non-Q-wave myocardial infarction randomly assigned to an invasive as compared with a conservative management strategy. Veterans Affairs Non-Q-Wave Infarction Strategies in Hospital (VANQWISH) Trial Investigators. N Engl J Med 338(25): 1785–1792

26. The Fragmin and Fast Revascularisation during InStability in Coronary artery disease Investigators 1999 Invasive compared with non-invasive treatment in unstable coronary-artery disease: FRISC II prospective randomised multicentre study. Lancet 354(9180): 708–715

27. The TACTICS-TIMI 18 Investigators, Cannon CP, Weintraub WS, Demopoulos LA et al. 2001 Comparison of early invasive and conservative strategies in patients with unstable coronary syndromes treated with the glycoprotein IIb/IIIa inhibitor tirofiban. N Engl J Med 344(25): 1879–1887

28. Fox KA, Poole-Wilson PA, Henderson RA et al. 2002 Interventional versus conservative treatment for patients with unstable angina or non-ST-elevation myocardial infarction: the British Heart Foundation RITA 3 randomised trial. Randomized Intervention Trial of unstable Angina. Lancet 360(9335): 743–751

29. The ISIS-1 (First International Study of Infarct Survival) Collaborative Group 1986 Randomised trial of intravenous atenolol among 16 027 cases of suspected acute myocardial infarction. Lancet 2(8498): 57–66

30. Rutherford JD, Pfeffer MA, Moye LA et al. 1994 Effects of captopril on ischemic events after myocardial infarction. Results of the Survival and Ventricular Enlargement trial. SAVE Investigators. Circulation 90(4): 1731–1738

31. Yusuf S, Sleight P, Pogue J, Bosch J, Davies R, Dagenais G 2000 Effects of an angiotensin-converting-enzyme inhibitor, ramipril, on cardiovascular events in high-risk patients. The Heart Outcomes Prevention Evaluation Study Investigators. N Engl J Med 342(3): 145–153

32. Schwartz GG, Olsson AG, Ezekowitz MD et al. 2001 Effects of atorvastatin on early recurrent ischemic events in acute coronary syndromes: the MIRACL study: a randomized controlled trial. JAMA 285(13): 1711–1718

33. The Heart Protection Study Group 2002 MRC/BHF Heart Protection Study of cholesterol lowering with simvastatin in 20,536 high-risk individuals: a randomised placebo-controlled trial. Lancet 360(9326): 7–22

34. The 4S Group 1994 Randomised trial of cholesterol lowering in 4444 patients with coronary heart disease: the Scandinavian Simvastatin Survival Study (4S). Lancet 344(8934): 1383–1389

35. Sacks FM, Pfeffer MA, Moye LA et al. 1996 The effect of pravastatin on coronary events after myocardial infarction in patients with average cholesterol levels. Cholesterol and Recurrent Events (CARE) Trial investigators. N Engl J Med 335(14): 1001–1009

SELF-ASSESSMENT

Questions
1. What are the regulations with respect to driving following acute coronary syndromes?
2. What is the role of angiotensin II receptor blockers post myocardial infarction?
3. What is the TIMI (Thrombolysis In Myocardial Infarction) risk score?

Answers
1. Up-to-date information can be obtained from the DVLA (http://www.dvla.gov.uk). The current guidelines (August 2003) define acute coronary syndromes (including MI) for group 1 licences to include **all** three of the following: persistent or recurrent pain; troponin release positive, and ECG changes. In this case driving must stop for at least four weeks, although there is no need to notify the DVLA. After this period driving can recommence providing there are no other disqualifying conditions.

   For group 2 licences, **all** acute coronary syndromes are considered relevant and this disqualifies the individual from driving for at least six weeks. Re-licensing may be permitted if a suitable exercise test* is achieved and there are no other disqualifying conditions. Whilst angiography is not required for re-licensing, if performed specific guidelines are available from the DVLA site.

   Exercise testing: Need to complete three stages of the Bruce protocol or equivalent safely, without anti-anginal medication for 48 hours. The individual should remain free from signs of cardiovascular dysfunction (angina, syncope, hypotension, sustained ventricular tachycardia, and/or ECG ST segment change indicative of myocardial ischaemia (usually >2mm horizontal or down-sloping) during exercise or the recovery period.

2. Two recent studies have shed further light on this area: the OPTIMAAL study randomized patients with acute MI and heart failure to losartan (50 mg od) or captopril (50 mg tds). There was a non-significant difference in total mortality in favour of captopril, leading to the suggestion that ACE inhibitors should remain first-choice therapy after complicated acute myocardial infarction. Losartan was, however, better tolerated than captopril with fewer discontinuations. It has been suggested that the dose of losartan used in this study was too low. More recently the VALIANT study randomized patients (already on conventional therapy) with acute MI (day 0.5 to 10) and left ventricular dysfunction and/or clinical heart failure to valsartan, valsartan and captopril or captopril alone. Valsartan was as effective as captopril, but a combination of valsartan with captopril increased the rate of adverse events without improving survival.

   The impact on clinical practice is that the majority of patients post MI should still receive an ACE inhibitor (unless contraindicated), since there is now a wealth of data supporting their use. These recent studies have provided evidence to support early transfer to an angiotensin II receptor blocker in those patients who suffer undue ACE inhibitor related side-effects.

3. In patients with unstable angina/NSTEMI, the TIMI risk score is a simple validated prognostic scheme which categorizes a patient's risk of death and ischaemic events and provides a basis for therapeutic decision making. The TIMI risk score was derived from seven standard clinical characteristics routinely obtained during the initial medical evaluation of suspected ACS patients (Box 10.1) which were assigned a value of 1 when present and 0 when absent. Event rates increase significantly as the risk score increases.

Box 10.1: Components of the TIMI risk score

Age ≥ 65 years
At least 3 CAD risk factors
Significant coronary stenosis (e.g. prior coronary stenosis ≥50%)
ST-segment deviation
Severe anginal symptoms (e.g. 2 anginal events in last 24 h)
Use of aspirin in last 7 days
Elevated serum cardiac markers.

(adapted from Antman EM et al. *JAMA* 2000; 284: 835–842).

Valvular heart disease

11

J. Greenwood and J. Kurian

INTRODUCTION

Over the last 25 years there has been a significant increase in our understanding of the natural history of valvular heart disease. There have been major advances in cardiac imaging modalities, in particular echocardiography. Treatment options for both interventional cardiology and surgical procedures have also expanded during this period. Despite this dramatic increase in our knowledge and understanding, in many areas management decisions remain uncertain or controversial due to a paucity of large-scale multicentre trials.

Each of the following sections in this chapter includes a brief introduction to the aetiology and natural history of the condition, followed by the major presenting symptoms and signs. With regard to the investigation and treatment options, suggestions are based primarily around the ACC/AHA 'guidelines for management of patients with valvular heart disease'.[1] Like all guidelines these are not prescriptive; local availability of diagnostic equipment, and expertise of interventional cardiologists and surgeons, may dictate alternative investigation and treatment pathways.

AORTIC VALVE DISEASE

AORTIC STENOSIS

The normal aortic valve is composed of three leaflets, with a valve orifice area between 3.0 and 4.0 cm². The aortic valve area must be considerably reduced before it causes any significant haemodynamic change. An aortic valve with an area below 1.0 cm² is now considered severely stenosed, whilst 1.0–1.5cm² is considered moderate stenosis and areas above 1.5 cm² are considered mild stenosis.[1] However, these measurements need to be considered in the context of the patient's body habitus; in larger patients there may be severe obstruction in the presence of valve areas that would otherwise be considered to be only moderate stenosis. The transvalvular pressure gradient in the presence of severe stenosis is usually >50 mmHg, although the gradient is dependent on the left-ventricular (LV) function and lower gradients could be significant if the LV function is impaired.

Aetiology

This may be congenital. Bicuspid aortic valves (Fig. 11.1) cause turbulent flow leading to leaflet trauma with fibrosis and later calcification eventually leading to obstruction. It usually presents in the 4th or 5th decade of life.

Idiopathic or degenerative disease presents in the 6th or 7th decades of life caused by the deposition of calcium in the base of the valve along the flexion lines, immobilizing the cusps. It has similar pathophysiology to ischaemic heart disease with risk factors such as raised cholesterol and hypertension. The rate of progression of the disease may be slowed by modifying these risk factors.

Rheumatic disease involving the aortic valve often causes regurgitation as well as stenosis. The mitral valve nearly always shows stigmata of disease.

Rare causes, such as Pagets' disease of bone, end-stage renal failure and ochronosis (pigmentation of cartilage seen in association with alkaptonuria) can cause aortic stenosis (AS).

Obstruction to the LV outflow tract may also occur due to:

1. Supravalvular stenosis: obstruction above the valve coexists with idiopathic infantile hypercalcaemia (Williams' syndrome).
2. Subvalvular AS: due to a membranous diaphragm, fibrous ring or a long fibromuscular narrowing present below the level of the valve in the LV outflow tract.

Natural history and pathophysiology

The disease is characterized by a long latent period during which patients are asymptomatic. The morbidity and mortality during this period is very low. The average

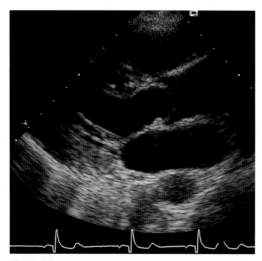

Figure 11.1
Parasternal long-axis 2-D echocardiographic view of the aortic valve showing reduced excursion and doming of the valve leaflets typical of bicuspid aortic valve stenosis

rate of reduction in valve area is around 0.12 cm^2/year, which equates to a gradient of 10–15 mmHg/year. The progression is more rapid in patients with calcific degenerative disease, although there are no indicators that help predict the rate of progression in an individual patient. Therapeutic decisions, particularly those related to surgery, are made on the basis of the presence or absence of symptoms and not on the absolute valve area or the pressure gradient.

Calcific AS is caused by focal lesions on the aortic side of the leaflet, which consist of deposits of protein, lipids and activated macrophages. These inflammatory cells release substances that facilitate the deposition of calcium, which causes obstruction to flow and increases the systolic wall stress and ventricular hypertrophy. A large pressure gradient can thus be sustained, without causing LV dilatation or decreasing the cardiac output, which allows the patient to remain asymptomatic until late in the disease process. Thus, the development of symptoms in a previously asymptomatic patient is a sign of decompensation and indicates the need for prompt investigation and, if appropriate, surgery.

Symptoms

Angina occurs in two-thirds of patients (only half of whom have coronary disease) as a result of an imbalance between the high O$_2$ demand, caused by increased afterload and myocardial hypertrophy, and a reduction in coronary blood flow due to the compression of epicardial vessels. Only 50% of patients survive 5 years once angina develops.

Exertional dizziness or syncope may be due to inappropriate ventricular baroreceptor responses, which cause peripheral vasodilatation leading to hypotension. Hypotension may also be caused by the inability of the ventricle to increase stroke volume with exertion because of the stenotic valve. Transient A-V block is sometimes seen due to extension of calcification from the valve into the conduction system. Survival is 50% at 3 years once syncope has occurred.

The development of heart failure is an ominous sign with only 50% of patients surviving 2 years. It may be due to either diastolic (non-compliant ventricle) or systolic dysfunction (tends to occur later).

Signs

There is a reduction in the rate and magnitude of rise in aortic pressure (producing the characteristic narrow pulse pressure). The upstroke of the carotid pulse is thus delayed and reduced (causing a 'slow rising' pulse). Vessel calcification in older patients can reduce arterial compliance and can negate these findings.

The S4 is prominent due to vigorous atrial contraction and reduced LV compliance. S2 is quiet or single due to calcification and immobility of the cusps with A2 becoming inaudible with increasing severity. There is sometimes the presence of paradoxical splitting of the second sound.

A systolic crescendo-decrescendo murmur is heard at the base and radiates into the carotids. The more severe the stenosis the longer the murmur with its peak later in systole. A systolic thrill may be palpable. Selective high frequency components radiate to the apex (Gallivardin phenomenon) with a quiet area between apex and base. The murmur may become softer later in the disease process when LV dysfunction develops.

Investigations

The main electrocardiogram (ECG) finding is LV hypertrophy (LVH), which is seen in 85% of patients who have critical AS. Progressive change in the ST segments and T waves suggest progression of hypertrophy. Chest X-ray (CXR) findings may be entirely normal.

Echocardiography

The diagnosis can be confirmed and the severity assessed by echocardiogram (echo):

- Aortic valve gradient using the modified Bernoulli equation: the peak velocity is measured across the valve and then is used in the formula $P = 4V^2$ (where P is the pressure gradient and V is the peak velocity) (see Fig. 11.2).
- Valve area can be calculated by the simplified continuity equation:

Aortic valve area = cross-sectional area LV outflow tract (LVOT) x velocity (LVOT)/ velocity (aorta)

- With better image resolution obtained by the latest generation echocardiographic machines the valve area can be planimetered, although there can be significant inter-observer and inter-study variability using this technique.

The echo also provides information regarding the LV size and function as well as the morphology and function of the other valves.

Exercise testing

In AS this test is unreliable in excluding the presence of coronary artery disease (CAD) and is only useful in obtaining an objective baseline regarding a patient's symptomatic state in those with vague symptoms or those that are asymptomatic. The test carries considerable risk in symptomatic patients and should *not* be performed.

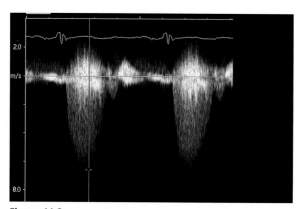

Figure 11.2
Continuous-wave Doppler recording across a severely stenosed aortic valve showing an instantaneous peak pressure gradient of approximately 170 mmHg

Angiography

The severity of stenosis can by assessed reliably by non-invasive methods but invasive measurements (e.g. Gorlin formula to calculate valve area using pressure gradient and cardiac output) may help clarify any discrepancy between the clinical and echocardiographic data. The valve gradient measured by echo is the maximum instantaneous gradient while that measured by the catheter at angiography is the peak-to-peak gradient (Fig. 11.3). The peak pressures in the aorta and the LV do not occur simultaneously and hence these two values are not the same. Echocardiography tends to overestimate the aortic gradient when compared with values obtained by catheterization. An additional reason for performing cardiac catheterization is the ability to delineate the coronary anatomy prior to aortic valve surgery in patients at risk of coronary artery disease.

The frequency of follow-up visits depends to a great degree on the severity of the valvular stenosis. A change in symptoms should prompt an earlier review, but in general patients with mild stenosis do not require more than an annual examination, whist those with moderate and severe stenosis without symptoms need to be seen more frequently. Patients with severe AS should have an annual echo, while those with moderate AS should have one every 2 years, and mild AS one every 5 years, as recommended by the AHA/ACC guidelines.[1]

Treatment

Medical

These patients are at relatively high risk of infective endocarditis and should receive antibiotic prophylaxis. In symptomatic patients the only effective therapy is surgical valve replacement.

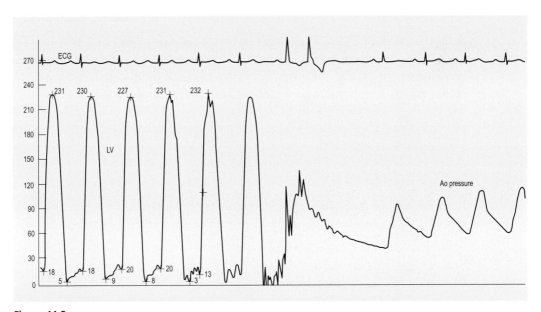

Figure 11.3
Pullback catheter pressure trace across an aortic valve showing a peak-to-peak pressure gradient in excess of 110 mmHg indicating severe stenosis
LV, left ventricular pressure; Ao, aorta

Surgical

Aortic valve replacement   This is indicated in:

1. Symptomatic patients with severe AS. These patients exhibit improvement in symptoms and survive longer following aortic valve replacement (AVR). AS is a pressure overload situation and patients may have LV impairment (the LV is unable to cope with the severity of stenosis) and a low transvalvular gradient as a result. Such patients often have an improvement in LV function after surgery (as AVR reduces the afterload on the LV). If the impairment in LV function is secondary to other causes, patients have a higher operative mortality and symptoms generally persist.
2. Patients with severe AS undergoing cardiac surgery (e.g. coronary artery bypass grafting (CABG), aortic surgery or other valve surgery) should have aortic valve replacement at the same time.
3. Decisions regarding AVR in asymptomatic patients are controversial. It has been suggested that patients with severe AS who have LV systolic dysfunction, an abnormal response to exercise, ventricular tachycardia or marked LVH (>15 mm) form a group of patients at high risk of sudden death and should have prophylactic AVR, although it is unusual for this patient group to be completely asymptomatic.

Prophylactic AVR for asymptomatic patients with mild or moderate stenosis but undergoing cardiac surgery for other indications is controversial.

Balloon valvotomy   This is useful in the treatment of adolescents and young adults. In older patients serious complications occur with a frequency in excess of 10%. The event free survival in older patients was shown to be 20% at 2 years and hence this procedure is no longer a treatment modality for older patients. It may still have a limited role in the older patient who is not a candidate for surgery or as a bridge to surgery.

Ross procedure   This consists of the native pulmonary valve and proximal pulmonary artery being harvested and positioned as a root replacement in the aortic position. The continuity between the right ventricle (RV) and distal pulmonary artery is then reconstructed with a pulmonary valve allograft. The autologous pulmonary valve for AVR has produced excellent results in children, infants and young adults. The procedure produces good haemodynamic characteristics, excellent longevity and negates the need for long-term anticoagulation.

AORTIC REGURGITATION

Incompetence of the aortic valve can occur due to disease of the aortic root, which prevents leaflet co-aptation, or due to disease of the leaflets themselves.

Aetiology

Pathology affecting the leaflets:

- endocarditis
- rheumatic fever
- anorectic drugs.

Pathology affecting the aortic root:

- anuloaortic ectasia
- Marfan's syndrome
- aortic dissection
- collagen vascular disease
- syphilis.

Natural history and pathophysiology

Acute aortic regurgitation

This is usually a surgical emergency (common causes are infective endocarditis and aortic dissection). The large regurgitant volume returning into a non-adapted LV causes a rise in the LV end-diastolic pressure and this leads on to pulmonary congestion and oedema. There is impaired cardiac output, which, together with the raised LV end-diastolic pressure, causes reduced coronary blood flow. Ischaemia is likely to worsen systolic function.

On auscultation the diastolic murmur is audible, S1 is soft but the large stroke volume seen in the compensated chronic state is absent and so the peripheral signs may not be marked. The large regurgitant volume causes the end diastolic pressure to rise rapidly and the mitral valve may close before the onset of systole, indicating the need for urgent surgery.

Chronic aortic regurgitation

This is a condition where there is combined volume and pressure overload on the LV. In the initial stages of the disease the patient remains asymptomatic as compensatory hypertrophy and an increased preload helps maintain normal ventricular function at rest. At a later date, the ventricular function declines due to a disproportionately high afterload or reduced contractility. This is the stage at which patients start to develop symptoms and is initially reversible. This progresses to an enlargement in the ventricular dimensions and the ventricular shape changes to a more spherical geometry. The LV systolic function and cavity dimensions are important determinants of long-term prognosis. The severity of symptoms, the severity of systolic dysfunction and the duration of dysfunction also affect long-term outcome.

Symptoms

Patients usually present with dyspnoea, orthopnoea and paroxysmal nocturnal dyspnoea (PND). Angina sometimes occurs (often at night) and associated with diaphoresis. This is said to be due to slowing of heart rate at night with the arterial diastolic pressures dropping to very low levels.

Signs

Precordial signs of aortic regurgitation (AR) are:

- a soft S1 (A2 also may be soft)
- a systolic ejection sound (increased forward flow volume)

- the regurgitant murmur is a high-pitched early diastolic murmur, heard best with the patient leaning forward, breath held in end-expiration. The severity of regurgitation correlates to the duration of the murmur, reaching an early peak in severe AR but lasting through most of diastole.
- Austin-Flint murmur which is a mid- and late-diastolic rumble heard at the apex (the regurgitant jet causes vibrations of the anterior mitral leaflet).

Peripheral signs in chronic severe AR include:

- collapsing pulse (Corrigan's pulse) with wide arterial pulse pressure
- head bobbing (de Musset's sign)
- pulsus bisferiens
- pulsating uvula (Muller's sign)
- femoral artery systolic murmur on proximal compression and diastolic murmur on distal compression (Duroziez sign). Pistol shot femorals – booming systolic and diastolic sounds over the femorals (Traube's sign)
- systolic plethora and diastolic blanching of the nail bed with mild pressure (Quincke's sign)
- systolic blood pressure in the leg >30 mmHg higher than the arm blood pressure (Hill's sign).

Investigations

The diagnosis can usually be made by physical examination. An ECG and CXR can help evaluate heart size and rhythm.

Echocardiography helps to confirm the diagnosis and severity, and assesses the aetiology (looking at valve morphology, and the dimensions and morphology of the aortic root).

Many echocardiographic parameters have been developed to assess the severity of AR, although each is associated with pitfalls:

1. Continuous-wave Doppler to obtain pressure half times (Fig. 11.4).

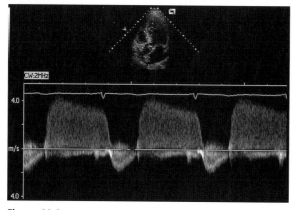

Figure 11.4
Apical four-chamber continuous-wave Doppler recording across a regurgitant aortic valve showing relatively high signal intensity in comparison to the antegrade signal

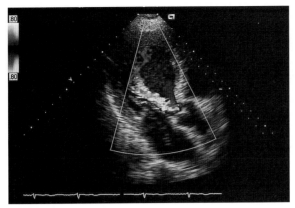

Figure 11.5
Apical 2-D view with colour Doppler showing a broad turbulent jet of aortic regurgitation (AR) into a dilated left ventrical

2. Colour Doppler to measure the width and length of the regurgitant jet (Fig. 11.5).
3. Calculation of the regurgitant fraction.
4. Calculation of the regurgitant orifice.

Serial echocardiography is recommended in patients with AR and new or changing symptoms. Asymptomatic patients with mild AR and little or no LV dilatation can be seen on a yearly basis and provided their symptoms remain stable, an echo can be performed every 2–3 years. Asymptomatic patients with more severe AR and LV dilatation but preserved systolic function, require a more careful physical examination every 6 months and an echo every 6–12 months, depending on severity of dilatation and stability of serial measurements. Angiography is indicated in patients who are due to undergo AVR and are at risk of CAD. It may also be used to assess LV function or degree of regurgitation when non-invasive tests are inconclusive.

Treatment

Medical

Medical treatment aims to reduce afterload by the use of peripheral vasodilators. This should reduce the amount of regurgitation and improve ventricular performance. This has been demonstrated in trials with nifedipine; ACE inhibitors have reported less consistent results. Vasodilator therapy is indicated in:

- symptomatic patients with severe AR in whom surgery is not recommended due to other factors
- asymptomatic patients with severe regurgitation and LV dilatation but normal LV function
- patients with hypertension and any degree of regurgitation
- patients with systolic dysfunction, which persists after AVR, should receive long-term ACE inhibitors.

Vasodilator therapy is not recommended for asymptomatic patients who have AR and a normal LV in the absence of hypertension. Patients with AR are at relatively high risk of endocarditis and should receive antibiotic prophylaxis.

Surgical

In the presence of severe AR, AVR is indicated in:

- patients with New York Heart Association (NYHA, see Ch. 12) Class III or IV symptoms
- patients with NYHA Class II symptoms in whom LV size increases or LV function declines
- asymptomatic patients when LV function declines (ejection fraction <50%) or dilatation is seen (end systolic dimension >55 mm). Smaller patients of either gender may develop symptoms with less dilatation, which can be corrected for by assessing body surface area
- coexisting aortic root dilatation >50 mm on echo, with regurgitation of any severity, should have aortic root reconstruction and AVR.

Follow-up for patients after aortic valve replacement   After AVR annual follow-up is usually adequate in asymptomatic patients. An initial echo after surgery is required but further studies are not mandated in patients with mechanical valves who have no evidence of dysfunction and have stable symptoms. Bioprostheses are at increased risk of deterioration after 5 years in the mitral position, and 8 years in the aortic position. Such patients should have annual echos. If there are signs suggesting prosthetic valve dysfunction an echo is required, and once AR has been detected further studies are required every 3–6 months.

Choice of valve   A mechanical valve has better structural integrity and longevity in patients <65 years old. However, they require anticoagulation, with the risks and side-effects of warfarin therapy. In patients >65 years a bioprosthesis has <10% deterioration over 10 years and does not need anticoagulation. Biological valves have a higher rate of deterioration if implanted in younger patients, those with renal failure on haemodialysis and patients with hypercalcaemia. The Ross procedure (described earlier) was developed to reduce some of these complications.

If patients need anticoagulation for another reason, e.g. atrial fibrillation (AF) or mechanical valve in another position, there is no benefit in using a biological valve. The risk of the patient developing endocarditis following valve replacement is identical irrespective of the type of valve implanted.

PULMONARY VALVE DISEASE

PULMONARY STENOSIS

Pulmonary stenosis (PS) is usually congenital in origin. Obstruction to the right ventricle (RV) can occur at:

- subvalvular level – hypertrophied infundibulum

- valvular level – thickening of the leaflets
- supravalvular – narrowing of the main pulmonary artery.

Valvular pulmonary stenosis is usually detected in childhood and is characterized by an ejection click and a systolic murmur. Progression of the stenosis is related to the initial gradient documented. Gradients in excess of 50 mmHg are considered severe and require treatment. The treatment of choice is percutaneous balloon valvotomy, which has excellent results.

PULMONARY REGURGITATION

Isolated pulmonary regurgitation (PR) causes RV volume overload and can be tolerated for many years.

Aetiology

- Dilatation of valve ring (e.g. pulmonary hypertension)
- Dilatation of pulmonary artery (e.g. connective tissue disorders such as Marfan's syndrome)
- Infective endocarditis
- Congenital abnormalities (including post-operative Tetralogy of Fallot).
- Carcinoid syndrome.

Symptoms and signs

The usual symptoms relate to the development of right-heart failure. The hyperdynamic RV produces a palpable pulsation in the left parasternal area. Systolic and diastolic thrills can be felt in the 2nd left intercostal space from the pulmonary artery. If patients have pulmonary hypertension a tap can be felt reflecting pulmonary valve closure.

On auscultation P2 can be soft if there is congenital absence of the valve, but is loud and widely split where PR is caused by pulmonary hypertension. The PR murmur is a diastolic low-pitched murmur best heard in the left 3rd and 4th intercostal spaces and is louder during inspiration.

Investigations

ECG and CXR findings are non-specific. Echocardiography shows RV dilatation and hypertrophy is seen in the presence of pulmonary hypertension. Pulse-wave and colour Doppler imaging can detect PR as diastolic flow disturbance in the RV outflow tract (RVOT). The extent of the flow disturbance provides a semi-quantitative estimate of PR, as does the intensity and shape of the continuous-wave Doppler velocity–time spectral output. Holodiastolic flow reversal in the main pulmonary artery may be present with significant PR. Abnormalities of the RVOT are associated with ventricular tachycardia and a 24-hour tape may be useful.

Treatment

PR is not usually severe enough to need specific treatment though the underlying condition may need treatment. Digoxin is useful for treating failure or dilatation. Primary or secondary PR that causes intractable right-heart failure may need valve replacement with a bioprosthesis.

MITRAL VALVE DISEASE

MITRAL STENOSIS

In developed countries, the commonest cause of mitral stenosis (MS) is rheumatic fever. It is more common in women, and there is usually a latent period of 20–40 years before the development of symptoms, after which the disease follows a progressive course. Ten-year survival of asymptomatic patients is in excess of 50%, but in the face of significantly limiting symptoms 10-year survival is 0–15%.

Aetiology

- Rheumatic fever is almost always the cause of mitral stenosis though the history may be difficult to obtain.
- Congenital MS is rare and seen in infants and young children.
- Other rare causes include malignant carcinoid, systemic lupus erythematosus (SLE), rheumatoid arthritis and methysergide therapy.

Natural history and pathophysiology

Rheumatic fever causes leaflet thickening and calcification and causes fusion of the valve apparatus. This can be of the commissures, chordae, cusps or a combination of these. This distortion of the valve apparatus causes valve area to be reduced resulting in the characteristic 'fish mouth' appearance of the mitral valve (MV) seen on echocardiography.

Symptoms

Normal mitral valve area is 4–6 cm^2; symptoms usually begin when the valve area approaches 1.5 cm^2 and become severe once the valve area is less than 1 cm^2 (which is an indication for intervention). Symptoms often present when the heart is stressed by an event such as pregnancy, infection or the onset of atrial fibrillation (AF). Symptoms occur as a result of increased left atrial (LA) pressure and decreased cardiac output due to obstruction of LV filling. They are typically those of left-heart failure (although the LV function is usually normal) and include fatigue, exertional dyspnoea, orthopnoea and paroxysmal nocturnal dyspnoea (PND). Occasionally there may be hoarseness of voice (recurrent laryngeal nerve compression by an enlarged LA), haemoptysis and additional symptoms of right-heart failure, as it is the RV that bears the burden of maintaining forward flow of blood through the mitral valve. Other complications include systemic emboli, recurrent chest infection, oesophageal/bronchial compression by the enlarged LA and infective endocarditis, although the latter is rare in pure mitral stenosis.

Signs

There may or may not be AF; a malar flush and cachexia are late signs. S1 is characteristically loud (as the MV is held open by the high LA pressure until it snaps shut due to LV systole) and produces the 'tapping' apex beat. There is a loud opening snap (OS) and as mitral stenosis worsens, the OS becomes closer to S2; an S2 to OS gap of < 0.11 seconds indicates tight stenosis. There is a low-pitched mid-diastolic murmur that increases in duration as the stenosis becomes more severe; in sinus rhythm (SR) there is pre-systolic accentuation of the murmur. Signs of pulmonary hypertension (loud P2, Graham Steell murmur (PR), RV heave, elevated jugular venous pressure (JVP), ascites, and oedema) indicate advanced disease.

Investigations

The ECG may show signs of LA enlargement, AF, and right axis deviation or other signs of RV hypertrophy.

A CXR may confirm LA enlargement with upper lobe diversion as a result of the raised pulmonary venous pressure.

A 2-D echo shows restricted opening of the mitral valve leaflets with a domed anterior leaflet and an immobile posterior leaflet in diastole (Fig. 11.6). Mitral-valve area (MVA) can be assessed by direct planimetry on the 2-D images or from the pressure half time (P1/2t) equation (MVA = 220/P1/2t) using Doppler (Fig. 11.7). Valve morphology may be

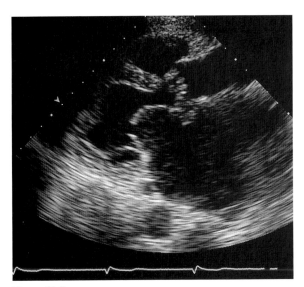

Figure 11.6
Parasternal long-axis 2-D echocardiographic view of the mitral valve showing doming of the valve leaflets in diastole and a large left atrium characteristic of rheumatic mitral stenosis

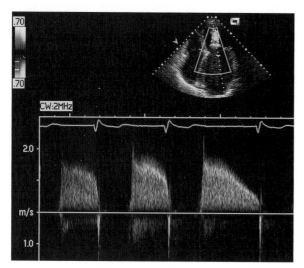

Figure 11.7
Apical four-chamber continuous-wave Doppler recording across a stenosed mitral valve in a patient with atrial fibrillation (AF). The pressure half time was calculated at 405 ms

better assessed by transoesophageal echo (TOE), which can give detailed information on the sub-valvular apparatus, the presence of thrombus in the LA or its appendage, and the degree of mitral regurgitation (MR). TOE is essential before attempting balloon valvotomy.

Cardiac catheterization (right and left) is advisable in patients in whom the symptoms and echocardiographic findings are discordant, who have other valve lesions (e.g. MR), angina (coronary angiography) or signs of severe pulmonary hypertension. There is a small subset of patients whose *resting* haemodynamics do not indicate the presence of moderate or severe disease but are symptomatic. However, the transmitral gradient is related to the square of the transvalvular flow rate, and exercise increases the flow and raises heart rate causing the diastolic filling time to reduce, both of which increase the LA pressure. In symptomatic patients a pulmonary artery pressure >60 mmHg, mean transmitral gradient >15 mmHg or a pulmonary artery wedge pressure (PAWP) ≥25 mmHg on *exertion* indicate haemodynamically significant mitral stenosis and should be considered for intervention.

Treatment

Medical

Anticoagulation is almost mandatory, especially if there is AF or an enlarged LA. Ventricular rate control (digoxin, beta-blockers, rate reducing calcium antagonists) is important, and can significantly improve symptoms. This is due to the fact that as the heart rate increases the amount of time available for LV filling in diastole decreases, which exacerbates the effect of the stenosis. Diuretics can provide symptomatic relief as they reduce preload and pulmonary venous congestion. The risk of endocarditis in MS is lower than that of MR, but antibiotic prophylaxis is still recommended.

Percutaneous and surgical intervention

Percutaneous balloon mitral valvotomy   Percutaneous commissurotomy became a feasible option in 1984 with the development of the Inoue balloon (Fig. 11.8). It is now considered the treatment of choice for pure symptomatic mitral stenosis. Numerous series have reported excellent long-term outcome with a low incidence of complications, with at least equivalent outcomes to that of open surgical valvotomy. An experienced operator is the key factor, in whose hands 80–95% of patients should have a successful procedure (defined as a post-procedure mitral valve area >1.5 cm^2 and a decrease in LA pressure to ≤18 mmHg) (Figs 11.9 & 11.10). There are a number of well-published selection criteria.[2]

Contraindications include:

- significant MR
- bilateral commissural calcification
- mobile thrombus, or thrombus in high-risk location (atrial septum, LA cavity, near the mitral valve orifice).

Relative contraindications include:

- unilateral commissural calcification
- thrombus confined to LA appendage.

Percutaneous balloon mitral valvotomy can be performed in any age group (best results are obtained in the young) and can also be considered in the elderly unsuitable for cardiac surgery as a palliative procedure even if the valve morphology is considered unsuitable. The procedure can also be performed in pregnancy (usually the 2nd trimester) to improve maternal haemodynamics, with data now from approximately 100 patients showing it is efficacious for both mother and foetus. Finally, repeat valvotomy for restenosis can be

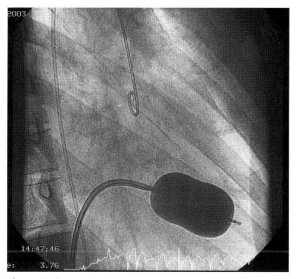

Figure 11.8
Percutaneous balloon mitral valvotomy, showing a 28 mm Inoue balloon inflated across the mitral valve

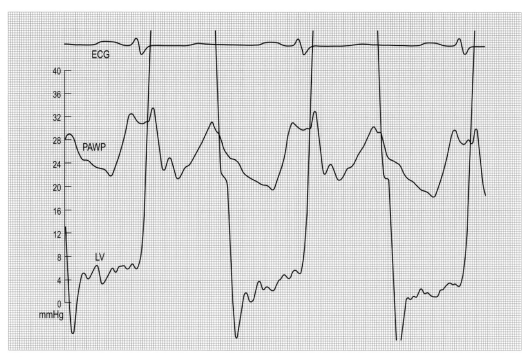

Figure 11.9
Left and right heart haemodynamic study in a patient with mitral stenosis. End diastolic trans-mitral gradient of 24 mmHg
LV, left-ventricular pressure; PAWP, pulmonary artery wedge pressure

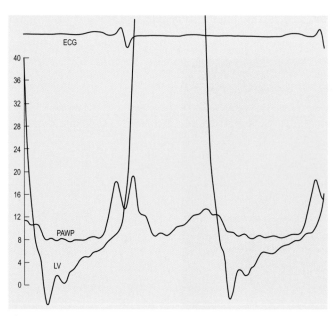

Figure 11.10
Left and right heart haemodynamic study in the same patient as Figure 11.9 following percutaneous balloon mitral valvotomy. The trans-mitral gradient has been reduced to <10 mmHg

performed (restenosis rates have been quoted at 40% at 7 years), but the results are often less satisfactory due to the increased valve deformity, fibrosis and calcification.

Open mitral valvotomy (commissurotomy)   Performed via a median sternotomy on cardiopulmonary bypass. It in used in patients who have had a previous closed valvotomy or in whom there are features of MR, calcification, thrombus or concern about the sub-valvular apparatus.

Mitral valve replacement   Performed in symptomatic patients with severe mitral stenosis unsuitable for valvotomy. In healthy young patients mitral valve replacement (MVR) has a risk of <5%, which increases to 10–20% in those with co-existent medical problems and pulmonary hypertension. For those patients with NYHA functional Class III symptoms, MVR results in excellent symptomatic improvement and surgery should not be delayed until progression to Class IV symptoms, as operative mortality is high and long-term outcome sub-optimal.

Patients who have had a successful procedure should have a baseline echo. Patients who have undergone percutaneous balloon valvotomy have a higher incidence of recurrent symptoms at 1–2 years if the initial morphology was unfavourable. Such patients need an annual echo and physical examination. Patients who have had MVR with a bioprosthesis are at increased risk of deterioration of the prosthesis after 5 years. Such patients need to be followed up with an annual echo.

MITRAL VALVE PROLAPSE

Mitral valve prolapse (MVP) has been quoted to occur in 2–6% of the population, but it is often overdiagnosed. Generally it carries a benign prognosis, and, although it can progress to significant MR, the age-adjusted survival rates are similar to normal individuals.[3]

Symptoms

Patients are usually entirely asymptomatic, often presenting as an incidental finding on auscultation. Risk of sudden death and endocarditis are low. Previously, MVP has been considered to be associated with embolic neurological events, although this association is now in doubt.

Signs

The principle auscultatory feature is a mid-systolic click (sudden tensing of the mitral apparatus as the leaflets prolapse into the LA in systole) with a late systolic murmur loudest at the apex. The click and the murmur occur later in systole (nearer S2) by manoeuvres that increase LV end-diastolic volume (e.g. squatting), reduce myocardial contractility or increase afterload.

Investigations

On 2-D echo, systolic displacement of one or both mitral leaflets >2 mm posterior to a line joining the annular hinge points in the parasternal long-axis view, and leaflet thickness >5 mm suggest MVP. Leaflet redundancy or an eccentric high-velocity jet of MR in late systole also suggests MVP. Serial echos are not usually necessary in the asymptomatic patient with MVP, unless there are clinical indications of worsening MR.

Medical treatment

Reassurance is usually all that is required, and, unfortunately, many patients are overdiagnosed as having MVP. For those with definite MVP, antibiotic prophylaxis is recommended for procedures associated with bacteraemia.

MITRAL REGURGITATION

Abnormalities of the mitral valvular apparatus and of the leaflets themselves can lead to mitral regurgitation (MR). 'Functional MR' occurs due to other causes such as annular dilatation or malalignment of the papillary muscles.

Aetiology

Causes due to the valve include:

- rheumatic heart disease
- endocarditis
- papillary muscle ischaemia or rupture
- MVR.

Functional causes include:

- dilated cardiomyopathy
- myocardial infarction – causes wall motion abnormalities affecting papillary muscle function.

Symptoms

Acute severe mitral regurgitation

Symptoms include acute dyspnoea, orthopnoea and PND due to pulmonary congestion. Patients may be symptomatically hypotensive as forward stoke volume and cardiac output are reduced.

Chronic mitral regurgitation

Patients are often entirely asymptomatic, even on exertion. The increase in LV end-diastolic volume permits an increase in total stroke volume and hence forward cardiac output. Increased preload and reduced/normal afterload (as the LV unloads into the LA) facilitates LV ejection. The gradual increase in LV and LA sizes allows accommodation of the regurgitant volume at a low filling pressure. This compensated phase of MR may last for many years before the burden of the volume overload results in LV dysfunction.

Signs

- Cardiac enlargement (displaced hyperdynamic apex).
- A pansystolic apical murmur that radiates to the axilla.
- A mid-diastolic murmur and apical S3 suggests MR is severe (rapid diastolic filling of the LV by the large volume of blood in the LA).

NB. In acute MR the LV has not had time to dilate and the apical impulse may be neither displaced nor hyperdynamic, the murmur is often less intense and may not be pansystolic.

Investigations

ECG and CXR confirm cardiac rhythm and size. The most important investigation is the echo, although it only gives a semi-quantitative estimate of severity, as the jet size seen on colour Doppler represents flow velocity rather than volume (Figs 11.11 & 11.12). Echocardiography also gives information on LV enlargement and any regional wall motion abnormality. Most importantly it gives detailed anatomical information about the mitral-valve leaflets and the sub-valvular apparatus. Echocardiography should be performed early to give baseline information, and if valve morphology and regurgitation severity are in question, TOE should be undertaken. For patients with mild or moderate MR, annual follow-up is usually sufficient. In severe MR (even if asymptomatic) follow-up is recommended 6 monthly (clinically and echocardiographically) to assess symptoms or transition to asymptomatic LV dysfunction.

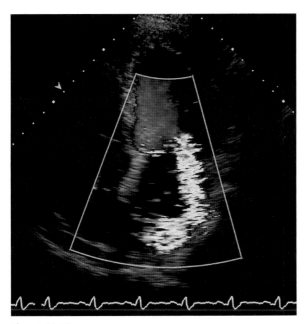

Figure 11.11
Colour Doppler image in the apical four-chamber view showing a broad jet of mitral regurgitation extending to the back wall of the left atrium

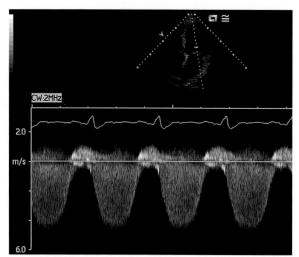

Figure 11.12
Continuous-wave Doppler recording of the mitral regurgitant jet seen in Figure 11.11

Right- and left-heart catheterization (with or without exercise) is necessary when there is a discrepancy between clinical and non-invasive findings. In patients with risk factors for CAD or in whom it is suspected that the MR is ischaemic in origin, coronary angiography should be performed. The size of the 'v' wave in the PAWP trace depends on the severity of MR and the size of the LA. In severe cases the 'v' wave might exceed 50 mmHg and increase sharply with effort (Fig. 11.13).

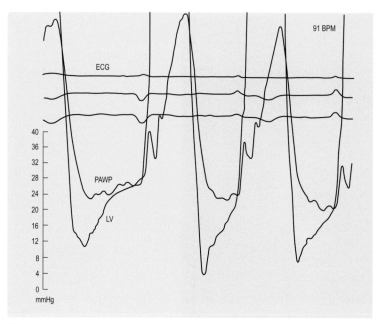

Figure 11.13
Left and right heart haemodynamic study in a patient with mitral regurgitation. Giant 'v' waves are present in the PAWP trace. (LV, left ventricular pressure; PAWP, pulmonary artery wedge pressure)

Treatment

Medical

There is no generally accepted medical therapy. Vasodilatation (ACE inhibitors) will increase cardiac output (CO) and decrease LV filling pressure in acute MR, but there is no apparent benefit to long-term use in chronic MR, especially in asymptomatic individuals. No study has shown that they reduce or delay the need for surgery or improve outcome. Diuretics and heart rate control (beta-blockers, digoxin, rate-slowing calcium antagonists) can be useful especially in AF. Anticoagulation should be implemented (INR 2–3) if AF develops or there is co-existent MS. Antibiotic prophylaxis is important, as the risk of endocarditis is greater than that of MS.

Surgical

MR progresses insidiously and can lead to irreversible LV dysfunction in the absence of significant symptoms. In MR the loading conditions are favourable to LV emptying (preload is increased and afterload is normal or low) which means that in the face of normal muscle function the ejection fraction should be super-normal. LV performance can be assessed from the diameter of the LV cavity at end systole, which is less dependent on preload than is ejection fraction. Patients should be referred for surgery if more than mild symptoms develop, once the end-systolic dimension exceeds 45 mm, or the ejection fraction falls towards 60% (even if asymptomatic) (Box 11.1). Following MVR the LV is prevented from emptying part of the stroke volume into the LA causing the afterload to increase, which actually causes a decrease in ejection fraction. Hence, the need for surgery before there is evidence of LV systolic dysfunction.

Mitral-valve repair has lower operative mortality, better functional results and fewer complications than MV replacement. It is the procedure of choice when the valve is suitable and surgical expertise available, as it avoids the potential for prosthetic valve failure and the need for anticoagulation if the patient is in sinus rhythm. The importance

---

Box 11.1: Major indications for surgery in non-ischaemic severe mitral regurgitation

Acute symptomatic mitral regurgitation (MR)

NYHA functional Class II, III, IV with normal left-ventricular (LV) function (ejection fraction >60% and end-systolic dimension <45 mm)

Symptomatic/asymptomatic with mild LV dysfunction, ejection fraction 50–60%, and/or end-systolic dimension 45–55 mm

Symptomatic/asymptomatic with moderate LV dysfunction, ejection fraction 30–50%, and/or end-systolic dimension 50–55 mm

Asymptomatic patients with preserved LV and AF

Asymptomatic patients with preserved LV and pulmonary hypertension (PHT) (pulmonary artery systolic >50 mmHg at rest or 60 mmHg with exercise)

Patients with severe LV dysfunction in whom chordal preservation is likely

Asymptomatic patients with chronic MR and preserved LV function in whom MV repair is likely

of the mitral-valve apparatus in maintaining LV function has only recently been appreciated, and attempts should be made to conserve the chordal structures and their connections in both MV repair and replacement. This has been shown to lead to better post-operative LV function and survival than in cases where the mitral apparatus is removed.

Repair is the preferred surgical technique in patients with:
- papillary muscle rupture due to ischaemia
- perforation of a leaflet due to endocarditis
- annular dilatation
- MR due to mitral valve prolapse.

TRICUSPID VALVE DISEASE

TRICUSPID STENOSIS

This is almost always rheumatic in origin, but other causes include congenital atresia, right atrial tumours, carcinoid syndrome, endocarditis and endomyocardial fibrosis. The morphological changes are similar to mitral stenosis (which usually co-exists), with shortening of the chordae and fusion at the commissures, although valvular calcification is rare. It is usually associated with a grossly enlarged right atrium (RA) and congestion of the liver and spleen.

Symptoms and signs

Symptoms are typically of a low cardiac output state, with lethargy and fatigue being prominent. Abdominal swelling due to organomegaly and ascites is common. Other physical signs include a prominent a-wave in the JVP (if in SR), and an opening snap and mid-diastolic murmur, which may be mistaken for mitral stenosis. The auscultatory findings are augmented by manoeuvres that increase tricuspid valve flow, such as inspiration, leg raising and squatting.

Investigation and treatment

The diagnosis is usually easily made by 2-D and Doppler echocardiography, and can be confirmed by right-heart catheterization. The management is essentially surgical, although diuretics may relieve symptoms. Surgical treatment (considered in patients in whom the mean diastolic pressure gradient exceeds 5 mmHg and the tricuspid orifice is <2 cm^2) includes open valvotomy or tricuspid valve replacement (TVR). A large porcine bioprosthesis is preferable to a mechanical valve due to its high risk of thrombosis and the increased durability of a bioprosthesis in this position compared to the mitral and aortic positions.

TRICUSPID REGURGITATION

The most common cause of tricuspid regurgitation (TR) is secondary to RV dilatation, i.e. functional regurgitation rather than as a result of an intrinsic valve lesion. This can occur secondary to any cause of pulmonary hypertension (e.g. chronic cardiac or pulmonary vascular disease), RV infarction, and congenital heart disease. In general, an RV systolic pressure greater than 55 mmHg will cause functional TR. Intrinsic valvular regurgitation may be secondary to rheumatic fever, endocarditis (intravenous drug abuse), congenital heart disease (e.g. Ebstein's anomaly), carcinoid syndrome, myxomatous degeneration, cardiac tumours and connective-tissue disorders (including Marfan's syndrome and SLE).

Symptoms and signs

Symptoms relate to a decreased cardiac output (e.g. weakness, fatigue) and also the discomfort associated with signs of right-heart failure (ascites, painful hepatomegaly and peripheral oedema). General examination usually reveals cachexia, cyanosis, jaundice, AF, elevated JVP (prominent systolic v wave), hyperdynamic RV impulse, enlarged pulsatile liver, oedema and ascites. Auscultation often reveals an S3 (from RV filling) and possibly a loud P2 if the TR is secondary to pulmonary hypertension. The murmur may occur only in the early part of systole in the absence of pulmonary hypertension or if the TR is mild, but is usually high-pitched, pansystolic and loudest parasternally in the 4th intercostal space. The murmur is augmented by inspiration (Carvallo sign), exercise, leg raising, hepatic compression and the Mueller manoeuvre. Increased diastolic forward flow across the valve may cause a short early diastolic flow rumble.

Investigation and treatment

Echocardiography is important to confirm the diagnosis of TR and to estimate its severity, assess pulmonary artery pressure and RV function. The RA and RV are usually dilated and there may be evidence of RV diastolic overload with paradoxical motion of the ventricular septum. 2-D echocardiography can give detailed anatomical information regarding the tricuspid annulus, valve leaflets and RV function. Doppler echocardiography will demonstrate reversed flow from the RV to the RA and sometimes flow reversal in the inferior vena cava and hepatic veins. The peak velocity of the TR flow is useful in the non-invasive estimation of RV and pulmonary artery systolic pressures.

In the absence of pulmonary hypertension the TR may be well tolerated and not require surgical treatment. In patients with severe MS and pulmonary hypertension causing TR, relief of the MS and reduction of the pulmonary artery pressure may result in a substantial reduction in TR. The need and timing of surgery is controversial. When performed, the preferred surgical treatment for acquired TR secondary to annular dilatation usually takes the form of tricuspid annuloplasty, with or without insertion of a prosthetic ring. When organic disease of the valve produces TR sufficient to require surgery, tricuspid valve replacement is usually performed. This is usually with a porcine bioprosthesis (rather than a mechanical valve due to the high thrombotic risk), the durability of which is often greater than 10 years.

ENDOCARDITIS

Infective endocarditis (IE) is a microbial infection of the cardiac endothelial surface. The valves are commonly the site of infection and show the characteristic lesion or 'vegetation', which is a mass of platelets and fibrin containing microorganisms and inflammatory cells. The disease can be acute, which progresses rapidly over days to weeks with valve destruction and metastatic infection. Subacute IE on the other hand progresses over weeks and months with only mild toxicity and does not usually cause metastatic infection. The left side of the heart is more commonly affected, although when IE is caused by intravenous drug abuse it tends to infect the right heart valves.

Prosthetic valve endocarditis is referred to as 'early' when the symptoms start within 60 days of surgery or 'late' when it occurs after 60 days. The pathophysiology of prosthetic valve endocarditis (PVE) differs from that of native endocarditis, as in PVE the infection may spread beyond the valve ring into the annulus and periannular tissue and causes ring abscesses, septal abscesses and dehiscence of the prosthesis.

Patients with endocarditis present with symptoms that include fever, chills, sweats, weight loss, anorexia and malaise. Signs seen are a raised temperature, new or a changing murmur, splenomegaly, embolic events, neurological signs and the peripheral signs of endocarditis. The diagnosis is made using the major and minor criteria from the modified Duke's criteria.[4] IE can present very insidiously and hence needs a high index of suspicion in order that the diagnosis is not missed.

Echocardiography can detect valve lesions and assess the severity of valvular/paravalvular involvement. It can concomitantly assess LV function and associated abnormalities such as intra-cardiac shunts. TOE is better suited to study PVE and can provide more information regarding associated abnormalities in complex endocarditis.

Almost 80% of cases of IE are caused by streptococci and staphylococci. In early PVE, staphylococci are the usual causative organism. Late PVE usually follows a similar pattern to native valve endocarditis. Antibiotic treatment in endocarditis is guided by identifying the causative organism, usually from blood cultures. Recommended antibiotic regimes are available for most common infective organisms and most involve approximately 6 weeks of therapy.[5] It is vital that adequate numbers of blood samples are sent for culturing, prior to starting empiric antibiotic therapy.

Patients who develop complications of endocarditis have a better prognosis when treated by a combination of surgery and antibiotic therapy. Surgery is indicated in:

- patients with significant haemodynamic decompensation with surgically treatable valve disease and reasonable chance of making a good recovery, and patients with acute AR or MR who develop heart failure
- fungal endocarditis
- development of root abscess
- infection which persists after prolonged antibiotic treatment and causes valve dysfunction
- recurrent emboli or large (>10 mm) vegetations.

Patients with PVE are recommended surgery in the setting of:

- early prosthetic endocarditis
- fungal endocarditis
- dysfunction of valve causing heart failure
- paravalvular leak, fistula formation, or root abscess
- failure of medical therapy.

Antibiotic treatment after surgery depends on the length of previous treatment, the causative organism's susceptibility, and the presence of organisms in the vegetation. If the culture of native valve operative specimens is negative the total duration of therapy before and after surgery should be at least equal to a full course of treatment. When culture of the operated specimen is positive a further full course of treatment is needed after surgery. All patients with PVE should also get a further full course of antibiotic treatment after surgery.

References

1. Bonow RO, Carabello B, de Leon AC et al. 1998 ACC/AHA practice guidelines. Guidelines for management of patients with valvular heart disease: executive summary. Circulation 98: 1949–1984
2. Prendergast BD, Shaw TR, Iung B, Vahanian A, Northridge DB 2002 Contemporary criteria for the selection of patients for percutaneous balloon mitral valvuloplasty. Heart 87: 501–504
3. Freed LA, Levy D, Levine RA et al. 1999 Prevalence and clinical outcome of mitral-valve prolapse. N Engl J Med 341: 1–7
4. Li JS, Sexton DJ, Mick N et al. 2000 Proposed modifications to the Duke criteria for the diagnosis of infective endocarditis. Clin Infect Dis 30: 633–638
5. Working Party of the British Society for Antimicrobial Chemotherapy 1998 Antibiotic treatment of streptococcal, enterococcal and staphylococcal endocarditis. Heart 79: 207–210

Further reading

Braunwald E, Zipes DP, Libby P (eds) 2001 Heart disease: a textbook of cardiovascular medicine, 6th edn. WB Saunders, London

Horstkotte D, Follath F, Gutschik E et al. 2004 Guidelines on prevention, diagnosis and treatment of infective endocarditis executive summary: the task force on infective endocarditis of the European Society of Cardiology. Eur Heart J 25(3): 267–276

Vlessis AA, Bolling SF (eds) 1999 Endocarditis: a multidisciplinary approach to modern treatment. Futura Publishing Company, Inc., New York.

Zoghbi WA (ed.) 1998 Cardiology clinics: valvular heart disease, vol. 16 (no.3). WB Saunders, Philadelphia

Chronic heart failure

12

Rakesh Sharma and P. Kalra

INTRODUCTION

Despite progress in treatment, chronic heart failure (CHF) is still associated with a high morbidity and mortality (prognosis is much worse than that of many common types of cancer). When considering treatment the majority of evidence relates to patients with left-ventricular (LV) systolic dysfunction. Diastolic dysfunction, although common, has, until recently, received much less attention. The management of cardiogenic shock is discussed in Chapter 10.

DEFINITIONS

Many terms are used in the description of patients with heart failure, and heart failure itself has received many definitions. A commonly encountered definition of heart failure is 'a pathophysiological state in which an abnormality of cardiac function is responsible for the failure of the heart to pump blood at a rate commensurate with the requirements of the metabolizing tissues'.

In general, definitions recommended by the European Society of Cardiology will be utilized in this chapter.

CHF (see Box 12.1) is the most common form, often punctuated by acute exacerbations. A broad definition is required since there is no simple objective cut-off value of cardiac dysfunction that reliably identifies all patients.

Box 12.1: Definition of chronic heart failure (European Society of Cardiology Guidelines)

Criteria 1 and 2 required in all cases:

1. Symptoms of heart failure (see Table 12.2)
2. Objective evidence of resting cardiac dysfunction and (in cases where diagnosis in doubt)
3. Response to treatment directed towards heart failure (e.g. diuretics)

Acute heart failure is better replaced with the most applicable of the following terms:

- Acute pulmonary oedema; or
- Cardiogenic shock – hypotension, oliguria, cool peripheries, clouded sensorium.

Other terms include:

- Systolic – many patients also demonstrate abnormalities of diastolic function (since ischaemic heart disease is the commonest aetiology in the UK).
- Diastolic – presumed to be present when symptoms and signs of heart failure are seen in the setting of preserved resting LV systolic function. The latter is more common in the elderly and in particular those with a prior history of hypertension.
- Myocardial stunning – post-ischaemic contractile dysfunction that persists following reperfusion, in the absence of irreversible damage and despite the restoration of normal/near-normal coronary blood flow. This is reversible.
- Hibernation – chronic stage of myocardial ischaemia, often not accompanied by pain and in which myocardial contractility and metabolism and thereby ventricular function are reduced to match the impaired blood supply (may actually be reduced coronary vasodilator reserve). Likely to be related to repeated episodes of stunning. The key point here is that the LV dysfunction is often reversible, at least in part, following revascularization.

PATHOPHYSIOLOGY

In CHF the severity of LV function does *not* closely relate to symptom severity and functional limitation; CHF is more than merely a disorder of the heart. In addition to significant co-morbidity such as hypertension, diabetes and chronic lung disease that is typical of many cardiology patients, these patients demonstrate additional metabolic, respiratory, renal, haematological and skeletal muscle abnormalities.

An understanding of the pathophysiology of CHF is essential to appreciating the mechanism of action of many of today's proven therapies. Following an insult to the myocardium activated neurohormonal mechanisms play an important role in the maintenance of circulatory homeostasis. They can be divided into the vasoconstrictive, sodium retaining and the opposing vasodilatory, natriuretic systems (Box 12.2). When circulatory integrity is threatened (e.g. acute myocardial infarction) vasoconstriction and sodium (and, therefore, water) retention act to maintain blood pressure and tissue perfusion. In contrast, prolonged activation of the systems involved has deleterious effects on haemodynamics and loading conditions in the failing ventricle (enhanced afterload). Direct adverse effects on the heart are also seen. For example, angiotensin II directly induces cardiac myocyte necrosis and together with aldosterone adversely affects myocardial matrix structure. Prolonged activation of the sympathetic nervous system has deleterious effects on myocardial remodelling and fibrosis and may provoke malignant ventricular arrhythmias. Large-scale clinical trials have provided a wealth of evidence supporting therapeutic manipulation of activated neurohormonal systems leading to the introduction of the majority of therapies currently available for CHF patients.

> **Box 12.2: Summary of the major neurohormonal systems involved in vascular regulation and sodium and water homeostasis in chronic heart failure patients**
>
> **Vasoconstriction and sodium retention**
> Renin–angiotensin–aldosterone system
> Sympathetic nervous system
> Non-osmotic release of vasopressin
> Endothelin-1
> Thromboxane
>
> **Vasodilatation and natriuresis**
> Atrial natriuretic peptide (ANP, primarily released from the atria)
> Brain natriuretic peptide (BNP, released from both the atria and ventricles)
> Nitric oxide
> Vasodilatory prostaglandins

Other abnormalities, such as inflammation and cytokine activation (e.g. tumour necrosis factor, interleukin-6) characteristically seen in advanced heart failure may play a role in disease progression and in particular non-intentional weight-loss, an adverse prognostic marker. This is an area of intense research, but as yet the benefit of immunomodulatory or anabolic therapies is not established.

DIAGNOSIS AND ASSESSMENT

The diagnosis of CHF is not always straightforward, particularly in the elderly in whom co-morbidity is common. Many patients with CHF are not diagnosed as such. Many patients are given an inappropriate diagnosis of CHF. For example, not all patients with swollen ankles have CHF and caution should be exercised in mis-diagnosing CHF when this is the only feature. There is no single diagnostic test for CHF; diagnosis is based upon careful clinical assessment (history and examination) complemented by appropriate investigations (see below). Heart failure should **not** be the final diagnosis. The underlying aetiology (Table 12.1) and presence of exacerbating factors should be sought. It is important to identify potentially reversible causes.

The major symptoms and signs exhibited by patients with CHF are highlighted in Table 12.2. Many features have a low predictive value alone, but when found as a constellation the diagnosis can be made with greater confidence. Objective evidence of LV dysfunction is still required. Documentation of symptomatic limitation is valuable, and most utilize the New York Heart Association (NYHA) classification (Box 12.3). It is important to recognize that there is a relatively poor relation between symptoms and severity of cardiac dysfunction. Other abnormalities such as skeletal muscle dysfunction may have greater impact on exercise capacity.

Many physical signs have low positive predictive value and are not specific to CHF, whilst others are difficult to illicit and have poor reproducibility in non-specialists. Despite these limitations clinical assessment should not be replaced by investigations, which should be

Table 12.1: Chronic heart failure aetiology

Aetiology	Comment
Coronary artery disease	Around 65% of cases of CHF in UK
Idiopathic	No obvious aetiology – 'diagnosis by exclusion'
Primary valvular disease	MR commonly found *secondary* to dilated annulus in patients with dilated LV In patients with ischaemic cardiomyopathy MR seen as a consequence of papillary muscle dysfunction
Hypertension	May also co-exist with CAD
Viral	Often difficult to confirm with viral titres, etc. – diagnosis made on basis of history, normal coronary angiogram and negative other tests
Alcohol	Often reversible with abstinence
Tachycardia mediated	Uncontrolled tachycardia, e.g. AF, potentially reversible
Metabolic	Hyperthyroidism – may be reversible Hypothyroidism Acromegaly Haemachromatosis Diabetic – possibly independent of CAD
Toxins	Chemotherapeutic agents: doxorubicin, adriamycin, 5-fluorouracil, etc. Cocaine
Infective	Sepsis – generally reversible Common in ITU patients with multi-system failure Bacterial endocarditis
Infiltration	Sarcoid Amyloid – failure of thickening of LV wall during systole, grainy echo-bright appearance of myocardium
Nutritional	Common in developing countries, e.g. beri-beri
Associated with other inherited conditions	e.g. Fabry's Muscular dystrophies
Peripartum	

AF, atrial fibrillation; CAD, coronary artery disease; MR, mitral regurgitation; LV, left ventricular

Box 12.3: New York Heart Association (NYHA) classification

Level of activity limited by symptoms

NYHA Class I: Asymptomatic with ordinary activity

NYHA Class II: Symptoms resulting in slight limitation of ordinary activity

NYHA Class III: Symptoms on minimal exertion, e.g. walking around house

NYHA Class IV: Inability to carry out any physical activity or symptoms at rest

Increasing symptomatic limitation is associated with poorer prognosis: 1-year mortality is around 50–60% for patients in NYHA Class IV, 15–30% for those in class II or III, and around 5% for patients in NYHA class I

Table 12.2: Symptoms and signs seen in patients with chronic heart failure

Symptoms	Comment
Exertional dyspnoea	Quantify by NYHA class
Orthopnoea	
Paroxysmal nocturnal dyspnoea	
Swollen ankles	Not specific – caution should be exercised in misdiagnosing CHF when this is the only feature
Lethargy	Often ignored
Muscle fatigue and exhaustion	Often ignored
Weight loss and muscle wasting	Poor prognostic feature
Dizziness	May relate to postural hypotension
Depression	Common and multifactorial
Signs	
General appearance, e.g. well or unwell?	Simple, but exceedingly important
Tachycardia	Non-specific Influenced by beta-blockers
Blood pressure	Low blood pressure and poor tissue perfusion in severe CHF
Peripheral oedema	Low positive predictive value In hospitalized or immobile patients do not forget sacral oedema
Hepatomegaly	Low positive predictive value
Jugular venous pressure	High predictive value but poor reproducibility between observers May still have severe CHF despite non-elevated JVP
Third heart sound	Present in more severe CHF Poor interobserver agreement
Pulmonary crepitations	Low positive predictive value
Apex beat	Displaced Character may be helpful, but again difficult to illicit
Murmurs	May be the cause, e.g. aortic stenosis, mitral and aortic regurgitation, or effect of heart failure, e.g. functional mitral regurgitation

Additional features may provide clues as to the underlying aetiology, e.g. angina, evidence of significant valvular disease

CHF, chronic heart failure; JVP, jugular venous pressure

considered as complementary. Physical signs will vary according to intensity of treatment and may of course change throughout the disease course.

INVESTIGATIONS

Investigations are directed towards:

- confirming the diagnosis of heart failure
- determining aetiology

- assessing prognosis
- identifying exacerbating factors.

All patients with suspected CHF should undergo a series of essential investigations (Table 12.3). The nature and extent of further investigations will be influenced by the age and general well-being of the patient and local facilities. Echocardiography is the main tool available in the UK for assessing cardiac structure and function. In many places echocardiography remains an under-resourced service, and is not freely available (particularly in primary care). Utilizing other tests to 'rule out' CHF first may reduce the burden on echo services. For example, patients with a completely normal ECG or normal concentration of brain natriuretic peptide (BNP or NT-BNP, see later) measured prior to initiation of treatment have an extremely low likelihood of CHF. Echo can, therefore, be reserved for patients who demonstrate an abnormality on either of these tests.

Since coronary artery disease (CAD) is the single most common aetiology of CHF within the UK, it is the authors' belief that coronary angiography should be considered (dictated by local resources) unless significant co-morbidity precludes consideration for revascularization or the disease is considered end-stage. The findings may have important implications not just with respect to revascularization (see Hibernation) but also to secondary prevention with drugs such as aspirin and statins. As yet no data exist to support such secondary prevention in patients with CHF without CAD. The presence and severity of underlying coronary artery disease is often underestimated in patients with CHF without the benefit of investigations such as angiography or myocardial perfusion imaging.

TREATMENT

GENERAL PRINCIPLES

Treatment should be tailored to improving quality of life as well as enhancing life expectancy. The relative importance of these aims will be decided on an individual patient basis and may change over time in the same patient. In some, palliative care will be the most appropriate therapeutic strategy and this should be discussed openly with all involved including the patient and carers.

Education of patients and their carers cannot be over emphasized, leading to more active roles in decision making and improving compliance. Monitoring of simple parameters such as weight can help identify early signs of decompensation; a compensatory increase in diuretic dose may break the spiral of decline and prevent hospitalization. Heart failure specialist nurses have an important role in education and monitoring of patients, particularly in the early stages following discharge when readmission rates are high (around 20% at 12 weeks). Patients with labile condition (e.g. recurrent decompensation) or significant co-morbidity (e.g. renal dysfunction) need particularly vigilant follow-up.

Much evidence for pharmacological interventions is derived from large randomized placebo-controlled trials. However, there are few direct comparisons between classes of

Table 12.3: Investigations for patients with suspected heart failure

Essential for all patients	Comment
ECG	A normal ECG is rare in heart failure – rhythm (e.g. AF) – LBBB – LVH – previous MI (e.g. Q waves) – prolongation of QRS duration – related to prognosis, severely symptomatic patients may benefit from resynchronization therapy
Chest X-ray	Poor relationship between CTR and LV function Exclude lung pathology Normal CTR – question the diagnosis
Blood tests	
Full blood count	Anaemia is an adverse prognosticator in established heart failure Correction (see text) may improve symptoms
Biochemical profile	Low sodium and renal dysfunction reflect a poorer prognosis
Liver function tests	Abnormalities may reflect hepatic congestion or provide clues to aetiology
Lipids	
Fasting glucose	
Thyroid function tests	Potentially reversible aetiology
Urinalysis	
Peak flow assessment	
Ideally for all patients	
BNP or NT-BNP	When normal has a high negative predictive value Powerful prognostic indicator May be useful in tailoring of therapy (see text)
Echocardiography	Non-invasive Routinely used for optimal diagnosis Valvular disease (primary or secondary) Chamber dimensions LVH Difficult to accurately quantify ejection fraction Physiological parameters may be measured
Additional tests	Determined on an individual basis
Cardiac catheterization	To assess burden of underlying CAD Concomitant right heart catheter may provide useful additional physiological data
Cardiopulmonary exercise testing	See Chapter 4 Desirable but not widely available Diagnostic and prognostic data Objective measure to assess change over time
Holter monitoring	Identification of symptomatic or asymptomatic arrhythmias
Other imaging	When poor image on echo, e.g. MRI, radionuclide angiography
Blood tests	Individual basis, e.g. ferritin, autoimmune profile, genetic studies
24-hour urine	Creatinine clearance (many patients will have low muscle bulk and serum creatinine may underestimate the degree of renal impairment)

AF, atrial fibrillation; CAD, coronary artery disease; CTR, cardiothoracic ratio; ECG, electrocardiogram; LBBB, left bundle branch block; LVH, left ventricular hypertrophy; MI, myocardial infarction; MRI, magnetic resonance imaging

drugs and most recommendations for lifestyle measures are derived from consensus opinion. The elderly (see below) and females have been dramatically underrepresented in most clinical studies, but on the whole clinical recommendations are the same. In women of child-bearing age discussion on risks of pregnancy (see Chapter 16) and potential teratogenic effect of drugs need careful consideration.

LIFESTYLE ADVICE

Applicable to all patients with CHF.

Smoking

Advice to stop smoking, particularly in those with CAD.

Alcohol

Abstinence if likely primary aetiology – may result in improvement or even complete recovery. Otherwise moderation (volume, pro-arrhythmogenic).

Fluids and salt

More important in advanced CHF – reduce salt intake and fluid restrict in most severe cases (around 1.5–2.0 l per day).

Vaccination

Vaccination against influenza and pneumococcus recommended for most patients.

Exercise training

Skeletal muscle deconditioning has an adverse effect on symptom limitation in CHF. Exercise training (aerobic and resistive) should be encouraged in all stable patients and may result in improved exercise capacity. Rehabilitation programmes offer integration of education, general support to carers and tailored exercise regimens but unfortunately are not yet freely available to CHF patients within the UK.

Driving regulations

It is important to maintain knowledge of updates and this can be obtained from www.dvla.gov.uk.

PHARMACOLOGY

Diuretics

Thiazides and loop diuretics

Why? Fluid retention is an important aspect of untreated heart failure. Since diuretics have been in routine use prior to the current era of mega trials there is less evidence for benefit on outcome, although meta-analyses suggest that this might be the case.

Who?   Diuretics are helpful for symptom relief in all stages of CHF. They should be used in combination with other proven therapies, namely ACE inhibitors and beta-blockers, since on their own may enhance neurohormonal activation.

Which diuretic?   Loop diuretics (e.g. furosemide or bumetanide) form the mainstay of therapy. The dose should be titrated according to the clinical status of the patient. Thiazides are generally used as singe agent in only the mildest cases, and are not effective as single agent when glomerular filtration rate is <30 ml/min. In more advanced CHF the addition of a thiazide (e.g. bendrofluazide 2.5 mg od) to a loop diuretic may result in a synergistic effect. Potassium level should be monitored accordingly.

Comments   In patients with labile CHF careful titration of diuretic dose may be required depending on fluid status and renal function. Informed patients may do this themselves (e.g. dictated by daily weights), but ideally via liaison with a specialist heart failure nurse.

During decompensation gut oedema may reduce absorption of tablets and thereby contribute to the downward clinical spiral. Whilst much higher doses of diuretics may break this cycle careful monitoring of renal function is required. Often the only acceptable and successful strategy is admission for intravenous therapy (or outpatient if facilities exist). The addition of metolazone can help in severe, resistant CHF but may result in large, rapid fluid shifts and the precipitation of worsening renal failure. It is the authors' belief that metolazone should not be prescribed *regularly* unless under specialist supervision with careful monitoring of electrolytes (unless for palliative care).

Spironolactone

Why?   Antagonism of aldosterone with spironolactone has beneficial effects on mortality (30% reduction) and morbidity (35% reduction in hospitalization, improved NYHA Class) in patients with severe CHF.

Who?   Severe heart failure – NYHA Class III or IV. Serum creatinine <221 µmol/l. On concomitant therapy with ACE inhibitor and loop diuretic (evidence pre-large scale beta-blocker use).

Dose?   Start at 25 mg od. Increase to 50 mg od if ongoing evidence of fluid retention. Halve to 12.5 mg od if hyperkalaemia develops.

Comments   Monitor creatinine and electrolytes. No significant problem with hyperkalaemia in major trial. Ten per cent gynaecomastia or breast pain in males, however, in general well tolerated.

ACE inhibitors

Why?   Angiotensin II is a powerful vasoconstrictor with adverse effects on myocardial remodelling, myocyte hypertrophy and matrix structure. ACE inhibitors improve mortality in patients with CHF. They also improve symptoms and reduce hospitalizations in patients with CHF and asymptomatic left-ventricular dysfunction.

Who? All patients with CHF due to LV systolic dysfunction. Patients with more severe heart failure derive even greater benefit. Concomitant use of NSAIDs should be avoided.

Dose? Initiation should be with low dose. Longer acting drugs may enhance compliance. A test dose is not required. The dose should be titrated up to that used in the major clinical trials or the manufacturers' or regulatory recommendations wherever possible (e.g. captopril 25–50 mg three times daily (tid), enalapril 10 mg bid, lisinopril 5–20 mg od, perindopril 4 mg od, ramipril 2.5–5 mg bid). However, low dose is considerably better than not receiving the drug.

Comments Renal function should be measured before starting an ACE inhibitor. It should be checked after 1–2 weeks and periodically thereafter. A small increase in creatinine is often seen (see Chapter 21), but this should not preclude continuation of therapy. It is particularly important to assess renal function if patients if become unwell from other causes resulting in fluid depletion, e.g. diarrhoea.

ACE inhibitors are often withdrawn as a consequence of dry cough. It is essential to confirm that this is secondary to the drug and not as a consequence of heart failure itself. In patients truly intolerant of ACE inhibitors or angiotensin receptor blockers, the vasodilator combination of isosorbide and hydralazine has been shown to improve outcome when compared to placebo. This combination is not as effective as ACE inhibitors.

Angiotensin-II receptor blockers (ARB)

Whilst current evidence does not support ARBs to be superior to ACE inhibitors, ARBs are better tolerated with reduced likelihood of discontinuation. The addition of valsartan to an ACE inhibitor and diuretic (VALHEFT) reduced hospitalizations secondary to worsening heart failure, without benefit on mortality. Post hoc analysis, however, suggested that the combination (small numbers of subjects) of ACE inhibitor, beta-blocker and ARB was actually detrimental to outcome. The recently published CHARM study had three arms and has added clarification to this important clinical question. Candesartan (target dose 32 mg daily) reduced cardiovascular morbidity and mortality in patients with symptomatic CHF and intolerance to ACE inhibitors (CHARM-alternative trial). The addition of candesartan to ACE inhibitor and conventional therapy (55% on beta-blockers) significantly reduced the composite primary outcome of cardiovascular death or hospital admission for CHF (CHARM-added trial). The use of candesartan in patients with CHF and preserved ejection fraction (>40%) did not result in improved mortality, but did result in preventing hospitalization for heart failure.

In summary, as an alternative to ACE inhibitors, ARBs should be reserved for patients who are truly intolerant of ACE inhibitors (approximately 15–20% generally secondary to cough). The addition of an ARB can be considered for symptomatic CHF patients already taking conventional therapy (few data available for patients also on spironolactone). Careful monitoring of renal function is advisable.

Beta-blockers

Why?   Beta-blockers antagonize detrimental effects of chronic catecholamine excess. There are beneficial effects on myocardial remodelling, myocyte hypertrophy, myocardial matrix and arrhythmias.

Who?   Beta-blockers confer mortality benefit and a reduction in hospitalizations in all classes of CHF. They have consistently been shown to reduce mortality by around 30% when added to patients receiving ACE inhibitors. They should be used in combination with diuretics and ACE inhibitors wherever possible. They should not be initiated during an episode of decompensation, where patients are receiving intravenous therapy. They can, however, be cautiously introduced early after stabilization (pre-discharge). They should be avoided in patients with high-degree heart block (unless paced) or severe reversible airways disease.

Dose   Two drugs are currently licensed for CHF in the UK: carvedilol (additional anti-oxidant and alpha-blocking properties) and bisoprolol. Initiation should be at low dose: 3.125 mg bid and 1.25 mg od, respectively. The dose should gradually be titrated towards target (bisoprolol 10 mg and carvedilol 50 mg per day).

Comment   Some patients exhibit a biphasic response with intial mild deterioration in symptoms followed by gradual improvement. It may be necessary to adjust diuretic dose accordingly. If patients deteriorate whilst on beta-blockers it is the authors' opinion that, wherever possible, treatment should be continued (clearly not in cardiogenic shock), although a temporary reduction in dose may occasionally be required.

Digoxin

This has negative chronotropic and weak positive inotropic effects. It may help to control ventricular rates in patients in atrial fibrillation, but its use should not preclude that of a beta-blocker. Digoxin does not seem to have a positive mortality benefit on CHF patients in sinus rhythm (in keeping with studies of other chronically administered positive inotropes). It has, however, been shown to reduce hospital admissions in patients with severe symptomatic heart failure despite full conventional therapy. It is usually prescribed at low dose (adjusted according to age and renal function).

Others

Calcium channel blockers

These are not routinely prescribed and may worsen CHF (short-acting dihydropyridines, verapamil, diltiazem). Long-acting dihydropyridines, e.g. amlodipine, can be used to treat concomitant hypertension and angina if required.

Aspirin

No specific evidence for benefit in patients with heart failure, without atherosclerotic disease. There is some concern that aspirin may reduce efficacy of ACE inhibitors. Aspirin is generally recommended for those CHF patients with CAD (or peripheral vascular disease).

Warfarin

> This treatment benefits CHF patients with atrial fibrillation. The general belief is that CHF patients in sinus rhythm with left-ventricular aneurysm or thrombus, or those with prior history of thromboembolic disease may benefit from long-term anticoagulation. Each patient should be considered on an individual basis since there are no randomized controlled studies.

Statins

> Patients with CHF and documented atherosclerotic disease should receive statins as indicated for persons without heart failure until further evidence is available (see Chapter 3). A prospective study is underway to evaluate the benefit of statins in patients with CHF not secondary to CAD.

Summary of drug management

> It is essential to increase compliance with drug regimens; education and simple dosing schedules (avoid tid prescriptions if possible) are paramount towards achieving this (Table 12.4). Most patients require a diuretic, and all patients with CHF secondary to LV systolic dysfunction will benefit from long-term ACE inhibitors and beta-blockers at the maximum tolerated dose. As ACE inhibitor dose is up titrated it is often possible to reduce diuretic dose.

> ACE inhibitors and beta-blockers remain under-prescribed in CHF. Beta-blockers were previously (erroneously) considered to be contraindicated in CHF. This belief will gradually change as experience in their use in this setting increases, allaying many unfounded fears. They should **not** be initiated during an acute episode of decompensation. Concerns exist over first dose hypotension with ACE inhibitors and potential adverse effects on renal function. The use of longer-acting agents, gradual titration and sensible monitoring can minimize these risks. Whilst all therapeutic interventions can be

Table 12.4: Pharmacological management of chronic heart failure – a summary

	Diuretic	ACE inhibitor	Beta-blocker	Spironolactone	Digoxin (in sinus rhythm)
Asymptomatic LV dysfunction	Not indicated	Indicated	Indicated post-MI	Not indicated	Not indicated
NYHA II	Indicated (loop or thiazide)	Indicated	Indicated	Not indicated	Not indicated
NYHA III–IV	Indicated (loop)	Indicated	Indicated	Indicated	May reduce hospitalization
End-stage CHF (NYHA IV)	Indicated (loop)	Indicated	Indicated	Indicated	May reduce hospitalization

CHF, chronic heart failure; LV, left ventricular; MI, myocardial infarction; NYHA, New York Heart Association

associated with adverse effects, it is important to place these in context of the proven benefits on mortality and quality of life; denying patients these therapies is more often likely to do more harm than good. The choice of ACE inhibitor and beta-blocker should be limited to those proven to be of benefit and licensed for use in CHF. Familiarity with the initiation and subsequent titration of a particular agent will add to the confidence of prescribing.

DIASTOLIC DYSFUNCTION

Whilst this is relatively common, there is little evidence regarding beneficial therapies. Diuretic therapy at low dose (try to avoid excessive lowering of preload) when there is evidence of fluid retention and aggressive treatment directed towards associated pathology, such as hypertension, is generally recommended. Beta-blockers, by lowering heart rate and increasing diastole, may be beneficial.

DEVICES

The indication for an implantable cardioverter defibrillator (ICD) in patients with CHF is rapidly expanding. ICDs and newer therapeutic device strategies aimed at electromechanical resynchronization (biventricular pacing) are discussed in Chapter 14.

SEQUELAE OF CHRONIC HEART FAILURE

- Renal impairment
- Anaemia
- Arrhythmia, e.g. atrial fibrillation, ventricular tachycardia
- Functional mitral regurgitation – secondary to dilation of mitral-valve annulus
- Embolic phenomena – secondary to atrial fibrillation or LV thrombus
- Weight loss and development of cachexia – poor prognostic feature.

CHF, anaemia and chronic kidney disease are intimately related, with each adversely affecting the other. Anaemia is an adverse prognostic indicator in CHF and contributes to limitation of functional capacity. There is much interest in correcting anaemia with a combination of erythropoietin and iron. Whilst prospective, large-scale studies are awaited intervention can be considered in those patients resistant to conventional neurohormonal antagonism who also have low haemoglobin levels.

HIBERNATION AND REVASCULARIZATION

Ischaemic heart disease is the principle cause of CHF in the Western world. Several small studies have demonstrated that revascularization can improve LV function and may confer symptomatic and even prognostic benefit. Whilst the mechanisms of hibernation remain poorly understood, several imaging techniques can be used to identify hibernating myocardium with reasonable specificity and sensitivity (myocardial perfusion imaging p. 58, stress echo p. 52, MRI p. 64 and PET p. 61). The choice of technique will depend upon local availability and expertise.

Current practice in the UK tends to target patients with ongoing ischaemic symptoms or severely limiting heart failure symptoms despite full conventional therapy. The potential degree of improvement in LV function is higher when 50% of the dysfunctional myocardium is deemed viable and amenable to revascularization. Whether a larger number of patients with milder symptoms may benefit from aggressive revascularization is unknown. HEART-UK is an ongoing randomized study comparing optimum medical therapy with or without complete revascularization. Whilst recruitment has been relatively slow, it is hoped that the results may provide clearer guidance on the management of many CHF patients.

CARDIAC TRANSPLANTATION

Currently in the UK approximately 200 cardiac transplants are performed each year in six adult transplant centres. The main limiting factor is donor scarcity. A rigorous selection process, to ensure that potentially reversible causes of ventricular dysfunction are corrected and specific contraindications are excluded, has contributed to the 80% 1-year and 70% 5-year survival rates now seen in transplanted patients. Orthotopic cardiac transplantation is generally performed; heterotopic operations, where the native heart is not removed, are now performed infrequently.

INDICATIONS AND CONTRAINDICATIONS

It is essential that close and early liaison with the local transplant centre occurs, since most candidates are considered on an individual basis (Box 12.4). An objective assessment of the severity of heart failure that involves evaluation of both cardiac function and symptom limitation is required. Selection based solely on ejection fraction is inadequate as it relates poorly to prognosis in this group of patients. Maximal exercise testing is a powerful discriminatory tool and should be performed whenever possible (see Chapter 4).

Box 12.4: Summary of major indications and contraindications for cardiac transplantation

Major indications

Advanced heart failure refractory to medical or conventional surgical management
Peak VO_2 < 14 ml/kg/min (provided the anaerobic threshold is achieved)
Patients dependent on inotropic agents (provided other organ function remains adequate)

Rarer indications

Severe ischaemia not amenable to revascularization.
Refractory life-threatening arrhythmias.

> **Box 12.4: (Cont'd) Summary of major indications and contraindications for cardiac transplantation**
>
> **Contraindications**
> Age >65 years
> *Irreversible* pulmonary hypertension (e.g. PVR > 4 Wood units) associated with particularly high perioperative risk
> Creatinine clearance of <50 ml/min (or <30 ml/min/m^2)
> Non-cardiac life-threatening disease
> Severe adverse psychosocial factors likely to prevent intensive follow-up protocol
>
> VO$_2$ = peak oxygen consumption
> PVR = pulmonary vascular resistance

POST-TRANSPLANT MANAGEMENT

Patients require life-long immunosuppression after transplantation. Most current regimens include ciclosporin, mycophenolate mofetil and prednisolone (the dose of the latter is gradually reduced and stopped). Acute rejection is an important cause of morbidity and occasional mortality and active surveillance with frequent endomyocardial biopsies is essential.

Immunosuppression is associated with complications:

- Renal impairment is frequent in patients on long-term ciclosporin therapy.
- Infections are a major cause of death post-transplantation and should be treated aggressively. Early infections (<1 month) tend to be bacterial (indwelling catheters and drains); from 1 to 6 months the risk is from opportunistic organisms, e.g. cytomegalovirus (CMV), pneumocystis, fungi; thereafter, community-acquired infections are the problem, often being more severe as a consequence of immunosuppression.
- Increased risk of neoplastic disorders, particularly of the lymphoid system and skin.
- Coronary artery disease (often diffuse and asymptomatic) in the transplanted heart (cardiac allograft vasculopathy (CAV)) occurs in 20–50% of patients at 5 years. CAV is an important cause of late allograft failure, and has a multifactorial aetiology. Conventional risk factors should be aggressively managed. Pravastatin is usually the cholesterol-lowering agent of choice as the incidence of severe adverse effects in transplanted patients (e.g. rhabdomyolysis) is less than that of other statins.

VENTRICULAR ASSIST DEVICES

Ventricular assist devices were initially developed to support patients in cardiogenic shock post cardiac surgery who were unable to be weaned from cardiopulmonary bypass. In a subgroup of patients with severe or rapidly deteriorating heart failure, circulatory support with a ventricular assist device may be required to maintain haemodynamic stability whilst on the transplant waiting list. In patients in whom cardiac transplantation is contraindicated because of a potentially reversible cause, such as renal impairment secondary to severe heart failure, a ventricular assist device may allow time for rehabilitation of the patient prior to listing. A recent study (REMATCH) demonstrated that the use of a LV assist device in patients with advanced heart failure, who were not candidates for transplantation, was associated with improved survival and quality of life at the expense of increased bleeding and infective complications. For LV assist devices, blood is pumped from either the left atrium or apex of the LV and returned to the ascending aorta. In right-ventricular assist devices, the blood is routed from the right atrium to the main pulmonary artery.

Early liaison with the local transplant centre is again recommended. With improved device technology and prospects of reduced bleeding and infective complications it is hoped that devices may become a long-term therapy and provide an alternative to transplantation, and even as a 'bridge to recovery' in certain cases of dilated cardiomyopathy.

Further reading

Cleland JGF, Swedberg K, Follath F et al. 2003 The EuroHeart Failure Survey programme - a survey on the quality of care among patients with heart failure in Europe Part 1: patient characteristics and diagnosis. Eur Heart J 24: 442–463

Remme WJ, Swedberg K, Task force for the diagnosis and treatment of chronic heart failure, European Society of Cardiology 2001 Guidelines for the diagnosis and treatment of chronic heart failure. Eur Heart J 22: 1527–1560

Rose EA, Gelijns AC, Moskowitz AJ et al. 2001 Randomized Evaluation of Mechanical Assistance for the Treatment of Congestive Heart Failure (REMATCH) Study Group. Long-term mechanical left ventricular assistance for end-stage heart failure. N Engl J Med 345: 1435–1443

SELF-ASSESSMENT

Questions
a. Which patients have an adverse prognosis and how can they be identified?
b. Is management the same in the elderly?
c. What should I do at clinical review?
d. Who should be referred for specialist advice?

Answers
a. It is important to readily identify patients with a particularly poor prognosis who may benefit from intensive treatment and follow-up. Mortality rates are high following admission to hospital with decompensated CHF (around 50% at 1 year) and this category of patient merits careful assessment. Cardiopulmonary exercise testing and plasma BNP concentrations are powerful prognostic indicators in CHF, but are not widely available in clinical use in the UK. Routine assessments available to all practitioners can provide useful data relating to severity of heart failure and prognosis:
   • NYHA Class (documented at each visit)
   • serum sodium and creatinine
   • plasma haemoglobin
   • QRS duration on ECG
   • body mass index.
b. Many studies have included patients with a mean age that is much lower than that seen in clinical practice. Significant co-morbidity, common in the elderly, is generally an exclusion criteria from randomized studies. Despite this, it is generally accepted that the therapeutic approach to systolic dysfunction in the elderly should be similar to that in younger CHF patients, whilst appreciating that tolerance of higher doses of drugs may be poorer and side-effects more common. Careful monitoring is vital and particular attention should be directed towards measures that may improve compliance. Similar principles apply to the elderly CHF patient as apply to older patients in general. The principle of 'start low and go slow' is of help when initiating ACE inhibitors and beta-blockers.
c. Patients with CHF are often under follow-up by several health-care professionals in primary and secondary care; communication between all involved is essential. The following would constitute the minimum assessment:
   • Functional capacity – NYHA class
   • Fluid status – examination (peripheral oedema, jugular venous pressure, lung crepitations), weight (including patient records), blood pressure (lying and standing), pulse rate and rhythm
   • Blood tests – biochemistry essential (other tests on individual basis, e.g. TFTs, haemoglobin). There is considerable interest in the use of BNP levels to monitor therapy or even titrate it (increase medication to reduce BNP levels towards normal range). More data are required before this becomes a clinical reality in the UK.
   • Review medication, doses and schedules, and side-effects. Discuss compliance and methods to increase it (e.g. flexible timing of diuretic).

- Serial echoes or chest X-rays are not usually required unless there is a marked change in the patient's clinical condition.

  The patient and carers should be encouraged to actively participate in their own management. In selected cases this may include monitoring of weight and titration of diuretics to maintain targets. A point of contact should be established whereby the patient can contact a health-care professional (ideally, heart-failure specialist nurse) if they have concerns or queries, and this might be effective in 'nipping symptomatic decline in the bud'.

d. This will be dictated by local facilities and expertise, but should include the following groups:
   - adverse prognosis (see above)
   - heart failure secondary to valvular disease
   - concomitant angina
   - other severe co-morbidity (particularly renal dysfunction)
   - hypotension pre-treatment
   - severe heart failure despite conventional therapies
   - young patients who are likely to require further detailed investigation.

Cardiomyopathies

13

P. Elliott and Rajesh Thaman

INTRODUCTION

Cardiomyopathies are diseases of the myocardium leading to cardiac dysfunction in the absence of pericardial, hypertensive, congenital, ischaemic or valvular diseases. The cardiomyopathies are classified into four types according to the predominant pathophysiological characteristics:

1. Dilated cardiomyopathy
2. Hypertrophic cardiomyopathy
3. Arrhythmogenic right-ventricular cardiomyopathy
4. Restrictive cardiomyopathy.

DILATED CARDIOMYOPATHY

DEFINITION

Dilated cardiomyopathy (DCM) is characterized by ventricular chamber dilatation, normal or reduced wall thickness and reduced systolic function of the left or both ventricles. The diagnosis excludes heart failure caused by coronary artery disease, hypertension, congenital, anatomical abnormalities, valvular or pericardial disease, acute myocarditis or arrhythmia.

PREVALENCE

DCM has an estimated prevalence of 30–40 cases per 100 000 and usually presents in the 4th to 5th decades, but can occur in childhood or old age. DCM is commoner in men than women and is 2.5 times commoner in blacks than whites.

AETIOLOGY

Many disease processes can ultimately lead to dilatation and reduced systolic function (Box 13.1). In most cases, however, the cause is unknown – idiopathic dilated

Box 13.1: Causes of DCM

Toxins
Alcohol
Drugs, e.g. anthracyclines, adriamycin, doxorubicin, bleomycin, zidovudine, didanosine, cocaine/amphetamines
Irradiation
Heavy metals, e.g. cobalt

Infections
Viral, e.g. Coxsackie B, echovirus, adenovirus, influenza, cytomegalovirus, Varicella zoster, HIV
Bacterial, e.g. diphtheria
Mycobacteria
Fungal
Parasitic, e.g. schistosomiasis, trichinosis, toxoplasmosis, *Trypanosoma cruzi*
Rickettsial, e.g. leptospirosis
Spirochaetal

Inflammatory
Connective tissue disorders
Sarcoidosis
Systemic lupus erythematosus
Scleroderma
Churg–Strauss

Metabolic and nutritional
Endocrine, e.g. thyrotoxicosis, acromegaly, Cushing's syndrome, phaeochromocytoma, haemochromatosis, diabetes mellitus
Deficiencies of thiamine, carnitine, and selenium

Others
Hypertensive heart disease
Sickle cell and chronic anaemias
Incessant tachyarrhythmia
Peripartum cardiomyopathy
Familial cardiomyopathies
Neuromuscular disorders, e.g. Duchenne muscular dystrophy, fascioscapulohumeral muscular dystrophy, Friedrich's ataxia
Other genetic abnormalities: mitochondrial DNA defects, X-linked cardiomyopathy

cardiomyopathy (IDCM). At least 25% of cases of IDCM are thought to have a familial origin. Some of the genetic mutations that result in DCM and their inheritance patterns are shown in Table 13.1. Viral and immunological mechanisms have also been implicated in the pathogenesis of IDCM. Evidence for viral involvement includes the demonstration of viral RNA in heart muscle and viral specific IgM antibodies in approximately one-third of patients; these, however, are also frequently found in unaffected controls. Evidence for immune mechanisms include autoantibodies against cellular components (e.g. adenine nucleotide translocator, beta-adrenoceptors, myosin, laminin, actin, tropomyosin and heat shock proteins), an association with human leukocyte antigen (HLA) class II phenotypes, inflammatory infiltrates and myocyte necrosis on myocardial biopsy.

Table 13.1: Recognized mutations causing DCM

Inheritance pattern	Chromosome	Gene	Skeletal myopathy
X linked	Xp21	Dystrophin	Duchenne/Becker muscular dystrophy
	Xq28	G4.5 (tafazzin)	Barth syndrome
	Xp28	Emerin	Emery-Dreifus
Autosomal dominant	15q14	Cardiac actin	No
	2q35	Desmin	Desmin myopathy
	5	δ-sarcoglycan	Limb girdle muscular dystrophy 2F
	1q32	Troponin T	No
	14q11	β-myosin heavy chain	Probably subclinical
	15q2	α-tropomyosin	?
	1q21	Laminin A/C	?
Mitochondrial	MtDNA	Mitochondrial respiratory chain	Mitochondrial myopathy

PATHOLOGY

The pathological features of dilated cardiomyopathy depend on the underlying cause. The features of IDCM are non-specific; myocytes tend to be pleomorphic and hypertrophied with enlarged and bizarrely shaped nuclei, interstitial fibrosis is common.

CLINICAL FEATURES

Most patients present with signs and symptoms of heart failure. Other features include chest pain in the absence of coronary artery disease, arrhythmias and embolic complications as a result of atrial arrhythmias, left-atrial enlargement or mural thrombi. Some patients are asymptomatic and are diagnosed after an incidental finding of cardiomegaly, atrial fibrillation or left bundle branch block (LBBB). Occasionally, sudden cardiac death is the first manifestation. Signs of heart failure are usually found at presentation. The apex beat may be displaced and dyskinetic, a third and fourth heart sound may be present and murmurs of mitral and tricuspid regurgitation are common.

INVESTIGATIONS

Electrocardiography

The electrocardiograph (ECG) is usually abnormal at presentation with sinus tachycardia, unexplained Q waves, varying degrees of atrioventricular (AV) block, atrial fibrillation (in 20–30%) and ventricular ectopy as frequent findings. LBBB is seen in 15–20%.

Echocardiography

DCM (Fig 13.1) is diagnosed when there is evidence of left-ventricular enlargement and reduced fractional shortening. Other abnormalities include atrioventricular valvular regurgitation, diastolic dysfunction, wall-motion abnormalities and occasionally left-ventricular (LV) thrombus.

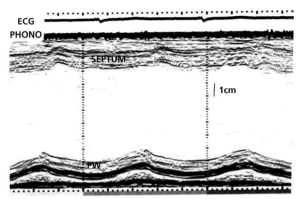

Figure 13.1
Dilated cardiomyopathy – parasternal long axis M-mode recording demonstrating dilated left ventricular cavity (left ventricular diastolic dimension approximately 7 cm), with markedly reduced fractional shortening in systole (PW = posterior wall)

Laboratory tests

All patients with DCM should undergo routine biochemical evaluation including full blood count, urea and electrolytes, blood glucose, liver and thyroid function tests. Additional blood tests such as serum ferritin, ACE levels, autoantibody profile, HIV serology, detection of viral specific antigens, specific DNA and gene analysis may be required in selected patients.

Metabolic exercise testing

Metabolic exercise testing provides an objective assessment of functional impairment and prognosis and is a useful way to examine the impact of the disease or treatment modalities over time.

24-hour Holter monitoring

The most common arrhythmias detected are supraventricular in particular atrial fibrillation and flutter. Non-sustained ventricular tachycardia is common but sustained ventricular tachycardia is rare.

Chest X-ray

Radiological abnormalities include cardiomegaly, atrial or biatrial enlargement, pleural effusions, interstitial oedema and alveolar oedema.

Cardiac catheterization

Cardiac catheterization should be performed in patients with signs, symptoms or risk factors for coronary artery disease. Left and right heart studies can provide prognostic information prior to cardiac transplantation. Endomyocardial biopsy may be useful when metabolic or storage disorders such as amyloid or sarcoidosis are suspected.

TREATMENT

See Chapter 12 for details of treatment of chronic heart failure.

HYPERTROPHIC CARDIOMYOPATHY

DEFINITION

Hypertrophic cardiomyopathy (HCM) is defined by the presence of left ventricular (LV) and/or right ventricular (RV) hypertrophy in the absence of a haemodynamic or systemic cause (e.g. aortic stenosis or hypertension).

PREVALENCE

The estimated prevalence of HCM is 1 in 500. Although hypertrophic cardiomyopathy can present at any age hypertrophy typically develops during adolescence. Young children and adults may occasionally present with LV hypertrophy in association with other diseases (e.g. Noonan syndrome, mitochondrial disorders, and metabolic disorders such as Fabry's).

AETIOLOGY

In the majority of cases HCM is a familial disorder with autosomal dominant inheritance. The disease is caused by mutations in genes encoding cardiac sarcomeric proteins. The most common mutations identified are in the genes encoding ß myosin heavy chain (chromosome 14), cardiac troponin T (chromosome 1) and the myosin-binding protein C (chromosome 11). Other genes affected include: cardiac troponin I (chromosome 19), regulatory (chromosome 12) and essential myosin light chains (chromosome 3), a-tropomyosin (chromosome 15) and cardiac actin (chromosome 15). Recently, mutations in the genes encoding the -2 subunit of cyclic AMP kinase gene (chromosome 7) have been identified in patients with HCM and Wolff–Parkinson–White syndrome.

PATHOPHYSIOLOGY

Microscopically HCM is characterized by myocyte hypertrophy and disarray, other characteristic features include fibrosis and narrowed intramural coronary arteries. Hypertrophy normally affects the interventricular septum more than the free or posterior walls (asymmetric septal hypertrophy). Concentric and apical hypertrophy is also described and right-sided involvement occurs in up to one-third of patients, although never in isolation. Global LV systolic function is usually normal or hyperdynamic at rest. One-third of patients have LV outflow tract obstruction (LVOTO) secondary to systolic anterior motion of the mitral valve. Diastolic dysfunction caused by abnormal LV relaxation and reduced LV compliance is common. A minority of patients have features resembling restrictive cardiomyopathy.

SYMPTOMS

The majority of patients remain asymptomatic or have mild symptoms only. When symptoms are present the most common are exertional with atypical chest pain, dyspnoea, palpitations, syncope and presyncope. Syncope/presyncope may be caused by paroxysmal arrhythmia, LVOTO, conduction system disease or abnormal vascular responses during exercise.

Examination

In most patients the physical examination is unremarkable. Patients may have a forceful LV impulse, rapid upstroke to the arterial pulse, a palpable left atrial beat, prominent 'a' wave in the jugular venous pressure and a fourth heart sound. In patients with LVOTO a mid–late systolic murmur can usually be heard. The intensity of this murmur can be increased by manoeuvres that decrease afterload or venous return such as standing, exercise, Valsalva or nitrates.

DIAGNOSIS

The ECG is abnormal in the majority of patients with HCM, although no specific changes are diagnostic. Left-axis deviation, criteria for LV hypertrophy with or without repolarization changes, left- and/or right-atrial enlargement and abnormal Q-waves are the most common features. The diagnosis of HCM depends on the echocardiographic demonstration of hypertrophy exceeding two standard deviations from the mean corrected for age, sex and height (see Fig. 13.2). Magnetic resonance imaging (MRI) is occasionally useful in patients with poor echocardiographic windows, patients with apical hypertrophy or to look for right-ventricular involvement.

TREATMENT OF SYMPTOMS

The treatment of symptoms depends on the presence or absence of LVOTO. In patients with a significant LVOTO (=30 mmHg) beta-blockers can be effective and are usually

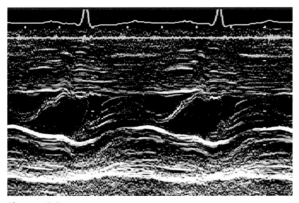

Figure 13.2
HCM – parasternal long axis M-mode demonstrating marked septal thickening, reduced left ventricular cavity size and systolic anterior motion of the mitral valve

tried first. Verapamil is also effective but can occasionally exacerbate LVOTO and should be used with caution. Disopyramide is probably a safer option but should be used with combination with low-dose beta-blockers or verapamil in order to prevent accelerated AV conduction. When drug therapy fails, surgery (septal myotomy–myectomy) guided by intraoperative transoesophageal echocardiography, alcohol septal ablation or dual chamber pacing should be considered. Surgery and alcohol septal ablation appear to have similar success rates (80%). Pacing has the lowest success rate and is usually reserved for patients that are either unsuitable or unwilling to undergo other treatments. In patients without significant LVOTO the treatment options are more limited, but beta-blockers and calcium channel antagonists can be effective in patients with chest pain, breathlessness or palpitations.

A small number (5–10%) of patients with HCM progress to an 'end-stage' characterized by wall thinning, cavity enlargement, and systolic impairment. In these patients treatment should include diuretics and ACE inhibitors.

MANAGEMENT OF SUPRAVENTRICULAR ARRHYTHMIA

Paroxysmal episodes of supraventricular tachycardias such as atrial fibrillation or flutter are common and are best treated with amiodarone or beta-blockers with Class III action, e.g. sotalol. Established atrial fibrillation/flutter should be cardioverted (after anticoagulation) but when restoration of sinus rhythm is not possible beta-blockers and calcium antagonists can be used to control the heart rate. Atrial fibrillation/flutter in HCM is associated with a significant risk of thromboembolism. All patients with sustained or frequent paroxysms and patients with left-atrial enlargement should be anticoagulated.

SUDDEN DEATH IN HYPERTROPHIC CARDIOMYOPATHY

Sudden death is the most common mode of death in patients with HCM and occurs most commonly in children and young adults. The overall sudden death rate is about 1%, although some individuals are at higher risk. Patients that have survived a cardiac arrest are at highest risk, most other patients at risk can be identified by non-invasive assessment, which should include history, echocardiography, 48-hour Holter and cardiopulmonary exercise testing. Established risk markers for sudden death include:

- non-sustained ventricular tachycardia (3 consecutive beats at a rate of 120 beats/min or more lasting for less than 30 seconds)
- LV wall thickness of ≥30 mm
- abnormal blood pressure response in those under 40 years of age
- family history of premature sudden cardiac death and unexplained syncope.

Patients with none of the above risk factors have <1% estimated annual risk of sudden death. Patients that have two or more of the above risk factors are at greatest risk (4–6% annual risk of sudden death) and should be offered some form of prophylactic therapy. Amiodarone has been used extensively in the past to treat risk but evidence increasingly shows that the implantable cardioverter defibrillator (ICD) is more effective. Risk stratification is problematic in those patients with a single risk factor and, at present, treatment is determined by the strength of the individual risk factor.

SCREENING

All first-degree relatives of patients with hypertrophic cardiomyopathy should be referred for screening. Current screening methods rely on ECG and echocardiography. In the near future genetic testing will prevent the need for continued clinical review and may identify patients at risk from sudden death prior to the onset of hypertrophy.

ARRHYTHMOGENIC RIGHT-VENTRICULAR CARDIOMYOPATHY

DEFINITION AND PREVALENCE

Arrhythmogenic right-ventricular cardiomyopathy (ARVC) is a primary abnormality of the myocardium characterized by progressive loss of myocytes, fatty infiltration and replacement fibrosis occurring predominantly in the right ventricle. The prevalence is estimated at 1 in 5000–10 000.

AETIOLOGY AND PATHOLOGY

ARVC is a familial condition; the mode of inheritance is mostly autosomal dominant with variable penetrance and incomplete expression. Pathologically ARVC is characterized by the replacement of myocytes with adipose and fibrous tissue. Although the condition mainly affects localized areas of the right ventricle, diffuse RV and LV involvement are also seen.

CLINICAL PRESENTATION

The age of onset of the disease is variable, but commonly ARVC manifests with ventricular arrhythmias during adolescence and early adulthood. Later in life heart failure predominates. Many cases are diagnosed at post-mortem examination after sudden death.

DIAGNOSIS

A definite diagnosis of ARVC requires the histological finding of transmural fibrofatty replacement of the RV myocardium at post mortem, or endomyocardial biopsy. Diagnosis by endomyocardial biopsy is difficult, however, because the disease is segmental and can be missed. ECG abnormalities tend to be subtle, abnormal findings include complete or partial right bundle branch block (RBBB) and repolarization abnormalities in the right precordial leads (normal <12 years of age). Epsilon waves (postexcitation electrical potentials that occur at the end of the QRS complex and at the beginning of the ST segment) are highly specific for ARVC but are found in a minority of cases only. Abnormalities are often more prominent on signal averaged ECG (SAECG) than standard 12-lead ECG. Patients with ARVC are prone to ventricular tachycardia, which usually has an LBBB pattern. On echocardiography, RV dilatation, hypokinesia and small aneurysms in the RV free wall may be seen. Magnetic resonance imaging (MRI) is the imaging modality of choice and may show infiltration and fibro fatty deposits. A normal MRI, however, does not exclude the diagnosis, as subtle abnormalities may not be detected.

TREATMENT

Treatment is warranted in symptomatic patients or those at risk of sudden death. Antiarrhythmic drugs can be used to suppress atrial and ventricular arrhythmias. Sotalol and amiodarone are the agents of choice. Patients who develop right- or left-sided heart failure may benefit from ACE inhibitors and diuretics. Patients who are at risk from thromboembolism will require anticoagulation.

SUDDEN DEATH

Patients who have had a previous cardiac arrest or those with symptomatic non-sustained or sustained ventricular tachycardia are at greatest risk. These patients should be treated with an ICD. Other risk factors may include:

- unexplained syncope
- strong family history of sudden death
- QRS dispersion >140 ms on SAECG
- globally reduced RV or LV function
- RV hypokinesis and enlarged RV chamber.

The presence of a number of these risk factors in an individual patient may also warrant prophylactic therapy.

RESTRICTIVE CARDIOMYOPATHY

Restrictive cardiomyopathy (RCM) is characterized by restrictive diastolic filling pattern, normal or near normal wall thickness and normal systolic function. Prevalence is unknown.

AETIOLOGY

RCM may be idiopathic or associated with other diseases (Box 13.2).

PATHOPHYSIOLOGY

RCM generally results from endocardial or myocardial fibrosis and infiltration. This leads to decreased ventricular compliance and filling, failure of the ventricle to relax during

Box 13.2: Causes of restrictive cardiomyopathy

Idiopathic

Endomyocardial disease, e.g. endomyocardial fibrosis, hypereosinophilic syndrome, carcinoid, metastasis, radiation damage

Loeffler's endocarditis

Infiltrative disease: amyloid, sarcoid, systemic sclerosis

Storage disorders: haemachromatosis, glycogen storage disorders (e.g. Gaucher's disease, Fabry's), mucopolysaccharidoses, inborn errors of metabolism

Drugs: anthracycline toxicity

diastole, increased end-diastolic ventricular pressures and bi-atrial enlargement. Other features may include myocyte hypertrophy in amyloidosis and the storage disorders, non-caseating granulomata in sarcoidosis, iron deposits in haemochromatosis and mural thrombi in endomyocardial fibrosis. Some apparently idiopathic cases have myocardial disarray; recently sarcomeric gene mutations (troponin I) have been identified in some of these.

CLINICAL PRESENTATION

RCM usually presents with gradual onset heart failure; right-sided findings frequently predominate. Atrial fibrillation is common and ventricular arrhythmias or heart block may be present in advanced cases.

DIAGNOSIS

The ECG may be normal, non-specific ST and T segment changes are sometimes seen and small voltages may be seen in amyloid. The chest X-ray may show a normal or slightly enlarged heart with atrial enlargement. On echocardiography the ventricular cavity size is usually normal (can be increased in amyloid and sarcoidosis) with an abnormal filling pattern and biatrial enlargement. Myocardial wall thickness is usually normal, but may be increased and have a bright speckled appearance in amyloidosis. Systolic function is usually normal. MRI can be useful in some patients.

TREATMENT

RCM is usually in its advanced stages before it is clinically recognized. The prognosis is poor with a 2-year mortality of 35–50%. The aims of medical therapy are to improve symptoms of heart failure, treat arrhythmias and prevent systemic thrombus. Diuresis may help with symptomatic relief, while ACE inhibitors may be of benefit with LV dysfunction. Pacemakers are indicated for patients with conduction disease and cardiac transplantation may be an option in selected cases. Vasodilators should be used cautiously because they may cause hypotension.

Further reading

Franz WM, Muller OJ, Katus HA 2001 Cardiomyopathies: from genetics to the prospect of treatment. Lancet 358: 1627–1637

Gemayel C, Pelliccia A, Thompson PD 2001 Arrhythmogenic right ventricular cardiomyopathy. J Am Coll Cardiol 38: 1773–1781

Julian DG, Camm AJ, Fox KM, Hall RJC, Poole-Wilson PA (eds) 1996 Diseases of the heart. Saunders, London

Maron BJ 2002 Hypertrophic cardiomyopathy: a systematic review. JAMA 287: 1308–1320

McKenna WJ, Behr ER 2002 Hypertrophic cardiomyopathy: management, risk stratification and prevention of sudden death. Heart 87: 169–176

Topol EJ (ed.) 2002 Textbook of cardiovascular medicine, 2nd edn. Lippincott Williams & Wilkins, Cleveland, Ohio

SELF-ASSESSMENT

Questions

1. A 32-year-old man presents with a 1-year history of central chest tightness and exertional dyspnoea. He occasionally feels 'light headed' if he stands up too quickly and over the last 5 years admits to having had three presyncopal episodes. He has no other relevant past medical history, and takes no regular medications. His father died at the age of 52 after a myocardial infarction and his mother is in good health. He has two children aged 15 and 17 years; both are in good health. His grandfather died in his early thirties, but he is unaware of the circumstances. On physical examination he was normotensive, there was a soft systolic murmur heard at the left sternal edge radiating into the mitral and aortic areas, the rest of the examination was unremarkable. Routine blood tests were normal, a coronary angiogram performed showed no significant coronary artery disease (see Fig. 13.3 for ECG). Echocardiography demonstrated an enlarged left atrium, systolic anterior motion of the anterior mitral valve leaflet against the septum and a thickened interventricular septum.

   a. What is the diagnosis?
   b. What are the possible causes of the presyncopal episodes?
   c. How would you risk stratify this patient?

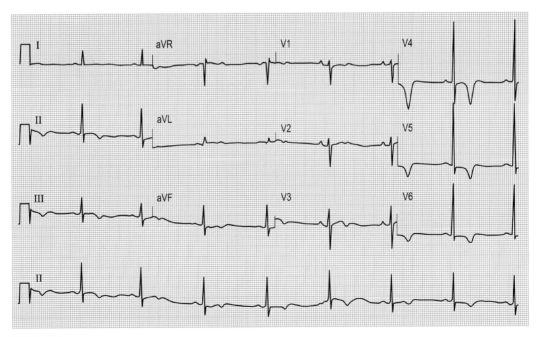

Figure 13.3

2. A 15-year-old boy has been referred to you by his general practitioner after having had a dizzy spell. He is otherwise fit and well with no other medical problems. On closer questioning he tells you that his brother died several years ago at the age of 17 years.
   a. What would you do next?
   b. What does the ECG show and what is the likely diagnosis (Fig. 13.4)?
   c. How would you confirm the diagnosis and what tests would you perform next?
   d. On exercise testing the following is seen (Fig. 13.5), what would your management be in the long term?

Answers
1. a. Hypertrophic cardiomyopathy
   b. Presyncope or syncope may be a result of dynamic LV outflow tract obstruction, abnormal vascular responses or arrhythmias
   c. Most patients at risk of sudden death can be identified by non-invasive evaluation that should include echocardiography, 48-hour Holter and exercise testing. Risk markers include:
      • non-sustained ventricular tachycardia
      • LV wall thickness ≥30 mm
      • abnormal blood pressure response in those under 40 years of age
      • family history of premature sudden cardiac death and unexplained syncope.

Patients with none of the above risk factors have <1% estimated annual risk of sudden death. Patients that have two or more of the above risk factors are at greatest risk (4–6% annual risk of sudden death).

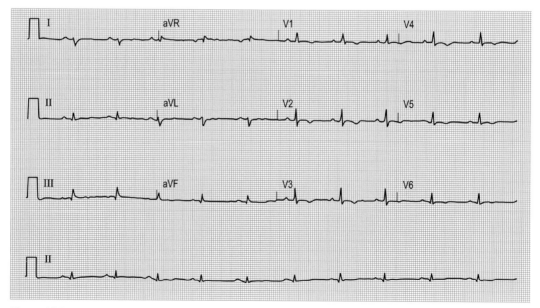

Figure 13.4

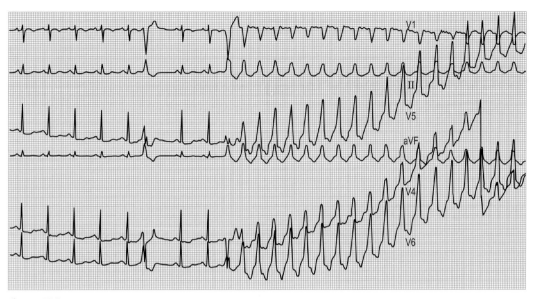

Figure 13.5

2. a. Initially it would be helpful to obtain the results of his brother's post mortem, and an extensive family history should be taken. An ECG should also be obtained.
   b. The ECG shows repolarization changes in the right sided leads characteristic of ARVC.
   c. The diagnosis can be confirmed on echocardiography and MRI. He should also undergo Holter monitoring and exercise testing.
   d. This patient has exercise-induced ventricular tachycardia and therefore requires an ICD. A beta-blocker or amiodarone may also be considered.

Electrophysiology and arrhythmias

14

P. Roberts and A. Yue

INTRODUCTION

In 1901, Einthoven adapted and developed the use of the string Galvanometer that led to the widespread use of the human electrocardiogram (ECG). With a better understanding of the normal cardiac conduction system and the introduction of intravascular catheters to record electrical events, the era of clinical cardiac electrophysiology was born. Programmed electrical stimulation, endocardial catheter mapping, radiofrequency ablation and implantable devices have changed the face of electrophysiology.

PATHOPHYSIOLOGY

Knowledge of the normal cardiac conduction system, cardiac action potential and cellular electrophysiology is essential for understanding the mechanisms of bradycardias and tachycardias and thus, their appropriate management.

NORMAL CARDIAC CONDUCTION SYSTEM AND CELLULAR ELECTROPHYSIOLOGY

Normal conduction system

Normal cardiac contraction relies on the conduction of electrical impulses in a coordinated fashion down the specialized conduction system:

- Sinoatrial node (SA node)
- Atrioventricular (AV) node
- His bundle
- Bundle branches, fascicles, and Purkinje network.

The sinus beat originates in the SA node, a focus of automatic cells at the junction between the superior vena cava and the right atrium. An electrical impulse then propagates through the atrial myocardium to the AV node, which is found in the anteromedial right atrium. The His bundle splits into the three fascicles: 1) the right bundle branch, 2) the anterior division of the left bundle branch, and 3) the posterior division of the left bundle branch (Fig. 14.1).

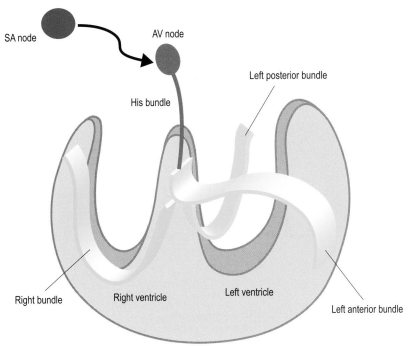

Figure 14.1
The normal cardiac conduction system

Blood supply

- SA node: from right coronary artery (55%), circumflex artery (35%), both (10%)
- AV node: from posterior descending artery of the right coronary artery (80%), circumflex artery (10%), both (10%)
- His bundle and bundle branches: from both posterior descending artery and left anterior descending artery.

Normal automaticity

This is defined as the ability of a cell to depolarize itself to a threshold and to generate an action potential. It is characteristic of the specialized conducting system. The SA node generally has the fastest intrinsic rate of spontaneous depolarization. The automaticity of the SA and AV nodes is affected by sympathetic/parasympathetic tone.

Cardiac action potential

The cardiac action potential reflects the change of transmembrane voltage with time. Ion channels are transmembrane proteins that respond to stimuli, such as a change in voltage across the cell membrane to allow specific ions to cross the cell membrane to generate the action potential (Fig. 14.2).

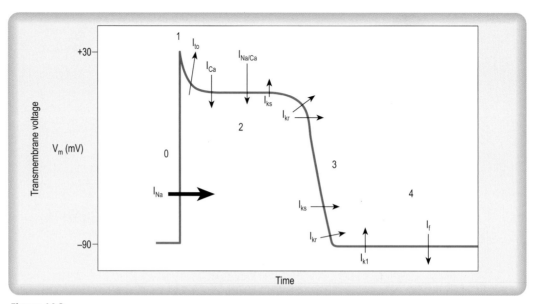

Figure 14.2

The cardiac action potential from the ventricular myocyte

Phase 0: During membrane depolarization, there is a net influx of sodium ions (in ventricular myocardium) or calcium ions (in pacemaker cells) into the cardiac cell, with an approximate rapid change in resting membrane potential from –90 to +30 mV.

Phase 1: This activates a transient outward repolarizing potassium current I_{t0}.

Phase 2: The plateau phase of action potential that follows is complex, owing to a multitude of current components that contribute at the same time. Of particular importance are the L- and T- type calcium currents, and the sodium–calcium exchange currents, which cause a net influx of calcium ions.

Phase 3: Repolarization occurs with an efflux of potassium out of the cell through the I_{ks} and I_{kr} currents.

Phase 4: During diastole, a predominantly outward potassium current, inward rectifier, I_{k1}, maintains the resting membrane potential at about –90 mV. The gradual decay of I_{k1} and activation of a slow inward sodium current, pacemaker current I_f, eventually result in membrane depolarization and reinitiation of the action potential

MECHANISMS OF ARRHYTHMIAS

There are three mechanisms for arrhythmogenesis: automaticity, triggered activity, and abnormal conduction.

Abnormal automaticity refers to disorders of impulse formation both from cells of the specialized conduction system and cells without normal intrinsic automaticity, e.g. sinus tachycardia, sinus bradycardia and ectopic atrial tachycardia. It accounts for 10% of tachyarrhythmias and often occurs in the setting of acutely ill patients, e.g. on ICU.

Triggered activity refers to arrhythmias that are initiated by after-depolarizations. These are caused by leakage of positive ions into cells producing a deflection in phase 3–4 of the action potential.

Disorders of impulse conduction include: conduction block caused by fibrotic degeneration or ischaemia, and reentry mechanisms.

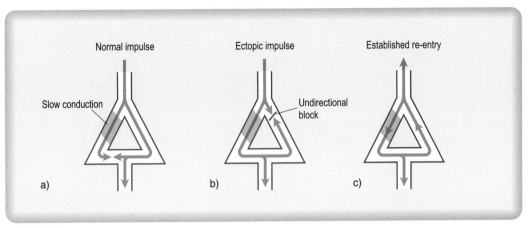

Figure 14.3
The conditions of re-entry mechanism. (a) A normal impulse enters a circuit with two pathways in which conduction velocities are different. (b) A critically timed premature ectopic impulse enters the circuit, encounters the refractory period of the faster pathway (unidirectional block), but conducts normally down the slower pathway. (c) The impulse from the slower pathway conducts retrogradely up the faster pathway following the recovery of refractoriness, and enters the slow pathway again, thus completing the reentry circuit

Re-entry is the principal mechanism for most forms of supraventricular tachycardia mediated by the AV node or an accessory pathway, and monomorphic ventricular tachycardia. There are three requirements for reentry arrhythmias (Fig. 14.3):

1. Two distinct conduction pathways (with slow conduction in one limb)
2. Unidirectional block
3. A critically timed ectopic impulse.

ANTIARRHYTHMIC DRUGS

The Vaughan Williams classification of antiarrhythmic drugs is based on the physiological effects of the drugs and is the most accepted classification in clinical practice (Table 14.1).

Antiarrhythmic therapy is effective in controlling a large variety of arrhythmias. However, lessons from past clinical trials have shown that the proarrhythmic risk of these medications may outweigh the benefits. An example is the use of flecainide to suppress ventricular ectopics post myocardial infarction in the Cardiac Arrhythmia Suppression Trial (CAST). The increased mortality in the flecainide arm means it is now contraindicated in patients with coronary artery disease and impaired ventricular function.

BASIC ELECTROPHYSIOLOGICAL STUDY

Aims

- To establish the mechanism of an arrhythmia
- To define prognosis/stratify risk of sudden death
- To guide treatment.

Table 14.1: Vaughan Williams classification of antiarrhythmic drug actions

Class	Action	Drug
I	Sodium channel blockade	IA: disopyramide, quinidine, procainamide IB: lidocaine, mexiletine, tocainide IC: flecainide, propafenone
II	Beta-blockade	Beta-blockers
III	Potassium channel blockade	Amiodarone* Sotalol* Dofetilide/azimilide
IV	Calcium channel blockade	Calcium channel blockers

*Other class properties present

The indications for electrophysiology study (EPS) are generally divided into three categories: tachycardias, bradycardias and syncope.

EPS procedure

Patients are studied using local anaesthesia and sedation. Insulated catheters with 2 to 24 electrodes are introduced into the heart from the venous system (usually femoral/subclavian veins). A standard study uses four catheters: high right atrium, His bundle, coronary sinus (enables left atrial and ventricular activation to be studied), and right ventricular apex (Fig. 14.4).

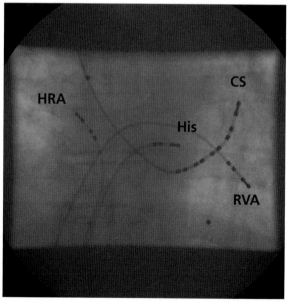

Figure 14.4
Image of an electrophysiological study. There are catheters in the high right atrium (HRA), His bundle (His), right ventricular apex (RVA) and coronary sinus (CS)

The functions of the AV node and SA node are observed with atrial and ventricular pacing, with the introduction of premature beats. Preexcitation and concealed retrograde VA (ventricle to atrium) conduction may be seen.

An attempt to induce tachycardia is made. In the atrium, drive-train pacing with one to four extrastimuli, incremental pacing and burst pacing are performed. To induce ventricular arrhythmias, progressive introduction of up to three extrastimuli are made at the right ventricular apex and outflow tract. Isoprenaline injections may be given to facilitate arrhythmia induction.

Following tachycardia induction, the response to further pacing manoeuvres and termination characteristics are tested.

RADIOFREQUENCY ABLATION

Early catheter ablation techniques using high-energy DC shocks have been superseded by radiofrequency (RF) energy. When applied with deflectable catheters, it has become an ideal technique for delivering localized heat energy to inactivate small areas of electrically active tissue. All arrhythmias apart from ventricular fibrillation may be amenable to RF ablation.

Techniques of RF ablation

For arrhythmias originating in the left heart, a retrograde trans-aortic approach or the transseptal technique may be used. A combination of local electrogram appearance and fluoroscopy are used to target anatomically, the delivery of RF energy. Usually, energy delivery to a critical area of a reentrant circuit or an automatic focus with a target temperature of 55–65°C for 30 seconds is used. Success rates exceed 95% for AV nodal modification and accessory pathway mediated tachycardias.

Complications of RF ablation

These include:

- Complete heart block (1% for AV nodal modification)
- Cardiac tamponade (<1%)
- Thromboembolic events (<1% for left-sided procedures).

BRADYCARDIAS

Patients with bradycardias may be asymptomatic, but they may also present with pre-syncope or syncope. The evaluation for pacemaker therapy hinges on history, physical examination and the resting 12-lead ECG. Some patients may require ambulatory monitoring.

Bradycardias may be caused by abnormalities in:

- sinus node function
- atrioventricular conduction
- intraventricular conduction.

SINUS NODE DYSFUNCTION

Approximately 50% of permanent pacemakers are implanted for sinus node dysfunction. It may be caused by abnormal automaticity, conduction, or both. Commonest causes are idiopathic degeneration and acute coronary syndromes (up to 30% of myocardial infarctions).

It is a complex syndrome of clinical manifestations. These may include:

- inappropriate sinus bradycardia
- chronotropic incompetence – this may lead to fatigue and poor exercise tolerance
- sinus pauses/exit blocks/arrests – sinus pauses of up to 3 s without symptoms need not be treated
- tachycardia-bradycardia syndrome – it is the most frequently symptomatic form of sinus node dysfunction.

Sinus node dysfunction is associated with a mortality that is related to the underlying pathological process, e.g. coronary artery disease. It carries with it a better prognosis than atrioventricular node dysfunction. Whilst pacing for sinus node dysfunction improves symptoms there is little evidence to suggest that it improves mortality.

ATRIOVENTRICULAR CONDUCTION DISTURBANCES

These are usually classified into first-, second-, or third-degree atrioventricular blocks. Idiopathic fibrosis is the most likely cause. Inferior (14%) or anterior (2%) myocardial infarctions not uncommonly result in atrioventricular block. A variety of drug effects, metabolic disturbances, and infiltrative diseases may also be responsible.

First-degree atrioventricular block

This is defined as a PR interval of more than 200 ms in adults. Conduction block in the specialized conduction system may occur anywhere from the atrium to the infra-His level. Pacing is not required.

Second-degree atrioventricular block

It is divided into type 1 (Wenckebach) and type 2 (Mobitz type II), although higher degree of atrioventricular block may also occur, resulting in 2 to 1 conduction. In type 1, atrioventricular block commonly occurs at the AV node level, whereas type 2 block involves the His bundle or below.

Third-degree atrioventricular block

This is characterized by complete dissociation of atrial and ventricular activity.

INTRAVENTRICULAR CONDUCTION DISTURBANCES

These abnormalities lie in the bundle branches, fascicles, and the Purkinje system. Therefore, conduction block at this level may result in:

- right (RBBB) or left bundle branch block (LBBB)
- left-anterior or posterior hemiblock
- intraventricular conduction defect.

Bifascicular block refers to LBBB, or RBBB in association with left-anterior or posterior hemiblock. Measurement of the HV (His to ventricle) interval at EPS represents conduction in the remaining fascicle, and when prolonged, this suggests a high risk of complete heart block. For example, an extremely prolonged HV interval (>100 ms) carries a 25% risk of developing complete heart block over 2 years.

TREATMENT OF BRADYCARDIAS

It is important to treat the underlying cause if it is reversible, e.g. drugs, ischaemia, metabolic disturbances. Atropine may serve as a temporary measure, and is effective in vagotonic states and following myocardial infarctions. Temporary and permanent cardiac pacing may also be used (see below).

PACEMAKERS

INDICATIONS FOR TEMPORARY TRANSVENOUS PACING

Acute inferior myocardial infarction

- Type 1 or 2 second degree AV block with broad QRS complexes
- Complete heart block
- Alternating LBBB and RBBB.

Acute anterior myocardial infarction

- All types of second-degree AV block
- Complete heart block
- Trifascicular block (left axis deviation, RBBB and first degree block)
- Alternating LBBB and RBBB.

Bradycardia with haemodynamic compromise

Temporary pacing my be used as a bridge to permanent pacing or whilst treating reversible systemic disturbances.

Ventricular tachycardia

Temporary pacing at a fast base rate is useful in treatment of bradycardia-dependent polymorphic ventricular arrhythmias as in long QT syndrome. Overdrive pacing may be used to terminate monomorphic ventricular tachycardia.

Temporary pacing for general anaesthesia

It is most important to take into account any previous symptoms of presyncope or syncope. The incidence of perioperative complete AV block in an asymptomatic patient with bifascicular block and first-degree AV block is low, and temporary pacing is generally not required.

PERMANENT CARDIAC PACING

Pacemaker technology and indications have evolved dramatically since the first implant in 1958. Current pacing systems have extensive programmability including rate adaptability, hysteresis, mode-switching, and algorithms for preventing atrial fibrillation. There is now substantial clinical evidence showing benefits of resynchronization pacing therapy in patients with heart failure and bundle branch block. Ongoing trials are investigating the potential benefits of multisite and overdrive pacing in patients with atrial fibrillation.

Pacemaker system

The pulse generator usually has a lithium–iodine battery and contains circuits for controlling timing, output, and sensing parameters. Passive fixation leads have a tine mechanism that anchors the lead tips between the endocardial trabeculations. Active fixation leads have a screw-in mechanism. Active fixation leads may be selected in the following circumstances:

- In post-operative patients where the atrial appendage has been excised
- In patients with dilated ventricles
- Where inadequate thresholds are obtained in conventional positions.

Most leads have a steroid eluting tip to reduce the acute inflammatory response and rise in pacing threshold following lead implantation (exit block).

In a conventional dual chamber pacing system, the ventricular lead tip is positioned at the right ventricular apex and the atrial lead in the right atrial appendage. The pulse generator is usually inserted in the prepectoral pocket contralateral to the patient's dominant side to reduce interference with everyday activities.

PACEMAKER CODING

The original three-letter coding has now extended to five letters in line with recent advances in technology. It is developed by the North American Society of Pacing and Electrophysiology (NASPE) and the British Pacing and Electrophysiology Group (BPEG) (see Table 14.2).

Indications for permanent pacing

These guidelines have recently been revised by the American College of Cardiology (ACC) American Heart Association Task Force (AHA) (see Table 14.3).

Table 14.2: BPEG/NASPE generic pacemaker code

Position Category	I Chamber paced	II Chamber sensed	III Response to sensing	IV Programmability	V Antiarrhythmic function
	O (none) A (atrium) V (ventricle) D (dual) S (single)	O (none) A (atrium) V (ventricle) D (dual) S (single)	O (none) T (triggered) I (inhibited) D (dual)	O (none) P (single programmability) M (multiprogrammable) C (communicating) R (rate modulation)	O (none) P (pacing) S (shock) D (dual)

Table 14.3: Indications for permanent pacing (modified from ACC/AHA guidelines)

Acquired AV block	Class I	Third-degree AV block associated with symptoms due to bradycardia, asystole of >3 s or escape rate <40 bpm Second-degree block with symptomatic bradycardia
	Class II	Asymptomatic third-degree AV block or type II second-degree block Asymptomatic type I second-degree block with infra-His block
	Class III	Asymptomatic first-degree block AV block expected to resolve, e.g. drug toxicity
Chronic bifascicular and trifascicular block	Class I	Intermittent third-degree AV block Type II second-degree AV block
	Class II	Syncope not proved to be due to AV block, e.g. VT Incidental finding of infra-His block
	Class III	Asymptomatic with or without first-degree AV block
After acute phase of myocardial infarction	Class I	Persistent third-degree AV block Persistent second-degree AV block with bundle branch block or symptoms Transient second or third-degree AV block with bundle branch block
	Class II	Persistent second-degree AV block at nodal level Transient AV block without bundle branch block
	Class III	Persistent first-degree AV block
Sinus node dysfunction	Class I	Documented bradycardia with symptoms Chronotropic incompetence with symptoms
	Class II	Symptoms and bradycardia <40 bpm but not correlated
	Class III	Asymptomatic bradycardia Symptoms documented not due to bradycardia Symptoms from non-essential drug therapy
Carotid sinus syndrome and neurocardiogenic syncope	Class I	Syncope caused by carotid stimulation with >3 s asystole
	Class II	Syncope with cardioinhibitory response without clear precipitants Syncope with cardioinhibitory response in tilt table testing
	Class III	Cardioinhibitory response without severe symptoms

Class I indications are considered necessary and acceptable. Class II indications are generally accepted but there is a divergence in opinion. Class III conditions are indications not recommended for pacing.

Rate-responsive pacing

This is a form of physiological pacing that attempts to mimic sinus node function. Pacing rate increases in response to metabolic demand and exercise. The most commonly used sensing parameters are:

- Motion sensors – body vibration with physical activity
- Physiological sensors – e.g. minute ventilation, changes in thoracic impedance
- QT interval – which shortens with exercise.

Pacemaker mode selection

Debates continue regarding selection of the optimal pacing mode for specific patient groups. The superiority of rate-adaptive pacing (VVIR) over fixed-rate pacing (VVI) is well established in terms of quality of life and exercise performance. Recent clinical trials comparing physiological pacing (AAIR or DDDR) with ventricular pacing (VVIR) have failed to demonstrate any significant difference in quality of life, incidence of stroke, or mortality between the two groups. Figure 14.5 demonstrates the ECG of a patient with a DDDR pacemaker.

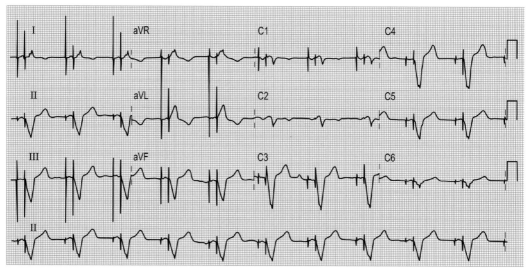

Figure 14.5
12-lead electrocardiograph showing normal dual chamber pacing

Complications of cardiac pacing

Procedure related

- Pacemaker pocket haematoma (<1% require surgical evacuation).

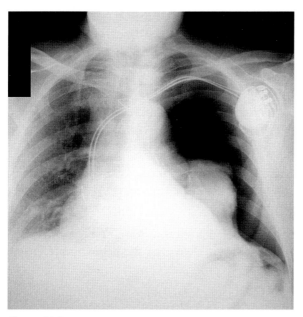

Figure 14.6
Chest X-ray showing a large pneumothorax following permanent pacemaker implantation

- Pneumothorax (Fig. 14.6). This can be managed conservatively if the patient is asymptomatic and the pneumothorax is small. A larger pneumothorax (>20%) that is associated with worsening symptoms should be treated with a chest drain (<1%).
- Cardiac perforation. Inadvertent perforation of the right ventricular wall during pacing wire manipulation is not uncommon. Generally, this is of no clinical consequence. However, cardiac tamponade should be suspected if a patient suffers chest pain or becomes hypotensive following pacemaker implantation (approx 0.1%).
- Diaphragmatic stimulation. The left phrenic nerve may be stimulated by apical placements of LV or RV leads. This can be avoided by screening the diaphragms during pacing at maximum voltage at the time of the implant.
- Lead dislodgement. Confirmed by failure to sense or capture during a pacing check. This may not always be obvious on a chest X-ray (<1% with ventricular leads and slightly higher with atrial leads).
- Pacemaker pocket infection (<1%). This is a potentially very serious complication leading to infective endocarditis. The only symptom may be pocket site tenderness or swelling. Any pocket erosion exposing the pacemaker or pus formation implies whole system infection. It is mandatory that the pacemaker and leads be extracted.

Pacemaker system malfunction

Pacemaker syndrome   This is caused by atrial contraction against a closed tricuspid or mitral valve in a patient with a single-chamber ventricular pacing system. Patients may experience dyspnoea, syncope, bloating or malaise. The pacing system should be upgraded to a dual chamber device.

Pacemaker-mediated tachycardia   Several forms of tachycardia may occur due to inadequate pacemaker programming, such as ventricular tracking of a rapid atrial rate, or oversensing of the atrial lead secondary to retrograde VA conduction or myopotentials.

Pacemakers and the environment

MRI   Strong magnetic fields may cause torque forces and pacemaker malfunction. Pacemakers may be inhibited or programming may be reset. MRI is generally avoided in patients with pacemakers.

DC cardioversion   Defibrillation pads should be placed as far apart as possible from the generator to avoid damage or reset of the device. The pacemaker should be checked after the procedure to ensure normal function.

Diathermy   Bipolar diathermy can be safely used if it is not applied to the region of the pulse generator. The pacemaker should be checked after the procedure to ensure normal function

Mobile phones   They may cause pacemaker interference and inhibition. Users are advised to hold the phones on the opposite side to the pacemakers.

Driving   Patients are allowed to drive 1 week after an implantation of a pacemaker, provided the pacemaker checks are satisfactory. They should inform the Driving and Vehicle Licensing Agency (DVLA) and the driving license is renewable every 3 years.

Pacemaker follow-up   Most patients will have their pacemakers checked 4 weeks after implantation and then subsequently at 6–12 months. As the device nears the end of its battery life, the frequency of pacemaker checks may be increased.

SUPRAVENTRICULAR TACHYCARDIAS

Supraventricular tachycardias have a diverse range of arrhythmia mechanisms. Conceptually, they can be more simply divided into three categories according to the mechanisms:

1. AV nodal reentry tachycardias
2. Accessory-pathway-mediated tachycardias
   a. Wolff–Parkinson–White syndrome
   b. concealed accessory pathway
3. 'Atrial' tachycardias
   a. atrial fibrillation and flutter
   b. ectopic atrial tachycardia
   c. sinus node reentry.

ATRIOVENTRICULAR NODAL RE-ENTRY TACHYCARDIA (AVNRT)

Clinical features

This mechanism is the most common cause of paroxysmal narrow complex tachycardia (80% of cases). The underlying substrate is present from birth. Younger females in particular are affected. Palpitations and anxiety are common presenting complaints. This condition is not life threatening unless there is co-existing structural heart disease.

Pathophysiology

The re-entry circuit involves atrial tissue surrounding the AV node. It mediates the tachycardia via two pathways:

1. The slow pathway – which has slow conduction velocity but a short refractory period
2. The fast pathway – which has fast conduction velocity but a long refractory period.

A critically timed extrastimulus triggers the tachycardia if it arrives in the circuit causing antegrade conduction in one limb and retrograde conduction in the other limb. In typical atrioventricular nodal re-entry tachycardia (AVNRT) (90%), the antegrade limb is the slow pathway and the retrograde limb the fast pathway (see Fig. 14.7). On the surface ECG, the retrograde P waves are not generally seen, as they lie within the QRS complexes (see Fig. 14.8).

Treatment

Drugs that modify AV nodal conduction such as Class I agents, beta-blockers and calcium antagonists may help relieve symptoms. Patients with frequent symptoms can now be referred for catheter ablation. Success rate approaches 95%. The risk of AV block (1%) is higher than other ablation procedures due to proximity to the AV node.

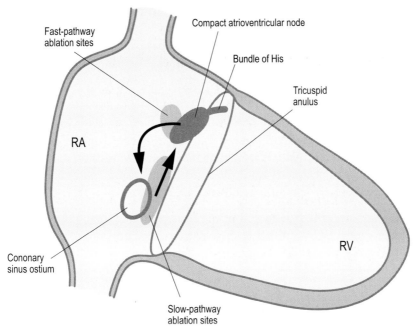

Figure 14.7
Diagram showing the atrioventricular nodal re-entry tachycardia (AVNRT) circuit. The anatomical sites for slow and fast pathway ablation are also highlighted

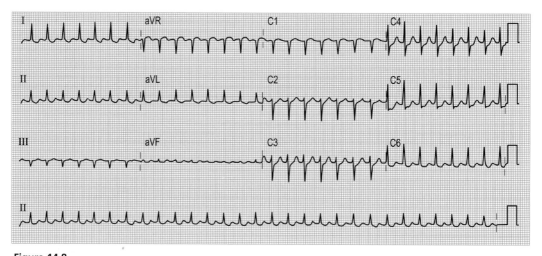

Figure 14.8
12-lead electrocardiograph (ECG) showing atrioventricular nodal re-entry tachycardia (AVNRT). Retrograde P waves are not visible in this ECG

ACCESSORY-PATHWAY-MEDIATED TACHYCARDIA

Clinical features

This is the second most common form of narrow complex tachycardia. Although the accessory pathways are present from birth, symptoms may not occur until adulthood. Usually, the resting ECG is normal, suggesting that the pathway conducts in the retrograde direction only (concealed accessory pathway). If pre-excitation is present on the ECG (short PR and delta wave) (Fig. 14.9), the pathway conducts in the antegrade direction as well (Wolff–Parkinson–White syndrome).

Pathophysiology

The accessory pathways are muscle bundles traversing the AV groove, thus connecting atrial and ventricular myocardium. They may occur anywhere on the mitral or tricuspid rings. In Wolff–Parkinson–White it is possible to locate the position of the pathway on the basis of the ECG appearance. Multiple accessory pathways may be present in 10% of cases, and are particularly common in Ebstein's anomaly.

In 90% of cases, antegrade conduction of the reentry circuit occurs through the AV node and retrograde conduction via the accessory pathway (orthodromic tachycardia) (Fig. 14.10). The reverse applies to antidromic tachycardia, which has a broad complex morphology.

Treatment

In the absence of pre-excitation on the ECG, patients with atrioventricular tachycardia may be treated as for those with AV nodal reentry. In Wolff–Parkinson–White syndrome, Class I or III drugs are preferred as these drugs slow conduction in the accessory pathway.

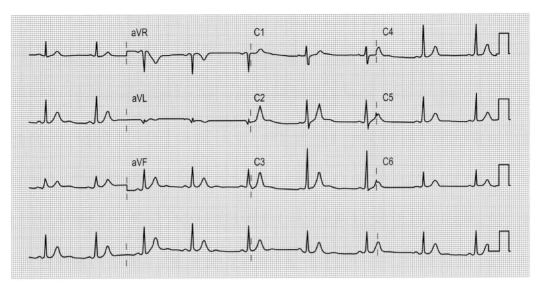

Figure 14.9
12-lead electrocardiograph showing pre-excitation in Wolff–Parkinson–White syndrome. Note the delta waves and short PR interval indicating pre-excitation

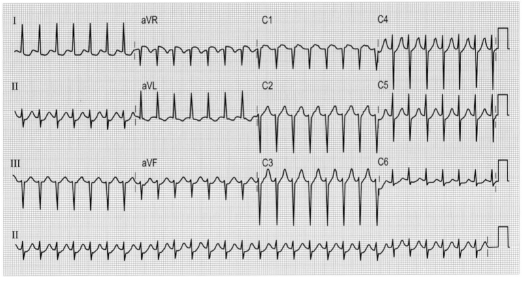

Figure 14.10
12-lead electrocardiograph showing atrioventricular re-entry tachycardia (AVRT) mediated by an accessory pathway. Retrograde P waves are visible during tachycardia

When atrial fibrillation occurs in Wolff–Parkinson–White syndrome, AV nodal slowing drugs such as digoxin, beta-blockers and diltiazem are contraindicated. The use of these drugs may predispose preferential antegrade conduction through the accessory pathway and extremely rapid ventricular response. Ventricular fibrillation may develop.

Catheter ablation is the treatment of choice in symptomatic patients (Fig. 14.11). Success rates are similar to AV nodal reentry tachycardia.

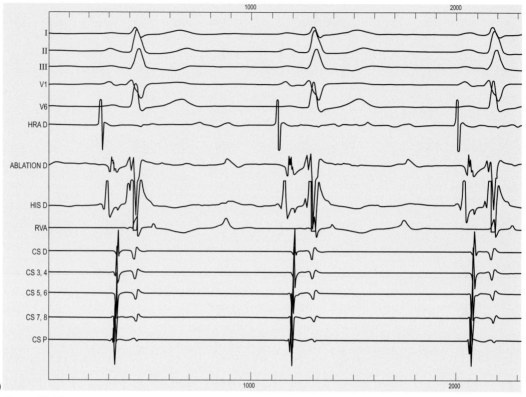

Figure 14.11
Radiofrequency ablation of accessory pathway in Wolff–Parkinson–White syndrome (paper speed 100 mm/s). (a) Pre ablation – note the pattern of activation in the coronary sinus (CS) electrograms. The A–V interval is shortest in the distal (D) electrograms compared to proximal (P) as the accessory pathway is in the left lateral region
HRA, high right atrium; RVA, right ventricular apex

ECTOPIC ATRIAL TACHYCARDIA

ECG shows a narrow complex tachycardia with abnormal or multiple P wave morphologies. The mechanism is abnormal automaticity. Response to drug therapy is poor. Verapamil may help in controlling heart rate. Catheter ablation is an option in selected cases with the use of advance mapping technologies.

ATRIAL FIBRILLATION

Atrial fibrillation (AF) is the most common sustained arrhythmia worldwide. The Framingham study showed that its prevalence increases with age, from approximately 0.5% of the general population to more than 10% of the population over the age of 80. It has significant impact on quality of life and is associated with heart failure and stroke.

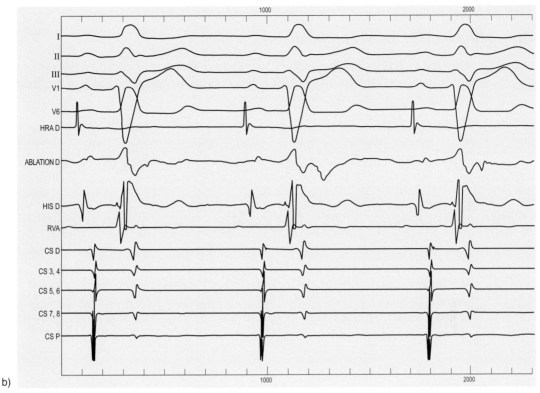

b)

Figure 14.11 (*Cont'd*)
Radiofrequency ablation of accessory pathway in Wolff–Parkinson–White syndrome (paper speed 100 mm/s). (b) Post ablation – the pattern of activation in coronary sinus is completely different as activation is now through the atrioventricular node

CLASSIFICATION

- Paroxysmal – spontaneous reversion to sinus rhythm without treatment
- Persistent – requires pharmacological or electrical therapy to restore sinus rhythm
- Permanent – sinus rhythm cannot be restored despite treatment.

PATHOPHYSIOLOGY

A variety of conditions are associated with atrial fibrillation, but the most common causes are hypertension, valvular heart disease, ischaemic heart disease and cardiac failure. It is now recognized that a subset of paroxysmal atrial fibrillation has a triggered mechanism. This is frequently due to ectopic focal atrial activity arising from the ostia of the pulmonary veins or other intracardiac structures. Thereafter, AF may be maintained by a reentry mechanism whereby multiple wavelets are perpetuated within the atria. Electrical and structural remodelling of the atria occurs which in turn predisposes and maintains further AF ('AF begets AF').

TREATMENT

Anticoagulation in atrial fibrillation (see Ch. 26)

Intra-atrial thrombus formation, especially in the left atrial appendage, may result in embolic stroke. The risk of stroke averages about 4% per year but is dependent on associated conditions.

The highest risk factors are patients with mitral valve disease, prosthetic heart valves and prior ischaemic attack or stroke, where anticoagulation with warfarin is absolutely indicated. Warfarin should also be considered (with a target INR 2–3) in the following groups:

- Hypertension
- Age >75 years
- Poor LV function
- Diabetes mellitus.

Patients are considered low risk if aged <65 years, without the above risk factors and have a structurally normal heart. They may be treated with aspirin instead. Paroxysmal AF has a similar risk of stroke as permanent AF, if the same risk factors are taken into account.

Rhythm control

In patients with new onset or symptomatic AF, it is desirable to restore and maintain sinus rhythm. The likelihood of restoration or maintenance of sinus rhythm is low in the following groups:

- Long duration (over 1 year)
- Large left atrium (over 4.5 cm)
- LV dysfunction
- Older age.

External DC cardioversion has a success rate of over 80%. Initial success rate is directly related to duration of atrial fibrillation. Of those successfully cardioverted only 50% will remain in sinus rhythm at 12 months. Anticoagulation with warfarin (target INR 2–3) for at least 3 weeks is advocated in AF lasting more than 48 hours prior to cardioversion. Atrial stunning is recognized after cardioversion and thromboembolism may occur in up to 10% of these patients. Therefore, anticoagulation is generally continued for a further 4 weeks.

Transoesophageal echocardiography may help to exclude patients from cardioversion if left atrial appendage thrombus is demonstrated.

Class IC antiarrhythmic drugs, flecainide and propafenone, are safe and effective agents for chemical cardioversion of AF in patients without structural heart disease. Amiodarone is a useful adjunct in cardioversion and maintenance of sinus rhythm. Most other drugs will only control rate.

Recently, RF ablation has been successful in selected patients with paroxysmal AF. Advanced mapping techniques allow precise localization of premature atrial activity to target focal ablation. Pulmonary vein isolation techniques empirically ablate one or all pulmonary veins and prevent the foci from conducting to the atrium to initiate AF (Fig. 14.12). Long-term success rates approximate 70%.

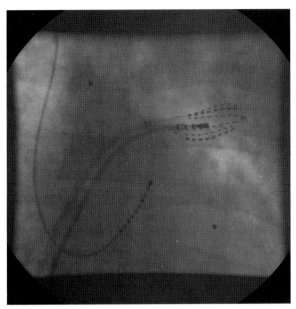

Figure 14.12
Pulmonary vein isolation using a basket catheter to guide ablation. Fluoroscopic image showing the basket catheter and an ablation catheter positioned within the left upper pulmonary vein. A coronary sinus catheter used for pacing during the procedure is also displayed

Rate control

Digoxin is frequently insufficient when used as a sole agent in ventricular rate control in AF, particularly during exercise. Combination therapy with a beta-blocker or verapamil provides much better rate control and symptomatic relief. In heart failure, a combination of digoxin with bisoprolol or carvedilol is warranted, whereas amiodarone can be considered in resistant cases.

Complete AV nodal ablation with catheter ablation is recommended when patients are severely symptomatic after failures in multiple drug therapy (Fig. 14.13). It is the most effective way of rate control and improving quality of life in these patients. However, there is a need for permanent pacing and a small risk of sudden death (about 2%) in the long term.

Electrical device therapy

Device-based therapy for AF includes specialized pacing devices and implantable atrial defibrillators. Dedicated AF pacing algorithms to prevent AF are beneficial to selected

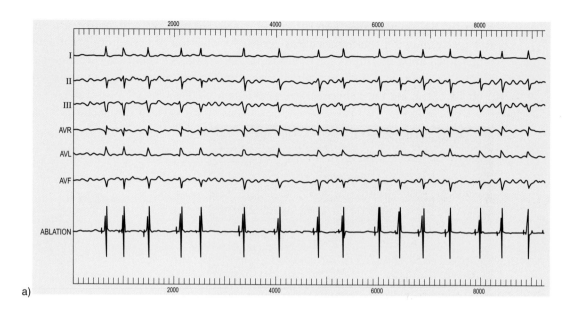

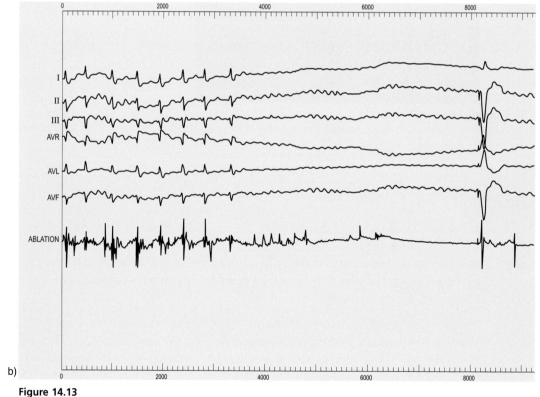

Figure 14.13
Induction of complete heart block in a patient with atrial fibrillation. (a) Pre-ablation – note the deflection in the ablation catheter before each ventricular electrogram representing the His electrogram
(b) While delivering radiofrequency energy complete heart block is induced and the patient is paced

patients only. Atrial defibrillators may reduce symptoms, hospital admissions, and quality of life but current experience is limited.

ATRIAL FLUTTER

Atrial flutters are intra-atrial macro re-entrant tachycardias. The flutter rates may vary between 250 to 350 bpm. Atrial flutter may have different morphologies.

CLASSIFICATION

- Typical atrial flutter
  – counterclockwise ('common flutter': 90%)
  – clockwise
- Atypical atrial flutter
- Surgical scar related atrial flutter (incisional tachycardia).

PATHOPHYSIOLOGY

Typical atrial flutter has the classical 'saw-tooth' baseline appearance on the surface ECG (Fig. 14.14). It results from a distinct anatomical re-entrant circuit. The impulse circulates in a caudal–cranial direction up the interatrial septum and down the right free wall in an anticlockwise manner. The narrow ridge of muscle isthmus between the tricuspid valve ring and the inferior vena cava (cavo-tricuspid isthmus) provides the slow conduction zone of the circuit (Fig. 14.15).

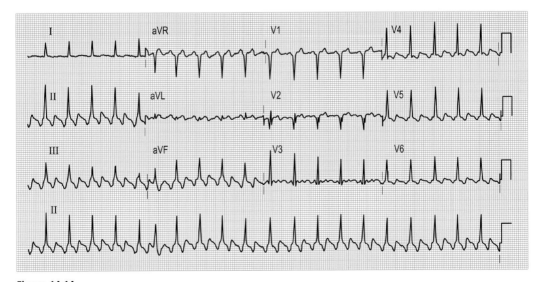

Figure 14.14
12-lead electrocardiograph showing typical anticlockwise atrial flutter (common flutter) identified by the negative flutter waves in the inferior leads

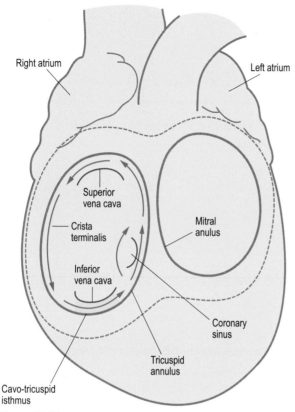

Figure 14.15
The typical atrial flutter circuit. The anatomical correlates of the circuit and the direction of the impulse are shown. The cavo-tricuspid isthmus (highlighted in yellow) is the site for catheter ablation

TREATMENT

Ablation across the cavo-tricuspid isthmus terminates atrial flutter (Fig. 14.16). Success rate exceeds 95%. Catheter ablation is therefore rapidly becoming the treatment of choice for atrial flutter.

VENTRICULAR TACHYCARDIA AND FIBRILLATION

Sudden cardiac death is most commonly due to ventricular tachyarrhythmias. Ventricular tachycardia (VT) is defined as three or more beats of tachycardia of more than 100 bpm originating from the ventricle (Fig. 14.17). Non-sustained VT refers to VT lasting less than 30 s. Sustained VT may degenerate into ventricular fibrillation (VF) resulting in death.

Monomorphic VT is an organized tachycardia with a re-entry mechanism often around scarred myocardium. Polymorphic VT is a disorganized tachycardia due to triggered activity and is probably sustained by re-entry mechanisms. Torsade de pointes refers to a

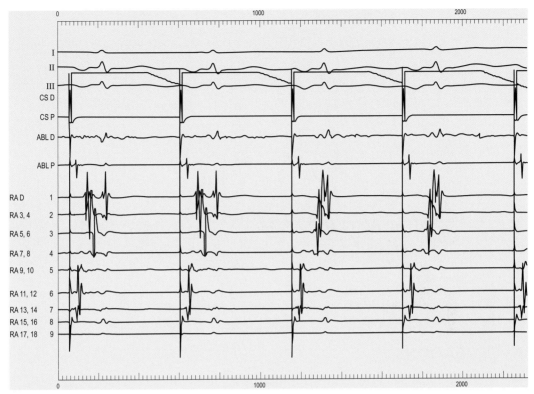

Figure 14.16
Atrial flutter ablation. The transition from normal conduction to conduction block across the cavo-tricuspid isthmus is identified by the change in the activation sequence in the right atrial electrograms with coronary sinus pacing. The first two beats show conduction across the isthmus with relatively early activation seen in the distal right atrial electrograms. The second two beats show a long delay in activation in the same electrograms as they have to be activated via the rest of the right atrium rather than across the isthmus

CS, coronary sinus; D, distal; P, proximal; ABL, ablation catheter; RA, right atrium

form of polymorphic VT with a characteristic 'twisting around the baseline' appearance on the ECG.

DIFFERENTIATION FROM SUPRAVENTRICULAR TACHYCARDIA

Many criteria exist with different complexity but are often impractical clinically. The most important characteristics of VT are:

- A–V dissociation. Visible independent atrial and ventricular activity at different rates.
- Capture beats. Occasional normal QRS complexes within a broad complex tachycardia due to intermittent AV node conduction.
- Fusion beats. Intermittent bizarre QRS complexes during tachycardia due to simultaneous atrial and ventricular activity.
- Extreme QRS axis: −90–180°.

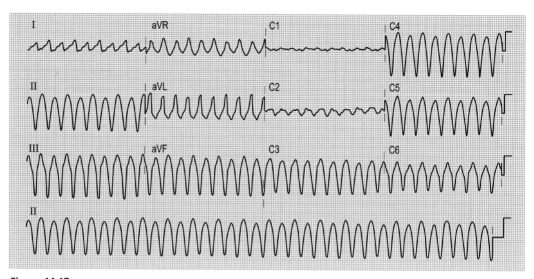

Figure 14.17
12-lead electrocardiograph showing monomorphic ventricular tachycardia. Note the broad complexes, abnormal axis and right bundle branch block morphology

INVESTIGATIONS

The initial aim is to identify the underlying disease substrate, such as ischaemic heart disease or cardiomyopathy. LV function assessment with echocardiography or ventriculography is essential for risk stratification. The electrophysiological study attempts to induce VT, so as to identify the mechanisms that may be amenable to ablation, and may provide prognostic information (Fig. 14.18).

TREATMENT

Pharmacological treatment

Drug therapy offers no significant protection for sudden cardiac death. However, antiarrhythmic drugs reduce patient symptoms and are effective in VT with a structurally normal heart.

Amiodarone is probably the safest agent. It carries a very low incidence of torsade de pointes. Intravenous lidocaine is now the second choice in peri-arrest situations due to the lack of supporting clinical evidence.

In torsade de pointes, the offending medication should be stopped, and intravenous magnesium and potassium considered. In refractory cases, the placement of a temporary pacemaker wire with overdrive pacing is most effective in suppressing tachycardia. Beta-blockers are given if no obvious cause of QT prolongation is identified.

Device therapy

See section on implantable cardioverter defibrillators (below).

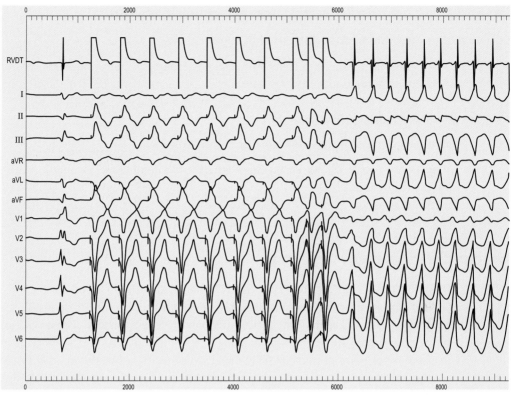

Figure 14.18
Ventricular tachycardia induced during an electrophysiological study. There are eight paced beats and then two extra stimuli delivered that induce ventricular tachycardia

Radiofrequency ablation therapy

Monomorphic VT due to reentry may be treatable with ablation. In ischaemic VT, success rates vary between 50 and 70%. Frequently, multiple morphologies of VTs are found in a patient, some of which may not be tolerated haemodynamically, making ablation difficult. Nevertheless, RF ablation is a useful adjunct to reduce symptoms and number of shocks in patients with implantable cardioverter defibrillators (ICDs).

VENTRICULAR TACHYCARDIA IN THE STRUCTURALLY NORMAL HEART

Certain forms of VT in the context of a structurally normal heart carry a more 'benign' outcome. They have specific ECG appearances during tachycardia and are highly amenable to catheter ablation treatment.

Right-ventricular outflow tract tachycardia

ECG: left bundle branch block pattern with inferior axis

Beta-blockers are usually effective.

Idiopathic left-ventricular tachycardia (fascicular tachycardia)

ECG: right bundle branch block pattern with superior axis

> This is caused by trigger activity from the posteroapical septum. It is responsive to beta-blockers or verapamil.

Bundle branch re-entry tachycardia

ECG: left bundle branch block pattern with superior axis

> This is common in idiopathic cardiomyopathy. It can be cured by ablation of the right bundle branch.

SUDDEN CARDIAC DEATH

> Sudden cardiac death presents a major public health problem. It is responsible for 50% of all cardiac deaths. The majority (80%) are due to coronary artery disease. Out-of-hospital resuscitation rates are very low, averaging 1 to 3% in most cities. A number of studies have focussed on primary prevention of sudden cardiac death by identifying risk factors. In this section, the sudden death syndromes with genetically based abnormalities are discussed.

HYPERTROPHIC CARDIOMYOPATHY (see Ch. 13)

> It is an inherited disorder of cardiac sarcomeric proteins leading to LV asymmetrical hypertrophy and dysfunction. Risk factors for sudden death are:
>
> - previous cardiac arrest
> - family history of sudden death
> - syncope
> - extreme LV hypertrophy (>3 cm)
> - documented nonsustained VT
> - cardiac troponin T mutation.
>
> In these subgroups of patients, the implantation of ICDs to prevent sudden death should be strongly considered.

LONG QT SYNDROME

> This familial disorder is characterized by QT prolongation on the ECG (Fig. 14.19) and polymorphic VT caused by specific cardiac ion channel mutations. There is currently no acceptable test for risk stratification. Traditional treatment options include beta-blockers, sympathetic denervation, and cardiac pacing. ICD is currently recommended in patients who have survived a cardiac arrest, but indications may be extended to others at high risk.

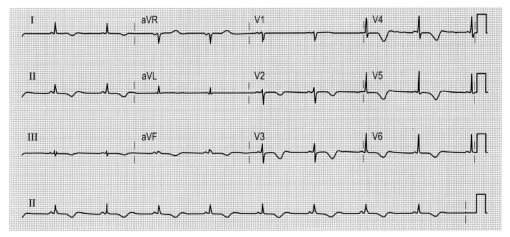

Figure 14.19
12-lead electrocardiograph showing abnormally prolonged QT duration

BRUGADA SYNDROME

This autosomal dominant disease is caused by mutations of the sodium channel gene resulting in abnormal cardiac repolarization. There is transient ST elevations in leads V1–V3 and partial RBBB.

EPSs are not useful in risk stratification. ICDs are recommended for:

- family history of sudden death
- syncope
- inducible ventricular arrhythmias.

ARRHYTHMOGENIC RIGHT-VENTRICULAR DYSPLASIA (see Ch. 13)

This is a cardiomyopathy whereby myocardium is replaced by fibro-fatty tissue. It predominantly involves the right ventricle but may progress to the left ventricle. The unique features on the ECG are the inverted T waves with epsilon waves in V1–V3. Investigations should include cardiac catheterization, echocardiography and magnetic resonance imaging. Only the ICD offers prevention of sudden death.

IMPLANTABLE CARDIOVERTER DEFIBRILLATORS (ICD)

It has been over 20 years since Mirowski implanted the first ICD in a human. The ICD is now a well-established therapy in the primary and secondary prevention of sudden cardiac death. The implantation procedure has simplified dramatically in the last decade from formal thoracotomy and placement of epicardial patches to one not too dissimilar to endocardial permanent pacemaker insertion (Fig. 14.20). Whilst the ICD does not prevent

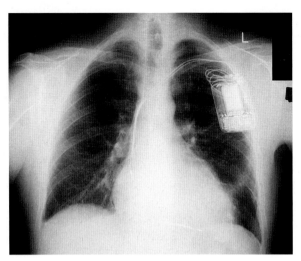

Figure 14.20
Chest X-ray showing a dual chamber implantable cardioverter defibrillator

the onset of ventricular arrhythmias, it promptly terminates them by means of antitachycardia pacing (Fig. 14.21) or shock delivery.

There is substantial evidence that ICDs reduce mortality in specific patient groups. The major clinical studies of ICD in the prevention of sudden cardiac death are summarized below.

SECONDARY PREVENTION STUDIES

Antiarrhythmics Versus Implantable Defibrillators Trial

The trial involved patients with previous myocardial infarction presenting with poorly tolerated VT or VF (syncope or cardiac arrest); LV ejection fraction was <40%. Over 1000 patients were randomized to ICD or drug therapy (amiodarone or sotalol). Significant mortality benefit in favour of ICD therapy was found (75% in ICD group vs. 64% in antiarrhythmic drug group survived).

The Cardiac Arrest Study Hamburg (CASH), and Canadian Implantable Defibrillator Study (CIDS) are similar prospective randomized trials showing similar mortality benefits of ICDs over drug therapy.

PRIMARY PREVENTION STUDIES

Multicenter Automatic Defibrillator Implantation Trial (MADIT)

The trial involved patients with prior myocardial infarction, ejection fraction of <35%, and spontaneous or inducible sustained VT. Two hundred patients were randomized to ICD or conventional therapy. The results were that ICD reduced overall mortality by 54%.

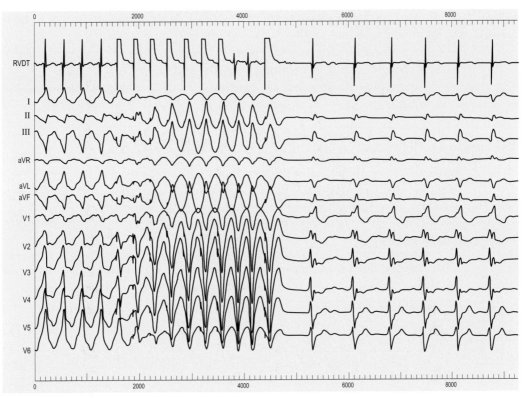

Figure 14.21
Diagram showing antitachycardia pacing. Ventricular tachycardia (VT) is successfully pace terminated by delivering nine bursts at a shorter interval than the VT. This successfully terminates the tachycardia

The results of the Multicenter Unsustained Tachycardia Trial (MUSTT) closely resemble those of MADIT, with significant mortality benefit in the ICD treatment arm.

Multicenter Automatic Defibrillator Implantation Trial II

This trial involved patients with prior MI, however, the ejection fraction was now <30%. Over 1200 patients were randomized to ICD or conventional therapy. Again ICDs reduced mortality, this time by 30%.

The results of MADIT II are particularly significant. For the first time, a simple risk stratification method (ejection fraction) for ICD implantation can now be applied to patients without the need for the EPS. The impact on reduction of sudden cardiac deaths in the general population at large is likely to be significant.

INDICATIONS FOR IMPLANTABLE CARDIOVERTER DEFIBRILLATORS

Guidelines for implantation of ICDs have been published by the American College of Cardiology and the European Society of Cardiology. At present, strong evidence supports the implantation of ICDs under the following conditions:

207

- Aborted sudden death or syncope due to VT or VF in the absence of acute myocardial infarction (<48 hours)
- Old myocardial infarction with poor LV function (EF<30%) and inducible VT or VF
- Syncope with poor LV function (EF<40%) and inducible VT or VF
- Non-sustained VT and with LV function (EF<40%) and inducible sustained VT or VF.

POTENTIAL PITFALLS AND SELECTION OF DEVICES

Implantation of ICDs carries the same inherent complications as in permanent pacing. In addition, there are potential specific complications associated with ICDs. These problems should always be referred to an electrophysiologist.

Inappropriate shocks

These may be due to supraventricular tachycardias, e.g. atrial fibrillation. Detection algorithms use tachycardia onset pattern or morphological changes. Careful programming can usually avoid inappropriate shocks.

Electrical storm

This is a recognized but poorly understood phenomenon in which episodes of recurrent VT or VF occur in rapid succession. Any reversible precipitating cause of VT should be corrected. Antiarrhythmic medication may need to be adjusted, and the ICD may need reprogramming.

Interaction with drug therapy

The concurrent use of antiarrhythmic therapy in ICD patients is sometimes essential to reduce the number of shocks. However, amiodarone may raise the defibrillation threshold. It is necessary to recheck the threshold after initiation of these drugs to ensure that the device can deliver therapy with an adequate safety margin.

Driving restrictions in the UK

ICD implantation in any patient permanently bars Group II driving. Group I drivers may resume driving 6 months following ICD implant if the device has not delivered shock therapy for 6 months and if no incapacity has resulted from device therapy in the preceding 5 years.

CARDIAC RESYNCHRONIZATION THERAPY

Many patients with heart failure remain symptomatic despite treatment with diuretics, ACE inhibitors, beta-blockers and spironolactone. Approximately 30–50% have intraventricular conduction defects, such as LBBB. This leads to discoordinated contraction of a dysfunctional left ventricle. Cardiac resynchronization therapy (CRT) involves biventricular pacing, with simultaneous left and right heart pacing. It is achieved by placement of a LV lead, usually into a left lateral cardiac vein via the coronary sinus, in addition to the conventional RV lead (Fig. 14.22 a, b).

Prospective randomized trials have demonstrated improvement in morbidity with CRT, however, mortality data are awaited. Many patients with indications for CRT will also be at high risk of sudden cardiac death. A number of devices are available that combine both features – CRT and ICDs.

SYNCOPE

Syncope is defined as sudden transient loss of consciousness due to loss of cerebral blood flow, followed by spontaneous recovery. It accounts for 6% of acute medical and 3% of casualty admissions.

Cardiovascular causes of syncope can be classified as:

- neurocardiogenic (vasovagal)
- carotid sinus syncope
- postural hypotension

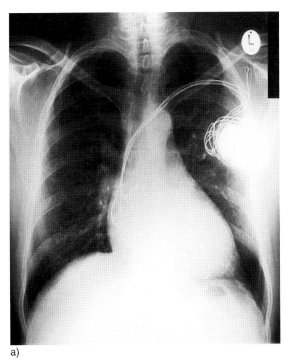
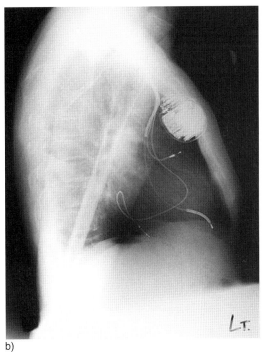

a)   b)

Figure 14.22
(a and b) Chest X-rays (frontal and lateral) showing a resynchronization implantable cardioverter defibrillator. The left-ventricular lead is implanted into the left posterolateral marginal vein

- situational syncope: micturition, coughing
- cardiac arrhythmias: sinus node disease, high grade AV conduction block, ventricular tachyarrhythmias
- structural heart disease: aortic stenosis, hypertrophic obstructive cardiomyopathy, mitral stenosis, severe cardiac ischaemia, pulmonary hypertension/embolism.

A detailed and focused history taking and clinical examination is paramount. During clinical evaluation it is important to look for postural hypotension and carotid sinus hypersensitivity with carotid sinus massage.

A 12-lead ECG may establish the diagnosis in 5% of cases. Echocardiography helps to rule out significant structural heart disease. However, 24-hour ambulatory ECG has a low diagnostic value unless symptoms occur daily or fortuitously whilst the patient is being monitored. Other important investigations include the tilt table test, EPS, and the implantable loop recorder. Generally, a pause of >3 s is felt to be significant (on ambulatory monitoring or carotid sinus massage) and may warrant consideration of a pacemaker.

TILT TABLE TEST

In a head-up tilt test, the table is angled at 70°. It is currently the investigation of choice for vasovagal syncope (Fig. 14.23). Unfortunately, the result is not reproducible in 15–25% making this test less useful in predicting efficacy of therapy. Haemodynamic responses to tilt testing are classified as shown below.

Type 1: mixed

- Heart rate more than 40 bpm without asystole for >3 s
- Blood pressure falls before heart rate.

Type 2A: cardioinhibitory

- Asystole for >3 s or heart rate lower than 40 bpm
- Blood pressure falls before heart rate.

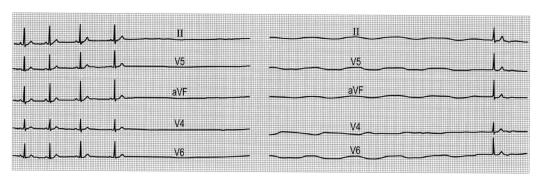

Figure 14.23
An electrocardiograph tracing showing a significant cardioinhibitory response to tilt table testing. Sudden bradycardia leading to asystole and syncope is demonstrated

Type 2B: cardioinhibitory

- Asystole for >3 s or heart rate lower than 40 bpm
- Blood pressure falls after heart rate.

Type 3: pure vasodepressor

- Heart rate does not fall more than 10%
- Blood pressure falls to cause syncope.

ELECTROPHYSIOLOGICAL STUDY

Electrophysiological study (EPS) is useful in patients suspected to have ventricular arrhythmias, such as ischaemic heart disease and cardiomyopathy. It is less sensitive in diagnosing sinus node dysfunction or AV nodal conduction abnormalities. Patients with a positive EPS have a higher mortality than those with a negative test. However, a negative EPS is not reassuring because it is still associated with significant mortality (approximately 7% in 2 years).

IMPLANTABLE LOOP RECORDER

An implantable loop recorder (ILR) is a small device with two sensing electrodes, and is able to record a single-lead electrogram. Implantation is in an infraclavicular pre-pectoral pocket. Manual activation of the device may record events up to 40 min before. Newer devices can be activated automatically by sudden bradycardia or tachycardia (Fig. 14.24). It is invaluable in the diagnosis in patients with infrequent syncope since the battery life lasts for 14–18 months.

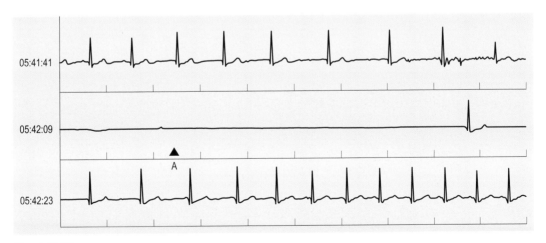

Figure 14.24
An electrocardiograph tracing from an implantable loop recorder. The patient activated the device when symptoms started (A). A significant pause has been documented followed by restoration of sinus rhythm

Further reading

Abraham WT 2002 Cardiac resynchronization therapy for heart failure: biventricular pacing and beyond. Curr Opin Cardiol 17(4): 346–352

Calkins H, Zipes DP 2001 Hypotension and syncope. In: Braunwald E, Zipes DP, Libby P. Heart disease: a textbook of cardiovascular medicine, 6th edn. WB Saunders, Philadelphia, pp. 932–940

Calkins H 2001 Radiofrequency catheter ablation of supraventricular arrhythmias. Heart 85: 594–600

Fogoros RN 1999 Electrophysiological testing, 3rd edn. Blackwell Science, Oxford

Fuster V, Ryden LE, Asinger RW et al. 2001 ACC/AHA/ESC guidelines for the management of patients with atrial fibrillation: executive summary: A report of the American College of Cardiology/American Heart Association Task Force on Practice Guidelines and the European Society of Cardiology Committee for Practice Guidelines and Policy Conferences. Circulation 104(17): 2118–2150

Hayes DL, Zipes DP 2001 Cardiac pacemakers and cardioverter-defibrillators. In: Braunwald E, Zipes DP, Libby P (eds) Heart disease: a textbook of cardiovascular medicine, 6th edn. WB Saunders, Philadelphia, pp. 775–814

Huikuri HV, Castellanos A, Myerburg RJ 2001 Sudden death due to cardiac arrhythmias. N Engl J Med 345(20): 1473–1482

Josephson ME 2002 Clinical cardiac electrophysiology: techniques and interpretations, 3rd edn. Lippincott Williams & Wilkins, Maryland

Moss AJ, Zareba W, Hall WJ et al. 2002 Prophylactic implantation of a defibrillator in patients with myocardial infarction and reduced ejection fraction. N Engl J Med 346(12): 877–883

Roden DM 2000 Antiarrhythmic drugs: from mechanisms to clinical practice. Heart 84: 339–346

Weigner MJ, Buxton AE 2001 Nonsustained ventricular tachycardia. A guide to the clinical significance and management. Med Clin North Am 85(2): 305–320

Wellens HJJ 2001 Ventricular tachycardia: diagnosis of broad QRS complex tachycardia. Heart 86: 579–585

SELF-ASSESSMENT

Questions

1. A 48-year-old man is admitted to the acute admissions ward with a 4-hour history of cardiac sounding chest pain. He has previously been fit and well apart from hypertension. He is haemodynamically stable. His pain has responded to diamorphine. His ECG shows an acute inferior myocardial infarction with 2:1 heart block.
   a. How are you going to manage his bradycardia?
   b. Would you thrombolyse him straight away?

He suddenly goes into complete heart block with a barely recordable blood pressure and he loses consciousness.

   c. What is you management?

He remains in complete heart block 7 days after admission.

   d. What would be your further management?

2. A 35-year-old male presents with a 5-year history of episodic palpitations. He presented to the A&E department 18 months previously with a syncopal episode following an alcohol binge. His general practitioner has sent him to you in outpatients for further management of his palpitations. Examination is normal. His 12-lead ECG is shown in Figure 14.25.
   a. What is the ECG diagnosis?
   b. What advice would you give him regarding his 'risk' and long-term prognosis?
   c. Which drugs would you consider in his management?

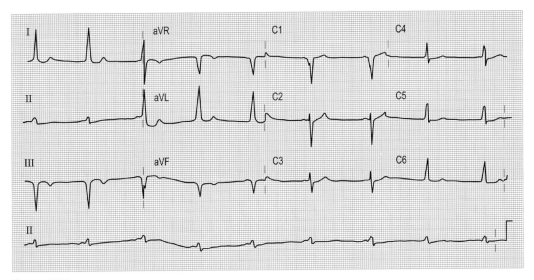

Figure 14.25

Answers

1. a. As he is asymptomatic and stable you should elect to monitor the rhythm carefully. If there was any evidence of deteriorating atrioventricular conduction (e.g. broad complexes or higher degree block) then you should consider temporary pacing.

   b. Thrombolysis should not be delayed for his 2:1 heart block. It is quite likely that his rhythm will improve with thrombolysis. If he had had an anterior myocardial infarction your management may be different. Thrombolysis should still, however, not be delayed. You would have a lower threshold for temporary pacing. Patients should be judged individually on their own merits. For example, a patient with an anterior MI and transient asymptomatic 2:1 heart block may be managed without a temporary pacing wire, but with a low threshold to place one if necessary. Complete heart block with an anterior myocardial infarction carries with it a very poor prognosis as it is generally associated with an extensive area of myocardial infarction and has a high incidence of cardiogenic shock.

   c. A bolus of atropine 1 mg may transiently improve the heart rate to allow siting of a temporary pacing wire. In this situation external pacing should be considered whilst the patient is prepared for a temporary pacing wire. The patient may need sedation with an intravenous benzodiazepine as he regains consciousness. If external pacing facilities are not available an adrenaline infusion may be appropriate. Intravenous isoprenaline should not be used.

2. a. His ECG shows pre-excitation with a short PR interval and delta waves. He, therefore, has Wolff-Parkinson-White syndrome (WPW).

   b. It is possible that his syncopal episode was a result of alcohol-induced atrial fibrillation with rapid antegrade conduction down the accessory pathway. The frequency of tachycardia in patients with WPW increases with age from 10% in the 20–39-year-old age group to 36% in those >60 years. Up to 30% of these tachycardias will be atrial fibrillation. It is impossible to directly assess risk as the antegrade properties of the pathway are unknown, i.e. the pathway may or may not have the ability to conduct rapidly during atrial fibrillation. However, as he has had a syncopal episode he must be at a significant risk. Therefore, he should be considered for further electrophysiological evaluation with a view to ablation.

   c. Drugs to be avoided are those that prolong conduction time and refractoriness of the atrioventricular node, i.e. verapamil, propanolol and digoxin. Drugs that prolong refractoriness of the pathway are preferred, i.e. class 1A and 1C drugs. Amiodarone or sotalol can be used as they prolong refractoriness of both the atrioventricular node and the pathway. This patient went on to have his pathway ablated. The point at which pre-excitation disappeared is shown in Figure 14.26.

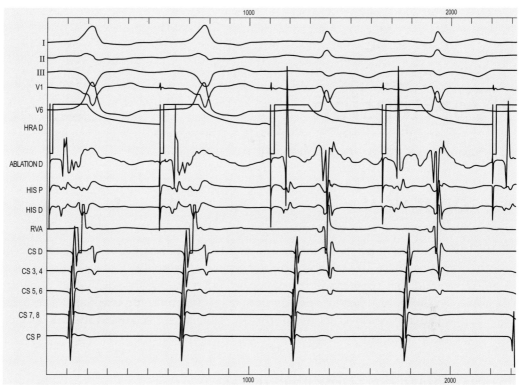

Figure 14.26
The first two beats with atrial pacing are preexcited. Note the surface electrocardiograph at the top of the image. In addition the pattern of activation in the coronary sinus electrograms shows a right-sided accessory pathway. The last two beats show sinus rhythm with conduction antegradely through the atrioventricular node

Hypertension

15

J. R. Wright and P. A. Kalra

INTRODUCTION

Hypertension is very common, and as it is a major risk factor for the development of cardiovascular disease it is the leading cause of morbidity and mortality in the Western world.[1] This chapter will review the definition and basic epidemiology of hypertension, the pathophysiology of and appropriate investigations for essential and secondary hypertension, as well as considering the rationale for treatment regimes, including the special situations of pregnancy-related hypertension and hypertensive crisis.

DEFINITION OF HYPERTENSION

Our current definition of hypertension arises from two main sources of evidence. Firstly, epidemiological studies have investigated the effects of different systolic and diastolic blood pressures within the general population, relating the different sub-sets of blood pressure to eventual cardiovascular events. The MRFIT study is just such an example.[2] This involved approximately 350 000 men who had no previous history of heart disease, and they were followed up for a mean period of over 11 years. Table 15.1 shows that the

Table 15.1: Baseline blood pressure and relative risk of mortality of men screened for MRFIT

Category of blood pressure	Percentage	Relative risk of IHD mortality	Relative risk of stroke mortality
Optimal	18.2%	1.00	1.00
Normal	24.5%	1.31	1.73
High normal	22.2%	1.61	2.14
Stage I hypertension	25.9%	2.33	3.58
Stage II hypertension	7.1%	3.20	6.90
Stage III hypertension	1.7%	4.64	9.66
Stage IV hypertension	0.4%	6.88	19.19

relative risk of mortality from ischaemic heart disease and stroke increased sequentially as blood pressure increased. Patients with a blood pressure of >180/110 mmHg had a 4.6-fold ischaemic heart disease (IHD) and almost 10-fold stroke mortality risk compared to patients with optimal blood pressure (Fig. 15.1).

Clinical trial data, incorporating therapeutic interventions for hypertension, also provide important evidence as blood pressure targets can be related to cardiovascular outcomes. In the Hypertension Optimal Treatment (HOT) study almost 19 000 patients with diastolic hypertension were randomized to one of three different diastolic blood pressure targets (<90, <85 and <80 mmHg).[3] Patients in the lowest blood pressure group were significantly less likely to suffer cardiovascular events.

There is now agreement that both systolic and diastolic hypertension are associated with increased likelihood of cardiovascular disease, and hence the blood pressure definitions shown in Table 15.2, which are derived from the Joint National Committee (JNC).[4] We now recognize optimal (<120/80 mmHg), normal (<130/85 mmHg) and high-normal blood pressure ranges; thereafter, hypertension is divided into three stages: stage 1 – mild (>140/90 mmHg) to stage 3 – severe (>180/110 mmHg). The JNC also recognize stage 4 hypertension (accelerated phase). This classification is of prognostic significance for morbidity and mortality.

Table 15.2: JNC VI stratification of hypertension[4]

Category of blood pressure	Systolic BP (mmHg)	Diastolic BP (mmHg)
Optimal	<120	<80
Normal	<130	<85
High normal	130–139	85–89
Stage I hypertension	140–159	90–99
Stage II hypertension	160–179	100–109
Stage III hypertension	>180	>110

DIAGNOSIS OF HYPERTENSION

This requires two or more elevated blood pressure readings on two or more separate occasions. Correct assessment of blood pressure with a sphygmomanometer necessitates the use of an appropriately sized cuff for the patient's arm circumference, and accurate recording of the Korotkoff sounds (IV and V). There is considerable diurnal variation in an individual's blood pressure; daytime variation is due to both physical and emotional activity. During the night, blood pressure falls by approximately 20% in line with decreased sympathetic nervous system (SNS) activity. Failure of this night time 'dip' is associated with left-ventricular hypertrophy (LVH). In view of this variation, accurate diagnosis of hypertension may require home monitoring and recording of blood pressure by the patient or the use of 24-hour ambulatory blood pressure monitoring (ABPM). The latter can provide the clinician with an immense amount of information. However, the equipment is expensive and, therefore, ABPM should be used in selected patients, such as in those with suspected white coat hypertension, for assessment of nocturnal variability in blood pressure and in the clinical trial setting.

EPIDEMIOLOGY AND AETIOLOGICAL CLASSIFICATION

At least 13% of the UK population and, because of genetic predisposition, as many as 25% of the US population, are affected by hypertension. Table 15.3 shows data from one study of over 12 000 UK adults (aged >16 years); even when using a cut-off blood pressure of >160/95 mmHg the prevalence of hypertension was found to be 19.5%.[5] The prevalence increased with age and was slightly greater in women.

Essential (primary) hypertension accounts for 90% of all hypertensive patients. The other 10% have secondary hypertension (Box 15.1) most commonly due to renal parenchymal disease (3%), renal artery disease (2%), primary hyperaldosteronism (2% – most often associated with bilateral adrenal hyperplasia) and drugs (2%). Rarer causes such as other endocrine disorders (e.g. phaeochromocytoma, Cushing's disease) and aortic co-arctation account for less than 1% of all cases. Pregnancy is a very common, but short-term, cause of secondary hypertension.

Table 15.3: Prevalence of hypertension in the UK adult population (hypertension defined as BP >160/95 mmHg or on treatment)

	All ages	Age (years)			
		45–54	55–64	65–74	>75
Men	18.6%	17.2%	34.9%	52.4%	51.8%
Women	20.2%	14.2%	33.9%	57.0%	66.5%

Box 15.1: Major causes of secondary hypertension

Endocrine – primary aldosteronism, Cushing's syndrome, phaeochromocytoma, hyperthyroidism, hyperparathyroidism, acromegaly, carcinoid

Renal – renal parenchymal disease (any type), renovascular disease

Co-arctation of the aorta

Pregnancy

Drugs – oral contraceptive pill, mineralocorticoids, glucocorticoids, non-steroidal anti-inflammatories, sympathomimetics (e.g. in cold remedies), erythropoietin, ciclosporin, monoamine oxidase inhibitors, alcohol and recreational drugs

Neurogenic hypertension – increased SNS activity, decreased parasympathetic nervous system activity, increased circulating renin levels

Neurological hypertension – increased intracranial pressure, spinal cord injury

Intravascular volume overload

PATHOGENESIS OF HYPERTENSION

ESSENTIAL (PRIMARY) HYPERTENSION

Genetic factors are thought to be important in essential hypertension and indeed a family history is often elicited. The SNS and renin–angiotensin system (RAS) both play an important role in the pathogenesis, but it is felt that the handling of sodium by the kidney may be one of the key factors in long-term blood pressure control (which in turn is affected by SNS, RAS, etc.). Other environmental factors may contribute to hypertension in those predisposed, and these are shown in Box 15.2.

Sympathetic nervous system

Overactivity of the SNS is seen in certain patient groups prone to hypertension, namely African-Americans, those with obesity and/or insulin resistance, and patients with excessive alcohol intake. Elevation in blood pressure occurs by an increase in peripheral vascular resistance, an increase in heart rate and by noradrenaline release from the adrenal medulla. Intra-renal vasoconstriction is also seen with a consequent drop in renal perfusion and stimulation of the RAS.

Renin–angiotensin system

Release of angiotensin II after RAS stimulation (Fig. 15.2) leads to increased renal sodium reabsorption via an effect on the proximal tubular cells. Angiotensin II also has direct vasoconstrictive effects on systemic blood vessels. Renal sodium reabsorption in the distal and collecting tubules is mediated by aldosterone. Although absolute renin activity is increased in only 20% of all hypertensive subjects, in many other patients with essential hypertension the renin level relative to total body sodium levels may be disproportionately raised.[6]

Renal sodium handling

There is evidence to suggest that blood pressure may be directly influenced by salt intake. Hypertension is highly prevalent in populations with a high sodium intake (e.g. >4 g or 180 mmol per day), such as those people living in Northern Japan and the South East of

---

Box 15.2: The major epidemiological risk factors for essential hypertension

Genetic/familial association
Increasing age
Male sex
African-American origin
Insulin resistance
Obesity
High alcohol intake
High emotional stress

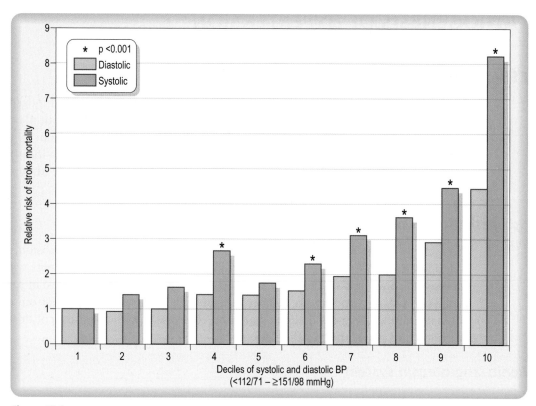

Figure 15.1
Relative risk of stroke mortality from Multiple Risk Factor Intervention Trial (MRFIT)

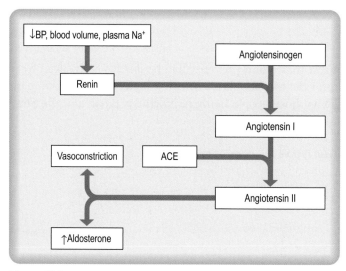

Figure 15.2
The renin–angiotensin system

the USA. Conversely, hypertension is almost unrecognized in populations who have minimal salt intake, such as Alaskan Eskimos and Amazon Indians.

Unifying hypothesis for pathogenesis of essential hypertension

The exact pathogenesis is undoubtedly complex and probably involves all of the above factors to a greater or lesser degree. It is hypothesized that the factors may be linked together as follows. Genetic factors predispose to increased SNS activity with consequent stimulation of the RAS and a rise in blood pressure. Initially, this rise may be corrected by renal autoregulatory mechanisms, afferent arteriolar vasoconstriction and tubulo-interstitial feedback. However, in time, glomerular ischaemia and intra-renal arteriosclerosis lead to renal damage and so to an acquired defect in sodium excretion.[7]

PATHOGENESIS OF RENAL-RELATED HYPERTENSION

There are several physical and hormonal factors which accompany the progressive nephron loss and structural changes of most chronic renal diseases. Increased renin release with stimulation of the RAS is likely in all disorders. A reduced sodium excretion often results from the fall in glomerular filtration rate (GFR), and hyperfiltration in remaining nephrons exacerbates a tendency to sodium retention by increasing the re-absorption of sodium. Clearly, in particular renal diseases one or other of these mechanisms may predominate (e.g. intense activation of the RAS in some patients with renal artery stenosis).

END ORGAN DAMAGE IN HYPERTENSION

CARDIOVASCULAR DISEASE

As previously stated, hypertension is a major risk factor for cardiovascular diseases, particularly coronary artery disease, stroke (Fig. 15.3) and peripheral vascular disease. LVH is a common accompaniment of long-standing hypertension (Fig. 15.4); it is associated with a risk of sudden death, but LVH can regress with time after optimal blood pressure control.

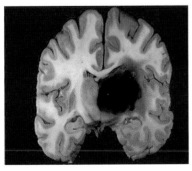

Figure 15.3
Consequences of hypertension: cerebral haemorrhage

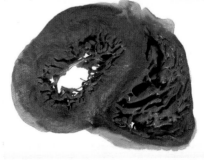

Figure 15.4
Consequences of hypertension: left-ventricular hypertrophy

RENAL DISEASE

The kidneys are at major risk of damage from hypertension; as discussed previously, several renal mechanisms contribute to the pathogenesis of hypertension, and so hypertensive renal injury is likely to exacerbate the hypertension. The first manifestation of renal damage is microalbuminuria (albumin excretion of 20–200 mg/day). With progressive injury persistent proteinuria (e.g. >0.5 g/day) may develop, and thereafter, impairment of renal function. Hypertensive renal injury is the second commonest cause (after diabetes) of end-stage renal disease (ESRD) in the USA. Figure 15.5 illustrates that increasing severity of hypertension is associated with progressively increasing relative risk of ESRD; patients with stage 3 hypertension are 12 times more likely to need dialysis than patients with optimal or normal blood pressure.

RETINOPATHY

The eyes are an important 'end organ' at risk of hypertensive injury (Fig. 15.6). Although moderate changes (e.g. arterio-venous nipping – grade 2 retinopathy) are seen in many patients, some patients are at risk of blindness from severe retinal ischaemia or haemorrhage.

INVESTIGATION OF THE PATIENT WITH HYPERTENSION

The investigation of the patient with hypertension has two main aims:

1. Search for secondary causes
2. Assessment of target organ damage.

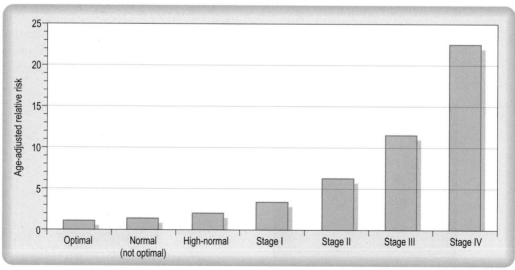

Figure 15.5
Relative risk of end-stage renal disease with increasing blood pressure

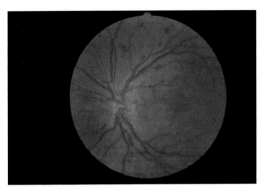

Figure 15.6
Consequences of hypertension: hypertensive retinopathy

In addition, ABPM may be indicated to confirm the diagnosis of hypertension as well as to assess the effect of treatment.

Clinical examination is important to assess some of the end organ effects of hypertension (e.g. retinopathy, LVH). In some cases of secondary hypertension the clinical examination will reveal important clues to underlying aetiology (e.g. radio-femoral delay in aortic co-arctation, classical appearance of Cushing's syndrome, or the presence of femoral, renal or epigastric bruits in patients with renal artery stenosis). However, the following basic investigations should be considered essential for all patients in whom hypertension proves difficult to control and in all young (age <50 years with no family history of hypertension) hypertensives:

- Biochemical profile (including calcium for rare cases of hyperparathyroidism, but especially potassium and renal function)
- Urine dipstick for proteinuria. If detectable, proceed to 24-hour urine collection for quantification of proteinuria (and creatinine clearance). Urinary dipstick should be performed at each clinic visit
- Chest X-ray
- Electrocardiogram (ECG) and echocardiogram (for LVH and cardiac function). If LVH is detected, follow-up echocardiography is advisable (e.g. 2 yearly)
- Renal ultrasound.

Other specific investigations may be indicated in individual cases, such as:

- Aldosterone:renin ratio
- 24-hour urinary catecholamine excretion
- Renal angiography.

In selecting patients for renal angiography, the highest degree of clinical suspicion of renovascular disease (RVD) will occur in patients with arterial bruits, ultrasonic discrepancy in renal size of >1.5 cm and evidence of co-morbid vascular disease. If a given patient has none of these three parameters, then RVD is highly unlikely – negative predictive value of 100% for significant renal artery stenosis.[8]

223

TREATMENT OF HYPERTENSION

The aim of hypertension treatment is to achieve the targets (recommended by the British Hypertension Society)[9] outlined in Table 15.4. For most patients a combination of pharmacological and lifestyle measures will be necessary. In all patients the lowering of blood pressure should be seen as a part of an overall reduction of cardiac risk, which includes advice on the complete cessation of smoking as well as cholesterol reduction below target levels. Drug compliance and regular follow-up of patients are of such fundamental importance that many centres now have hypertension nurse specialists leading clinics in an effort to improve patient education and overall hypertension management.

LIFESTYLE MEASURES

Of the many lifestyle measures advocated as part of a blood pressure lowering regimen, a graded weight-loss programme with realistic targets, remains the most beneficial.[10] An individually tailored exercise regime is usually appropriate, but a minority of patients are at risk of dangerous blood pressure elevations during exercise. Moderate alcohol consumption is known to be cardioprotective, but this effect depends on gender and race. Alcohol does stimulate the sympathetic nervous system and so excessive consumption should be discouraged. Salt restriction may be of some benefit to patients prone to salt-sensitive hypertension; however, such dietary restriction remains controversial for the general hypertensive population. Despite the importance of lifestyle changes, these are themselves unlikely to achieve optimal blood pressure targets in most patients, and so the vast majority of patients are likely to need pharmacological treatment as well.

PHARMACOLOGICAL MEASURES

A full discussion of the available therapeutic agents for treatment of hypertension is beyond the scope of this chapter. However, the mechanisms of action of the most commonly used groups of anti-hypertensive drugs are shown in Table 15.5, and several important considerations regarding drug therapy are worthy of emphasis:

- An understanding of the likely pathophysiology of a particular patient's hypertension enables selection of the most appropriate therapeutic agent to achieve control (e.g. diuretics, ACE inhibitors or angiotensin II receptor blockers in patients with sodium retention, beta-blockers or centrally-acting agents where increased SNS activity is important).

Table 15.4: Suggested blood pressure targets[9]

General population	<140/85 mmHg
Uncomplicated diabetic patients	<130/80 mmHg
Patients with proteinuria >1 g/day	<125/75 mmHg
Patients with renal impairment	<125/75 mmHg

Table 15.5: Mechanism of action of major classes of antihypertensive drugs

Drug class	Mechanism of action
Beta-blockers (β_1 and β_2), e.g. propanolol	Decrease heart rate, cardiac output, and central sympathetic outflow Relaxation of vascular smooth muscle
Calcium channel blockers, e.g. amlodipine	Vascular smooth muscle relaxation
Angiotensin converting enzyme (ACE) inhibitors, e.g. lisinopril	Inhibition of conversion of angiotensin I to angiotensin II
Angiotensin II receptor blockers, e.g. losartan	Blockade of angiotensin II receptors
Loop diuretics, e.g. frusemide	Decrease sodium, potassium and chloride absorption in the loop of Henlé
Thiazide diuretics, e.g. metolazone	Decrease sodium absorption in the distal tubule
Potassium sparing diuretics, e.g. spironolactone	Decrease sodium absorption in the collecting duct
α_1 blockers, e.g. doxazosin	Post-synaptic blockade at vascular smooth muscle causing relaxation
α_2 agonists, e.g. methlydopa	Decrease central sympathetic outflow
Imidazole agonist, e.g. moxonidine	Centrally-acting vasodilator

- Data from studies such as the UK Prospective Diabetes Studies (UKPDS) indicate that the use of several anti-hypertensive agents in combination is needed to achieve target blood pressure in many patients.[11]
- Certain classes of drugs are more effective in particular patient groups (Table 15.6).

SURGICAL AND INTERVENTIONAL MEASURES

In rare cases of endocrine hypertension (Cushing's disease, acromegaly, phaeochromocytoma) surgery may be necessary to control or cure hypertension. Renal revascularization by transluminal angioplasty with/without stenting (Fig. 15.7) can improve hypertension control in renovascular hypertension. Significant improvement in blood pressure may be expected after angioplasty in 80% of patients with fibromuscular disease and in 65% of cases with renal artery atheroma.[12]

SPECIFIC TYPES OF HYPERTENSION

WHITE-COAT HYPERTENSION

This phenomenon may account for 20% of patients with hypertensive blood pressure readings. Patients, often young women of low body weight, have raised blood pressure in

Table 15.6: Specific benefits to patient groups of differing classes of anti-hypertensive drugs

Patient group	Drug class	Reason
Uncomplicated	See Fig. 15.9 for current recommendations	Standard therapy
Elderly	Thiazide diuretics	Recommended first-line therapy
African-Americans	First-line – thiazide diuretics or calcium channel blockers	Because of genetic factors and salt-sensitivity these drugs are more likely to be effective than ACE inhibitors
Ischaemic heart disease and/or left-ventricular hypertrophy (LVH)	Beta-blockers, ACE inhibitors, angiotensin II receptor blockers and loop diuretics	With IHD and post MI and with LVH, beta-blockers and ACE inhibitors are of benefit, loop diuretics also recommended with LVH Recent studies have highlighted the benefits of angiotensin II blockers in patients with LVH[13]
Diabetics	ACE inhibitors and angiotensin II receptor blockers, non-dihydropyridine calcium channel blockers and α_1-blockers	ACE inhibitors and angiotensin II receptor blockers have anti-proteinuric effects to delay onset and progression of diabetic nephropathy
Non-diabetics with micro-albuminuria	ACE inhibitors and angiotensin II receptor blockers	ACE inhibitors and angiotensin II receptor blockers have anti-proteinuric effects
Hyperlipidaemia	ACE inhibitors, calcium channel blockers, alpha-blockers, low-dose diuretics	Improve lipid profile
Benign prostatic hypertrophy	α_1-blockers	Reduce sympathetic tone in the bladder
Hyperaldosteronism	Spironolactone	Potassium sparing diuretic
Renal failure	ACE inhibitors and angiotensin II receptor blockers	Antiproteinuric effect may delay progression of renal impairment

ACE, angiotensin converting enzyme; MI, myocardial infarction; LVH, left ventricular hypertrophy

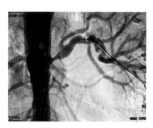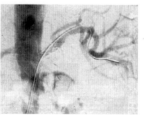

Figure 15.7
Secondary hypertension: atherosclerotic renal artery stenosis before (left) and after (right) revascularization with angioplasty and stenting.

the clinical setting, but normal 24-hour ambulatory blood pressure monitoring. Although many believe the condition to be of little consequence, white-coat hypertension has been associated with increased LV mass and LV diastolic dysfunction. It is important that such patients are followed up regularly with particular attention paid to the investigation of target organ damage.

ISOLATED SYSTOLIC HYPERTENSION

This is defined as systolic blood pressure of >140 mmHg, but with diastolic pressure of <90 mmHg. Isolated systolic hypertension ISH incidence increases with age and the condition increases the risk of myocardial infarction and especially stroke.[13] Aggressive treatment of blood pressure is warranted; particularly efficacious agents are calcium channel blockers, alpha-blockers and angiotensin II blockers.

HYPERTENSION IN PREGNANCY

This is defined as a blood pressure >140/90 mmHg or a rise of 25 mmHg of systolic and/or 15 mmHg of diastolic pressure above baseline (or first trimester) measurements. Hypertension affects approximately 10% of pregnancies. It may be classified into the following:

- Chronic hypertension – occurring before 20 weeks of pregnancy (usually pre-existing)
- Gestational hypertension – occurs after 20 weeks of pregnancy with no evidence of maternal organ dysfunction (43% of all pregnancy-related hypertension)
- Pre-eclampsia – occurs after 20 weeks of pregnancy with evidence of maternal organ dysfunction (34% of all pregnancy-related hypertension). Hypertension usually occurs with oedema and proteinuria but many other renal (and other organ) abnormalities can occur in complicated cases.

Treatment of pre-eclampsia involves placental delivery, as placental ischaemia is thought to be the major factor triggering and driving the pre-eclamptic process. It is important that management is jointly between physicians and obstetricians. Drug therapy of hypertension in pregnancy relies on the use of those few anti-hypertensive agents that are proven to be safe, and of no risk to the fetus or the mother. These include methyldopa and labetolol as first-line agents, with hydralazine, nifedipine and prazosin as second-line agents. A gradual reduction in blood pressure is required and for this reason, unless the level of blood pressure is immediately life-threatening, drugs should be given orally. Post-delivery follow-up is essential for all patients with pregnancy-related hypertension; blood pressure should have returned to normal within 3 months of delivery in most. Prompt investigations for an underlying cause are indicated for patients with persistent post-partum hypertension.

HYPERTENSIVE CRISIS

This is defined as a diastolic blood pressure of >130 mmHg with evidence of encephalopathy, LV failure or unstable angina. Hypertensive crisis is often confused with

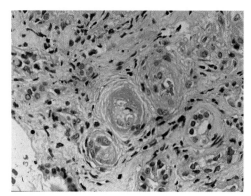

Figure 15.8
Consequences of hypertension: fibrinoid necrosis in renal arterioles

'malignant' or 'accelerated' hypertension but the latter is strictly defined as a diastolic blood pressure >120 mmHg with grade III or grade IV hypertensive retinopathy. Although both clinical scenarios require urgent lowering of blood pressure, malignant hypertension is associated with severe arteriolar injury in the retina and kidney. The renal biopsy finding of proliferative arteriolopathy with fibrinoid necrosis is characteristic (Fig. 15.8).

In hypertensive crisis the patient should be managed in hospital, and usually with intravenous agents. The aim of therapy is a gradual decrease of blood pressure (e.g. no more than 10 mmHg per hour). The avoidance of a sudden fall in blood pressure reduces the risk of acute renal failure, stroke, myocardial infarction and sudden death, which are predisposed to by overload of the autoregulatory mechanisms that control blood flow in vital organs (kidney, brain and heart).[14] The intravenous agents most often used to treat hypertensive crisis are labetolol, an adrenergic blocker, or sodium nitroprusside, a vasodilator. The previous use of sublingual nifedipine for rapid lowering of blood pressure in hypertensive crisis has been discontinued because of the risk of sudden death.

References

1. MacMahon S, Peto R, Cutler J et al. 1990 Blood pressure, stroke and coronary artery disease. Part 1, prolonged differences in blood pressure: prospective observational studies corrected for dilutional bias. Lancet 335(8692): 765–774
2. Kannel WB, Neaton JD, Wentworth D et al. 1982 Overall and coronary heart disease mortality rates in relation to major risk factors in 325,428 men screened for MRFIT. Multiple Risk Factor Intervention Trial. Am Heart J 112(4): 825–836
3. Hansson L, Zanchette A, Carruthers SG 1998 Effects of intensive blood pressure lowering and low-dose aspirin in patients with hypertension: principal results of the hypertension optimal treatment (HOT) randomised trial. Lancet 351(9118): 1755–1762
4. Joint National Committee on prevention, detection, evaluation and treatment of high blood pressure 1997 The sixth report of the Joint National Committee on prevention, detection, evaluation and treatment of high blood pressure. Arch Intern Med 157(21): 2413–2446
5. Colhoun HM, Dong W, Poulter NR 1998 Blood pressure screening, management and control in England, results from the health survey for England 1994. J Hypertens 16(6): 747–752

6. Sealey JE, Blumenfeld JD, Bell GM et al. 1998 On the renal basis for essential hypertension: nephron heterogeneity with discord renin secretion and sodium excretion causing a hypertensive vasoconstrictive-volume relationship. J Hypertens 6(10): 763–777

7. Johnson RJ, Schreiner GF 1997 Hypothesis: the role of acquired tubulointerstitial disease in the pathogenesis of salt-dependant hypertension. Kidney International 52(5): 1169–1179

8. Shurrab AE, Mamtora H, O'Donoghue D, Waldek S, Kalra PA 2001 Increasing the diagnostic yield of renal angiography for the diagnosis of atheromatous renovascular disease. Br J Radiol 74(879): 213–218

9. Williams B, Poulter NR, Brown MJ et al. 2004 Guidelines for management of hypertension: report of the Fourth working party of the British Hypertension Society. J Hum Hypertens 18: 139–185

10. Trials of hypertension prevention collaboration research group 1992 The effects of nonpharmacologic interventions on blood pressure of persons with high normal levels. J Am Med Assoc 267: 1213–1220

11. UK Prospective Diabetes Study Group 1998 Tight blood pressure control and risk of macrovascular and microvascular complications in Type 2 diabetes: UKPDS 38. BMJ 317(7160): 703–713

12. Plouin PF, Chatella G, Darne B, Raynaud A 1998 Blood pressure outcome of angioplasty in atherosclerotic renal artery stenosis: a randomised trial. Hypertension 31(3): 823–829

13. Kjeldsen SE, Dahlof B, Devereux RB et al. 2002 Effects of Losartan on cardiovascular morbidity and mortality in patients with isolated systemic hypertension and left ventricular hypertrophy: a Losartan Intervention for Endpoint Reduction (LIFE) substudy. J Am Med Assos 288(12): 1491–1498

14. Murphy C 1995 Hypertensive emergencies. Emerg Med Clin North Am 13: 973–1007

SELF-ASSESSMENT

Questions

1. A 42-year-old man is found to have a blood pressure of 170/96 mmHg during a routine physical examination at work. What would be the appropriate management of this patient?

2. A 22-year-old lady who is 39 weeks pregnant develops a BP of 180/115 mmHg. She has had dipstick trace of proteinuria since 36 weeks of pregnancy and has lower limb oedema. What is the appropriate management?

3. An 18-year-old male presents to casualty fitting with a blood pressure of 230/140 mmHg. What is the appropriate blood pressure management?

4. An overweight (BMI 35) 78-year-old lady presents with an upper respiratory tract infection to her general practitioner. During routine physical examination, her BP is noted to be 170/100 mmHg. You are asked to advise on management.

Answers

1. The first issue to consider is whether this reading is an isolated high reading or a reflection of hypertension. Repeated readings are necessary to confirm the diagnosis in a patient of this age as treatment may well be lifelong, and it will have implications for insurance and mortgage reasons. A 24-hour ABPM may also be useful to confirm hypertension. A careful family history and physical examination should be undertaken. In this age group, even in the absence of physical findings, investigation for an underlying cause is appropriate. Blood tests should include urea and electrolytes, calcium, parathyroid hormone level, thyroid function tests. Twenty-four-hour urine collections should be performed for proteinuria, creatinine clearance, catecholamines. A chest X-ray, electrocardiogram and renal ultrasound should also be performed. Any underlying cause should be referred to an appropriate specialist. Provided there are no contraindications, a beta-blocker or an ACE inhibitor or AIIR blocker would be the first-line management with either a calcium channel blocker or diuretic added as needed to achieve a BP <140/85 mmHg. In addition to drug use, attention to lifestyle measures, including weight loss, exercise and the cessation of smoking, is necessary. See Figure 15.9 for the current ABCD recommendations of the British Hypertension Society (BHS).

2. The diagnosis is pre-eclampsia and the essential management is to induce delivery. Placental delivery will remove the factors driving the pre-eclamptic process. It is important to note that the patient is at risk of eclampsia in the post-delivery period, and so close observation of the patient is appropriate after the delivery. Blood pressure management should involve the use of one of the agents known to be safe in pregnancy, e.g. labetolol or methyldopa, which may be given orally in the first instance. Follow-up of this patient is essential; if the hypertension persists beyond 3 months post-partum further investigation is required for an underlying cause, but only 2% of pre-eclamptic patients will have an underlying renal abnormality. The dipstick proteinuria should have disappeared by 12 months; persistent proteinuria beyond 1 year should prompt renal investigation. Recurrence of pre-eclampsia occurs

only in 5% of patients who present after 28 weeks' gestation and in 25% of those who present before 28 weeks' gestation; however gestational hypertension occurs in up to 40% of subsequent pregnancies.

3. The aim of blood pressure management in this case is the gradual reduction of blood pressure at no more than 10 mmHg per hour. Intravenous agents should be employed with the drugs of choice being either labetolol or sodium nitroprusside. During the follow-up period, this patient should be fully investigated for potential causes of secondary hypertension.

4. Repeated readings, at least two on two separate occasions, are required for a definite diagnosis. A weight-loss programme with realistic targets would be appropriate for this lady and a 3-month period should be allowed before pharmacological treatment is instituted. If blood pressure is not at target level (<140/85 mmHg) after this time then perhaps a thiazide diuretic would be appropriate first-line management.

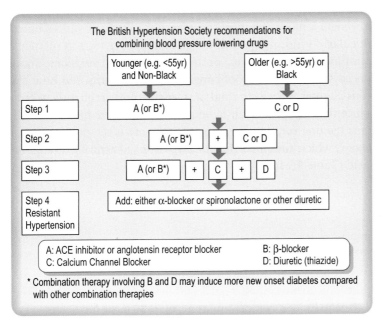

Figure 15.9
Recommendations for combining blood pressure lowering drugs/ABCD rule

Grown-up congenital heart disease

16

F. Walker and N. Velstrup

INTRODUCTION

So what do you need to know when you encounter an adult with congenital heart disease? This will become a more common occurrence thanks to advances in diagnosis, treatment and particularly surgical repair of congenital heart defects in infancy and childhood. Adult cardiologists, physicians, obstetricians, general surgeons, and family doctors alike will need some knowledge of congenital heart defects and how best to manage them. In this chapter we will try and answer the most frequently asked questions and, hopefully, reduce the trepidation felt by most who even hear mention of the word 'congenital'! Perhaps the first step in alleviating this anxiety is the provision of a 'congenital pictionary', which simplifies the language of paediatric cardiologists and specialists in the field (Table 16.1).

BACKGROUND

Approximately 8 per 1000 live births have congenital heart disease and 90% of these now survive to adulthood. This means an estimated 700 new cases are added to the books per region per year, with nine lesions comprising more than 80% of the defects (Table 16.2). Occasionally adults present de novo, but more often than not they will have been diagnosed in infancy or childhood (75% of cases). For those previously diagnosed, intervened or operated upon, follow-up will ideally have occurred regularly throughout childhood and adolescence at a specialist centre. Clearly those newly presenting in adulthood tend to have less severe lesions including atrial septal defects (ASDs), partial atrioventricular septal defects (AVSDs), partial anomalous pulmonary venous drainage (PAPVD), small ventricular septal defects (VSDs), co-arctation of the aorta (CoA), pulmonary stenosis (PS), small patent ductus arteriosus (PDA), Ebstein's anomaly, or uncommonly congenitally corrected transposition (ccTGA). Occasionally, an adult will present with Eisenmenger syndrome secondary to an undiagnosed duct, AVSD or VSD. The majority of patients will, however, be seeking follow-up for the residua and late sequelae of interventions or surgeries previously performed. We will discuss the individual lesions on a 'what you need to know' basis for this synoptic text.

Table 16.1: The congenital pictionary

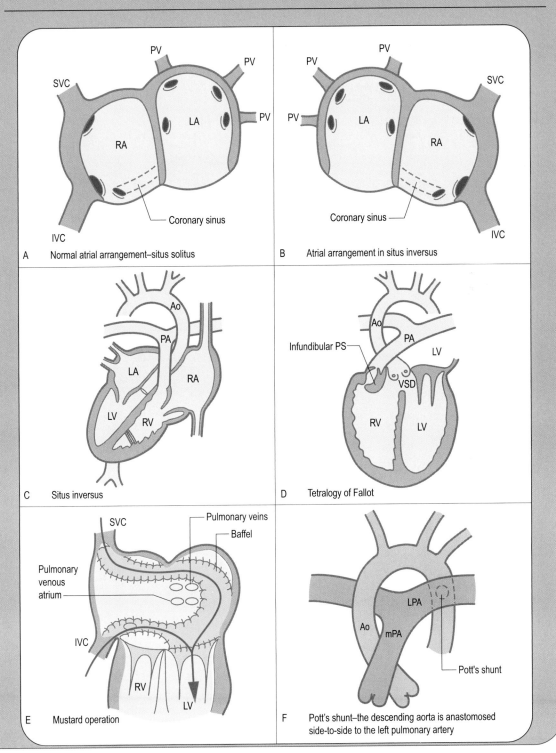

A Normal atrial arrangement–situs solitus

B Atrial arrangement in situs inversus

C Situs inversus

D Tetralogy of Fallot

E Mustard operation

F Pott's shunt–the descending aorta is anastomosed side-to-side to the left pulmonary artery

Table 16.1: (Cont'd) The congenital pictionary

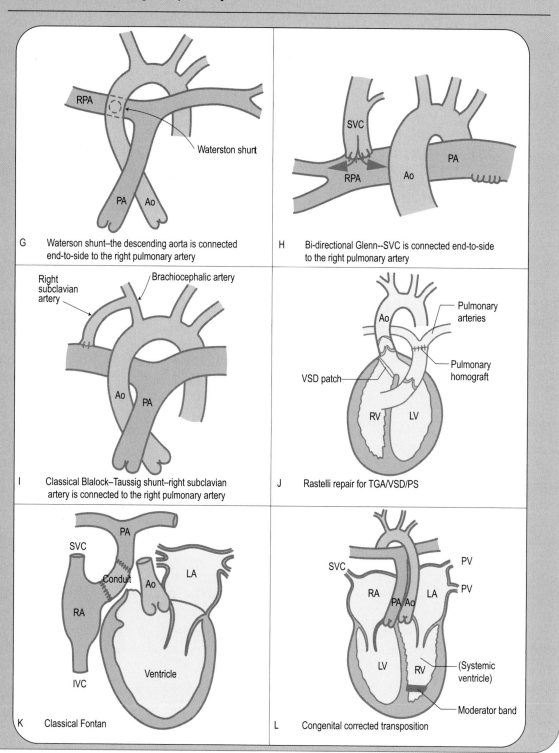

G   Waterson shunt–the descending aorta is connected end-to-side to the right pulmonary artery

H   Bi-directional Glenn--SVC is connected end-to-side to the right pulmonary artery

I   Classical Blalock–Taussig shunt–right subclavian artery is connected to the right pulmonary artery

J   Rastelli repair for TGA/VSD/PS

K   Classical Fontan

L   Congenital corrected transposition

Table 16.1: (Cont'd) The congenital pictionary

Left AV valve

What adult doctors call a mitral valve (MV), but this valve is morphologically quite different to a normal MV as there are usually multiple clefts. This abnormal valve is seen in atrioventricular septal defects with varying degrees of dysmorphology and dysfunction.

Baffles

A term used to describe the surgically created pathways that direct venous blood across the intra-atrial septum (IAS) to the mitral orifice and into left ventricle (LV) and pulmonary venous blood across the IAS to the tricuspid valve (TV) orifice and into right ventricle (RV), in those with a Mustard operation for TGA. Baffles are analogous to a pair of trousers with the legs coming in from inferior vena cava (IVC), superior vena cava (SVC) and the waistband attaching to the MV orifice. Baffles are made of pericardium in the Mustard repair or infoldings of the atrial myocardium in the Senning repair.

Table 16.2: Incidence of congenital heart lesions

Acyanotic lesions	Cyanotic lesions
VSD – 35%	TOF – 5%
ASD – 9%	TGA – 4%
PDA – 8%	Complex/miscellaneous – 20%
PS – 8%	
AS – 6%	
Co-arctation of the aorta – 6%	
AVSD – 3%	

GENETIC BASIS OF CONGENITAL HEART DISEASE

Emerging evidence supports the concept that genetic causes are common and often due to a single gene defect. Mutations at a single locus, however, may cause multiple different cardiac phenotypes.[1] The most important evidence for a genetic aetiology of congenital heart disease was the discovery of the association of conotruncal abnormalities with monosomy of a locus on chromosome 22. The acronym CATCH-22 was coined to encompass the spectrum of clinical manifestations in patients with deletions in this locus. More recently, patients with velo-cardio-facial syndrome (VCFS or Shprintzen syndrome) have been noted to share some manifestations with Di George. The cardiac manifestations include VSD (54%) and tetralogy of Fallot (TOF) (20%), often with a right aortic arch or arch vessel anomalies. Other types of congenital heart disease secondary to single gene defects are listed in Box 16.1.

Box 16.1: Congenital heart lesions of a genetic aetiology

CATCH-22 syndrome

Cardiac defects, **A**bnormal facies, **T**hymic hypoplasia, **C**left palate and **H**ypercalcaemia. Caused by 22q11 deletions.

Should be tested for in all patients with truncus arteriosus (20–30%), interrupted Ao arch (25–40%), absent pulmonary vein (PV) syndrome, isolated VSD (10%) tetralogy of Fallot (8%), any patient with congenital heart disease and absent thymus.

Supravalvular aortic stenosis (SVAS)
Elastin gene deletions chromosome 7 (7q11.23). May be familial with autosomal dominant inheritance, may occur as part of Williams syndrome and may be sporadic.

Holt-Oram syndrome (upper limb abnormalities + atrial septal defects/ventricular septal defects)
Unidentified gene defect chromosome 12 (12q21-q3). Autosomal dominant.

Familial atrioventricular septal defects
Unidentified gene defect (chromosome 21 not implicated).

Familial TAPVD (total anomalous pulmonary venous drainage)
Unidentified gene defect chromosome 4.

SPECIFIC CONGENITAL HEART LESIONS

VENTRICULAR SEPTAL DEFECT

Ventricular septal defects (VSDs) are the most common congenital heart defects. Most VSDs close spontaneously or are closed surgically in childhood. Ventricular septal defects are divided into four major groups according to their location in the ventricular septum (Fig. 16.1).

Adults with a VSD will have one of the following:

- A small haemodynamically insignificant VSD that poses an increased infective endocarditis risk
- A large Eisenmenger VSD (see section on Eisenmenger syndrome)
- A doubly committed subarterial VSD – the VSD is closed by a prolapsing aortic valve cusp. These patients need close follow-up as they often develop significant aortic regurgitation (AR).

With a small VSD there is often a palpable thrill at the left sternal edge and a loud pansystolic murmur. It is important to listen for aortic regurgitation. The electrocardiogram (ECG) and chest X-ray (CXR) are normal.

Intervention

The small VSD requires no treatment unless there have been more than two episodes of infective endocarditis, where some advocate closure. If there is volume loading of the left

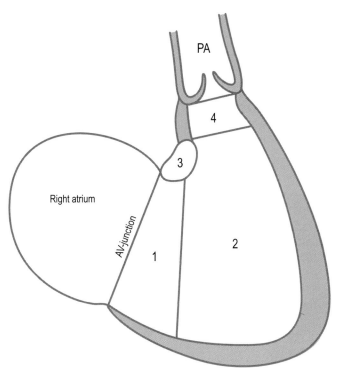

Figure 16.1
Diagram of the ventricular septum viewed from right ventricle, showing the position of the 4 main types of VSD.
Inlet VSDs (1), muscular VSDs (2), perimembranous VSDs (3), doubly committed VSDs (previously known as supracristal or outlet VSDs) (4).
PA, pulmonary artery; AV, atrioventricular

ventricle and or a Qp:Qs>1.5 the defect should be closed. The subarterial VSD causing aortic regurgitation should be closed. Percutaneous device closure of VSDs has been performed with success. If a VSD is present lifelong endocarditis prophylaxis is required.

ATRIAL SEPTAL DEFECT

There are three types of atrial septal defect (ASDs), all of which can present in adulthood:

- Secundum ASD – the commonest defect (75% of ASDs) in the area of the foramen ovale (Fig. 16.2).
- Primum defect or partial AVSD (15% of ASDs) – a defect in the atrial septum between the foramen ovale and the AV valves (Fig. 16.3).
- Sinus venosus ASD – bad terminology, as not a defect in the atrial septum but a communication created when the superior vena cava straddles the atrial septum, entering both left atrium (LA) and right atrium (RA). It is often associated with anomalous pulmonary veins (right pulmonary veins drain into superior vena cava (SVC) (Fig. 16.4).

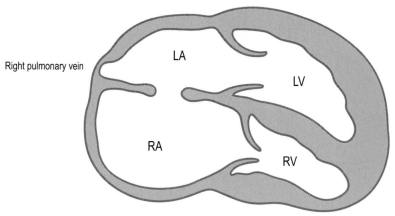

Figure 16.2
Anatomical diagram of secundum atrial septal defects

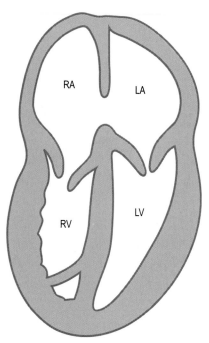

Figure 16.3
Anatomical diagram of primum atrial septal defects

The direction of blood flow across the defect is determined by the relative compliance of each ventricle. Normally the right ventricle is more compliant than the left therefore the shunt is left to right. Pulmonary blood flow (Qp) is, therefore, higher than systemic blood flow (Qs) and Qp/Qs is >1.

Symptoms are often insidious with increasing breathlessness, and reduced exercise tolerance. On examination of a patient with secundum ASD there is wide fixed splitting

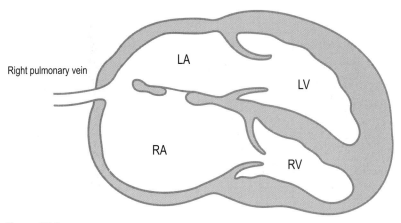

Figure 16.4
Anatomical diagram of sinus venosus atrial septal defects

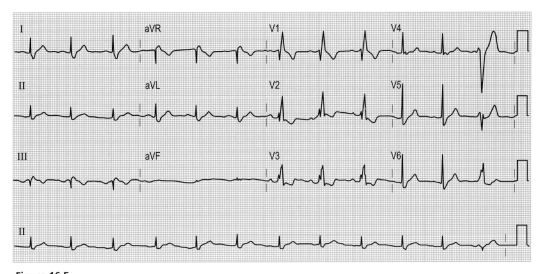

Figure 16.5
12-lead electrocardiogram in secundum atrial septal defects

of the second sound (does not vary with respiration) with a soft pulmonary ejection murmur. With a primum defect the systolic murmur of MR can also be heard.

The ECG will show right axis deviation (RAD), and partial right bundle branch block (RBBB) in secundum ASD (Fig. 16.5). In a primum defect there is often first-degree AV block and a superior axis (dominant S waves III and AVF) (Fig. 16.6). In sinus venosus defects there may be a coronary sinus rhythm with inverted P waves in AVF. The CXR will show an increased right heart size and large central pulmonary arteries (PAs). A transthoracic echo (TTE) will detect most secundum and primum ASDs (subcostal view best), but venosus defects are often only seen on transoesophageal echo (TOE).

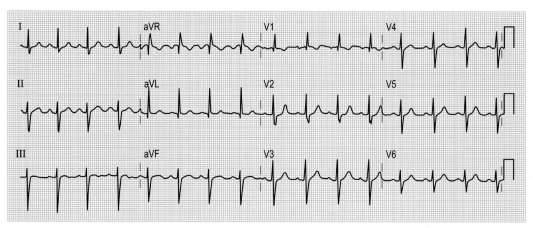

Figure 16.6
12-lead electrocardiogram in primum atrial septal defects

Intervention

Closure of a secundum ASD is indicated if the Qp:Qs is >1.5, or if there is evidence of volume loading of the right ventricle (RV). A large ASD may cause pulmonary hypertension over time, but atrial fibrillation and right heart failure are more common. Secundum defects can be closed surgically or percutaneously with a device.

Device closure of secundum defects is becoming increasingly popular with a recovery time of only 24–48 hours. The debate as to whether closure of a secundum ASD should be undertaken in those >40 years old, is ongoing. From surgical series it is known that if repair is left to the 4th or 5th decade the prevalence of late atrial arrhythmias and stroke is unchanged. Whether device closure alters this prevalence remains to be seen. There is, however, good evidence that closure of an ASD results in an objective improvement in exercise tolerance, even in those who are asymptomatic or only mildly symptomatic.[2] Surgery is necessary for primum or venosus defects. Endocarditis prophylaxis is not required for isolated ASD.

PULMONARY STENOSIS

Pulmonary stenosis (PS) is relatively common, especially in its mild and moderate forms. It can be subvalvar, valvar (most common) and supravalvar (associated with Williams syndrome). Patients may complain of breathlessness, exercise intolerance and if severe, symptoms of RV failure. There may be an RV heave +/– a thrill in the 2nd right intercostal space. S2 is split but not fixed (c.f ASD). A systolic click may be heard.

The ECG will show RAD +/– RV hypertrophy (RVH). The TTE will identify the level of the stenosis and Doppler echocardiography will provide an estimate of severity.

Intervention

If there is severe stenosis (angio pull-back gradient >50 mmHg at rest, RV systolic pressure >100 mmHg) intervention is indicated. Symptoms dictate whether less severe PS is intervened upon. Percutaneous balloon dilatation is safe and effective in relieving valvar PS.

PATENT DUCTUS ARTERIOSUS

A left-to-right shunt (Qp:Qs >1.5) through a PDA over time can cause pulmonary vascular disease and closure is indicated. A small haemodynamically insignificant PDA does not cause pulmonary hypertension (PHT) but closure should be considered if there has been an episode of infective endarteritis. Percutaneous device closure of a duct is safe and effective.

TETRALOGY OF FALLOT

Successful repair of tetralogy of Fallot (TOF) has been possible for over 20 years and there are now more adult patients with TOF than children. TOF comprises four lesions – VSD, RV outflow tract obstruction (RVOTO), RVH and an overriding aorta (Fig. 16.7). Most adult TOF patients will have been repaired in infancy/childhood. The older tetralogy patients will often have had prior Blalock–Taussig (BT) shunts. Definitive repair includes VSD patch closure, and resection of the RVOT obstruction. A transanular patch is often used to open up the RVOT, which results in important pulmonary regurgitation (PR).

On examination there is usually an ejection systolic murmur (ESM) in the pulmonary area +/– a diastolic murmur. Even in the presence of severe PR the diastolic murmur may be barely audible. Most operated TOF patients have RBBB on the ECG. QRS duration >180 ms is associated with an increased risk of sudden death.

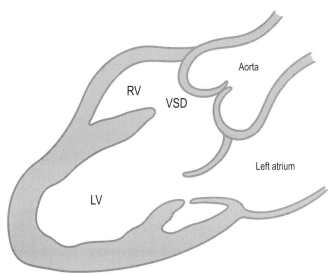

Figure 16.7
Anatomical diagram of tetralogy of Fallot (Parasternal long axis view)

Intervention

Late problems in TOF are related to RV dilatation and dysfunction secondary to PR. RV size/function, TV function and exercise capacity need surveillance over time. Follow-up should be in a specialist unit as the timing of pulmonary valve (PV) implant is critical to RV function and long-term outcome.

TRANSPOSITION OF THE GREAT ARTERIES

In transposition of the great arteries (TGA), the aorta comes off the RV and the pulmonary artery comes off the LV. These patients are cyanosed at birth and will have been operated on in childhood. The adult with repaired TGA will have undergone an atrial switch procedure (Mustard/Senning operations). A few patients are now reaching adulthood who have been repaired with the arterial switch operation. All should be followed in a specialist unit.

Mustard and Senning operations

Blood flow is redirected at atrial level. An atrial septectomy is performed and blood flow is directed with a baffle (Mustard) (Fig. 16.8) or by infoldings of the atrial walls themselves (Senning). On examination there will be a RV heave, single S2, and often a pansystolic murmur (PSM) of tricuspid regurgitation (TR). The ECG shows RAD and RVH (Fig. 16.9). Systemic RV dysfunction may occur over time and is treated as per LV dysfunction with ACE inhibitors, diuretics, etc. Referral for heart transplantation may be necessary if there is intractable heart failure despite optimal medical therapy. Bradyarrhythmias and atrial tachyarrhythmias are common. The baffles may obstruct insidiously causing either systemic or pulmonary venous pathway obstruction. SVC obstruction is in the main benign but both IVC obstruction and pulmonary venous pathway obstruction can be life threatening. These patients require follow-up and echo surveillance in a specialist unit.

Arterial switch

This operation corrects TGA by moving the aorta and pulmonary artery so the aorta arises from the LV and the PA from the RV. Because this operation requires re-implantation of the coronary arteries surveillance for ostial coronary stenosis is required. Any symptoms of breathlessness or chest pain must be taken seriously in these young adults. Supravalvar PS or AS and branch PA stenoses may be late complications.

CO-ARCTATION OF THE AORTA

Co-arctation of the aorta (CoA) is a narrowing of the aorta usually just distal to the left subclavian artery. CoA results in upper body hypertension. It is often associated with bicuspid aortic valve, VSD and intracranial berry aneurysms. CoA in childhood will have been repaired with a patch, subclavian flap repair, excision with end-to-end anastomosis or insertion of a Gortex tube graft. Hypertension can persist following successful repair especially if performed after the age of 5 years.

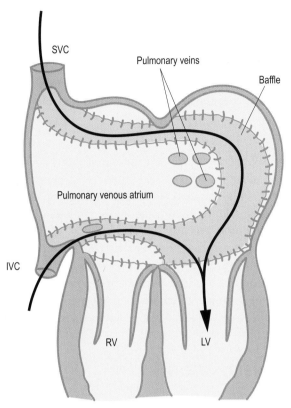

Figure 16.8
Anatomical diagram of Mustard operation

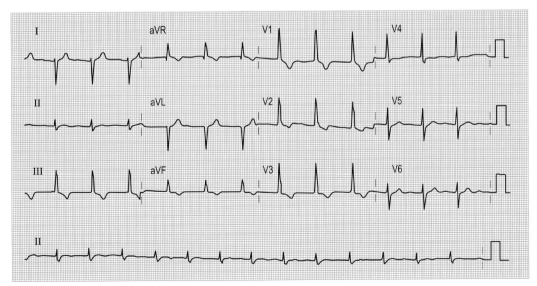

Figure 16.9
12-lead electrocardiogram of Mustard

Adults do present de novo, often with systemic hypertension (HT) or leg fatigue on exercise. The lower limb pulses are reduced in volume. Radiofemoral delay if present represents significant collateralization to the lower body. If there is a significant CoA lower limb BP will be less than upper limb BP (normal >20 mmHg higher). The ECG may show LVH. The CXR may show rib notching from large collaterals. On TTE the suprasternal window is best for visualizing the arch and descending aorta.

Intervention

Intervention on a native or previously operated CoA, is indicated if there is HT and or symptoms, with a descending Ao gradient on echo of >20 mmHg with diastolic flow continuation, or a pullback gradient across the CoA site at angiography of >20 mmHg. Percutaneous intervention with balloon dilatation and stenting is gaining acceptance as the treatment of first choice in re-CoA and more recently has also been used for the treatment of native CoA. Although surgery still has its place, there is a risk of spinal cord ischaemia (0.4%). CoA patients should be followed up at a specialist unit for surveillance for re-CoA and aneurysm formation. Hypertension resolves in 50% but should be treated aggressively if it persists, because all CoA patients have an increased incidence of premature cardiovascular disease and death over long-term follow-up. Endocarditis prophylaxis is required.

CONGENITALLY CORRECTED TRANSPOSITION

This would be easier to remember if called ventricular inversion (Fig. 16.10). There is atrio-ventricular discordance together with transposition of the great arteries. Of those with complex congenitally corrected transposition (ccTGA), the majority have VSD, PS or sub PS, or an Ebsteinoid TV and will usually have been diagnosed in childhood. If there is simple ccTGA (no associated anomalies) they may present as adults with a co-incidental murmur (systemic TR), breathlessness (RV dysfunction) or complete AV block (there is also a 2% risk per annum of developing complete AV block). A TTE will confirm the diagnosis. The main late complication is systemic RV dysfunction/failure. These patients should be followed in a specialist unit. Those who develop early RV dysfunction may need surgical intervention including TV replacement or consideration for a double switch operation (Senning + arterial switch).

EBSTEIN'S ANOMALY

This accounts for 0.5% of cases of congenital heart disease, most of which are sporadic. It is characterized by an apical displacement of the septal and often posterior leaflet attachments of the tricuspid valve from the AV ring (>8 mm/m^2 significant). The inlet portion of the right ventricle is, therefore, 'atrialized' and the RV is functionally small (Fig. 16.11). There will be varying degrees of TR (or exceptionally stenosis) and 80% have a communication at atrial level (ASD or patent foramen ovale (PFO)). Arrhythmia, congestive heart failure or cyanosis (right-to-left shunting across a PFO) is a common adult presentation. On examination the jugular venous pressure (JVP) is often normal

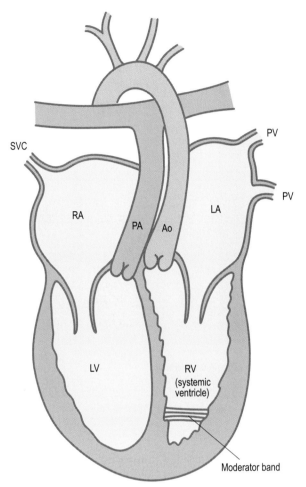

Figure 16.10
Anatomical diagram of congenitally corrected transposition

even when TR is severe (large compliant RA). S1 is widely split (long TV leaflets), as is S2 (late PV closure in presence of RBBB). S3 and S4 are often present. The ECG will show RBBB and tall broad P waves. First-degree AVB occurs in about 50% and a delta wave (Wolff–Parkinson–White – virtually always type B) is present in ~25%. TTE confirms the diagnosis.

Intervention

The most important predictors of outcome are New York Heart Association (NYHA) functional class, heart size, presence or absence of cyanosis, and presence or absence of paroxysmal atrial arrhythmias. Surgical intervention with tricuspid valve repair or replacement (bioprosthesis) is recommended if there is an increase in symptoms (NYHA Class III/IV), cyanosis, right-heart failure or resistant arrhythmias. This condition requires follow-up in a specialist unit where there is expertise in TV surgery.

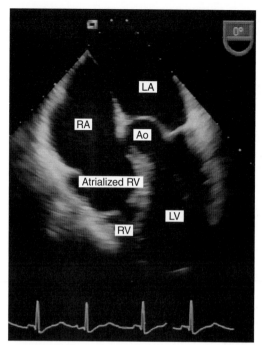

Figure 16.11
4 chamber apical transthoracic echo image of Ebstein's anomaly

FONTAN

The Fontan circulation is unique, with no right-sided pump and a passive flow of blood into the PAs. The 'true'/classic Fontan connection was a valved homograft between the right atrium (RA) and pulmonary artery (PA) (Fig. 16.12). The Fontan is used as a palliation for tricuspid atresia, pulmonary atresia, double inlet LV (DILV) and some forms of AVSD. There have been many modifications of the original operation, e.g. atrio-pulmonary Fontan, total cavo-pulmonary connection (TCPC), extra-cardiac conduit or lateral tunnel Fontan, but the physiological principles remain the same. Because pulmonary blood flow is passive, venous pressure is elevated (+8–10 cm) to provide sufficient hydrostatic pressure for forward flow through the non-pulsatile pulmonary circulation. Most atriopulmonary (AP) Fontan connections lead to the development of a huge RA (often >7cm) with a propensity for atrial arrhythmias (15–20% at 5 year follow-up) and thrombus formation (6–25%). Some patients will be de-saturated as they have a fenestration in the Fontan circuit (communication between RA and LA) allowing right-to-left shunting of blood. On examination S1 is normal, S2 is single and there should be no added sounds or murmurs.

Atrial arrhythmias are common and when present may precipitate cardiac failure and reduce long-term survival. The onset of atrial arrhythmias should prompt a full haemodynamic assessment to exclude obstruction (usually by thrombus) of the Fontan circuit (MRI or cardiac catheterization).

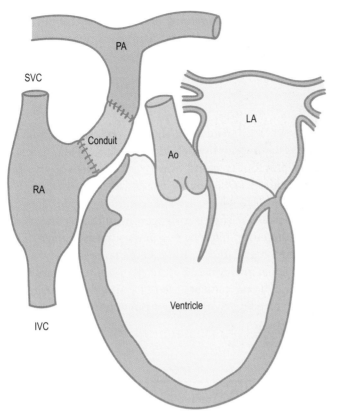

Figure 16.12
Anatomical diagram of classic Fontan

The onset of AF is considered an emergency and decompensation can occur rapidly. Prompt DC cardioversion should be performed with prior TOE, preferably in a specialist unit with a cardiac anaesthetist. These patients require specialist follow-up.

COMPLEX CYANOTIC HEART DISEASE

These patients are comprised of a heterogenous group of congenital lesions, from uni-ventricular hearts to defects where creation of a biventricular circulation was not possible, e.g. complete AVSD, pulmonary atresia/VSD with small or non-confluent PAs. Pulmonary blood flow is often dependent on surgically created shunts, e.g. BT shunts, central shunts. There is central cyanosis, which in itself is a multisystem disease affecting the cardiovascular, haematological, renal and musculoskeletal systems. Cyanotics may suffer from gout due to a low uric acid fractional excretion (a marker of abnormal renal function) and over-diuresis will exacerbate this problem. Skin sepsis and pustular acne is common, and wounds tend to heal poorly. Cerebral abscess must be considered in any cyanotic patient who presents with headache, vomiting, low-grade fever, apathy or focal neurology, as it more common in this patient group. Spontaneous venous and, less commonly, arterial thrombosis may occur, in part due to polycythaemia. Dehydration must, therefore, be avoided as should the combined oral contraceptive pill in female patients. The polycythaemia associated with chronic cyanosis is not comparable to polycythaemia rubra vera and is, therefore, not managed as such (see venesection).

EISENMENGER SYNDROME

Eisenmenger syndrome occurs when a left-to-right shunt is reversed secondary to pulmonary hypertension. Most commonly the defects are: a large VSD, patent ductus arteriosus or AVSD. Increased pulmonary blood flow over time leads to the development of pulmonary vascular disease and increased pulmonary vascular resistance (PVR). Such patients are cyanosed and clubbed. They have a RV heave, loud P2 and diastolic murmur of PR. Lowering peripheral vascular resistance is dangerous in these patients as right-to-left shunting is increased and, therefore, hypoxaemia and cyanosis worsen. The following conditions may, therefore, be life threatening in these patients: pregnancy, anaesthesia, drugs that lower peripheral vascular resistance, large changes in temperature (hot bath, sauna, etc.) or strenuous exercise. These patients are not routinely anti-coagulated because if anything they have a bleeding diathesis and pulmonary haemorrhage is often a terminal event.

References

1. Strauss AW 1998 The molecular basis of congenital cardiac disease. Semin Thorac Cardiovasc Surg Pediatr Card Surg Annu 1: 179–188
2. Brochu MC, Baril JF, Dore A, Juneau M, De Guise P, Mercier LA 2002 Improvement in exercise capacity in asymptomatic and mildly symptomatic adults after atrial septal defect percutaneous closure. Circulation 106(14): 1821–1826
3. Thorne SA 1998 Management of polycythaemia in adults with cyanotic congenital heart disease. Heart 79(4): 315–316
4. Guillebaud J, de Swiet M, Thorne SA et al. 2002 UK working party for pregnancy and contraception in women with heart disease. Personal communication
5. Siu SC, Sermer M, Colman JM et al. 2001 Prospective multicenter study of pregnancy outcomes in women with heart disease. Circulation 104(5): 515–521
6. Daliento L, Somerville J, Presbitero P et al. 1998 Eisenmenger syndrome. Factors relating to deterioration and death. Eur Heart J 19(12): 1845–1855

SELF-ASSESSMENT

Questions

a. Which patients should be considered for venesection?

b. What precautionary measures should be advised to patients with congenital heart disease around pregnancy?

c. What up-to-date assessment is advisable pre non-cardiac surgery?

Answers

a. Chronic hypoxaemia leads to increased erythrocyte production with an increase in haematocrit and blood viscosity. A very high haematocrit >0.65 does not result in an increased risk of arterial thrombosis, although venous thrombosis is more common. Venesection, once in vogue for this patient group, is no longer indicated unless there are hyperviscosity symptoms (headaches, blurred vision, lethargy and myalgia).[3] Chronic venesection can lead to iron deficiency anaemia with microcytosis, which has been associated with an increased arterial thromboembolic event rate. The benefits of venesection are transient and short-lived, but if indicated it should be performed with equal volume replacement (Gelofusine) and low-dose oral iron supplementation (200 mg once daily). Cyanotic patients with a normal haematocrit should be investigated to exclude anaemia.

b. As a general rule, any patient with congenital heart disease who wishes to become pregnant should receive specialist review prior to conception. Genetic counselling, assessment of functional status, maternal risk, and fetal risk need to be discussed. Counselling requires an understanding of the specific congenital defect, the nature of prior surgical correction and residua and sequelae. The risk of recurrence of congenital heart disease in the offspring needs to be discussed in the context of a 0.4–0.6% risk in the general population, and a 10-fold increased risk if a first-degree relative is affected. Left-heart obstructive lesions and those with 22q11 deletion have a higher recurrence rate. Using a modified version of the WHO classification for pregnancy (pWHO)[4], this can be translated into a lesion specific pWHO risk classification for pregnancy in women with heart disease.

In a prospective multicentre study of pregnancy outcomes in women with heart disease, the four predictors of maternal cardiac events identified were:

- Prior episode of heart failure, transient ischaemic attack (TIA), cerebrovascular accident (CVA) or arrhythmia
- NYHA Class $\geq$ II or cyanosis
- Left-heart obstruction (mitral valve area <2 cm^2, aortic valve area <1.5 cm^2, peak left ventricular outlet obstruction (LVOT) echo gradient >30 mmHg)
- Reduced LV function (ejection fraction <40%).

In the absence of any predictor the risk of a cardiac event is 5%, with one predictor the risk is 27%, and with more than one predictor the risk is 75%.[5]

For all but the simplest lesions, most pregnant women with congenital heart disease require specialist multidisciplinary care, with involvement of cardiologist, obstetrician, anaesthetist, geneticist and midwife.

c. As a general rule, patients with congenital heart disease undergoing any surgery should have an up-to-date clinical review. The operating team should know the nature of prior surgical correction, residua and sequelae. Specialist advice should be sought if in any doubt. Patients with pulmonary hypertension, cyanotic heart disease, Fontan circulations, Mustard or Senning repairs or those with any significant residua should undergo their operation in a cardiac unit, with a cardiac anaesthetist and cardiac ITU support.[6]

Aortic dissection

17

M. Dayer

INTRODUCTION

Aortic dissection is a tearing of the intima of the arterial wall, with blood passing from the true lumen of the aorta into the media. It cleaves the medial layer longitudinally and creates a false lumen; blood may later re-enter the true lumen through a different tear (Fig. 17.1). Dissection may occur at any point in the aorta, but usually arises just above the aortic sinuses or beyond the left subclavian artery. Dissection may be acute or chronic.

This condition is highly lethal. One of the earliest and best-recorded cases was the death of King George II in 1760. Death often results from the rupture of the aorta into the pericardium or left pleural space. Untreated, the mortality rate is thought to be around 1–2% per hour in the first 24 hours, although some estimates suggest that 35% of patients die within the first 15 minutes.

Although surgery may be required as a definitive management strategy, the immediate management is medical, and cardiologists often undertake long-term follow-up. Furthermore, stenting of dissecting thoracic aneurysms is emerging as an acceptable alternative to surgery in some situations. This chapter will primarily be concerned with the medical aspects of this condition, in particular diagnosis and initial management. Surgical options will be outlined, but not discussed in detail. The treatment of paediatric patients with the disease will not be covered and neither will the management of abdominal aortic aneurysms.

SCOPE OF THE PROBLEM

The true incidence is hard to estimate. Recent autopsy studies have found evidence of dissection in 1–3% of cases. Aortic dissection is two to three times more frequent than rupture of an abdominal aortic aneurysm. Three-quarters of cases occur between the ages of 40 and 70 years, with the peak incidence in the sixth and seventh decades. The male to female ratio is two to one. It is more common in the black population and less common in Asians than in the white population.

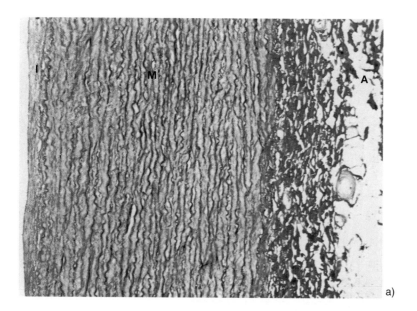

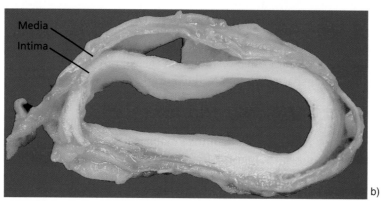

Figure 17.1
(a) Aorta at histological level (endothelium, etc.). From: Wheater PR, Burkitt HG and Daniels VG. Functional Histology, 2nd ed, with permission from Churchill Livingstone; I, intima; M, media; A, adventitia (b) Showing where the intima has been stripped from the media (see Fig. 17.2 for medial degeneration)

AETIOLOGY

Any condition that weakens the aortic wall may predispose to aortic dissection. Hypertension is the most common condition associated with aortic dissection, and is found in 72–80% of cases. Marfan's syndrome is also an important risk factor. This disorder leads to cystic medial degeneration (Fig. 17.2) and patients are at high risk of dissection from a young age; the syndrome accounts for between 5% and 9% of all aortic dissections. A bicuspid aortic valve is also a well-recognized association, and has been found in 7–14% of dissections. Cardiac intervention is another important cause. A more comprehensive list can be found in Box 17.1.

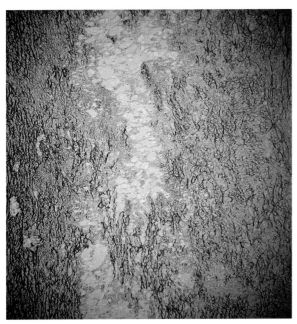

Figure 17.2
Cystic medial degeneration

Box 17.1 Predisposing factors

Common
Hypertension
Bicuspid aortic valve
Marfan's syndrome

Abnormalities of collagen/fibrillin
Ehler's–Danlos syndrome
Familial aortic dissection
Other fibrillinopathies

Iatrogenic
Cardiac catheterization
Previous cardiac surgery (aortic catheterization sites)
Intra-aortic balloon pump

Congenital
Co-arctation of the aorta
Patent ductus arteriosus

Vasculitides
Behcet's disease
Rheumatoid arthritis
Giant cell arteritis
Takayasu's arteritis

Pregnancy
Usually 3rd trimester, 50% of dissections in women
<40 years

Infections
Syphilis
Bacterial infection
Fungal infection

Drugs
Cocaine
Amphetamines

Trauma

Other
Annuloaortic ectasia

Table 17.1: *Classification of aortic dissection according to site involved*

Classification	Site involved
Stanford	
Type A	Any dissection involving the ascending aorta
Type B	Any dissection not involving the ascending aorta
De Bakey	
Type I	Any dissection originating in the ascending aorta that propagates at least to the aortic arch
Type II	Any dissection originating and confined to the ascending aorta
Type III	Any dissection originating in the descending aorta

CLASSIFICATION

There are two principal classifications of aortic dissection: the Stanford and the De Bakey classifications (Table 17.1 & Fig. 17.3). Both divide dissections into those affecting and not affecting the ascending aorta; the former generally require surgery. Other classifications exist.

CLINICAL FEATURES

Perhaps the biggest challenge in the management of aortic dissection is considering it as a diagnosis from the outset. Approximately one-third of patients with dissection are initially suspected to have other diagnoses, particularly acute coronary syndromes or pulmonary embolism. This is because aortic dissection may present in a myriad of ways.

SYMPTOMS

Severe pain is a characteristic symptom but is not universal. It typically has an abrupt onset and is often described as tearing, in contrast to ischaemic pain that tends to be dull and increases over time. With more proximal dissections the pain is located retrosternally, whereas with distal dissections it tends to be interscapular. As the dissection extends the pain may move. Although dissection may be painless, its absence is more commonly associated with chronic dissection.

Syncope is also common, being reported in approximately 10% of cases. This may be a consequence of pain, cardiac tamponade, dissection of the cerebral vessels, or hypotension secondary to haemorrhage.

SIGNS

On examination the most common findings include aortic regurgitation (30%), a pulse deficit (15%) and signs of a cerebrovascular accident or heart failure. Blood pressure is

| De Bakey | I | II | III |
| Stanford | A | A | A |

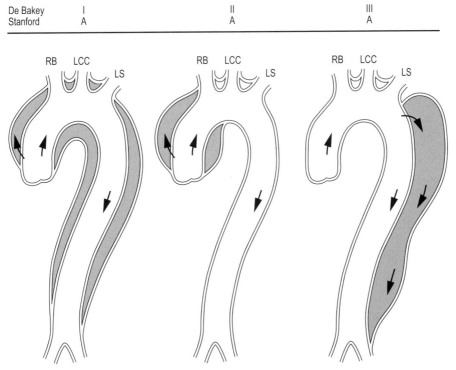

Figure 17.3
Schematic of aorta (ascending/arch/descending), with branch vessels showing classification of dissection RB, right brachiocephalic artery; LCC, left common carotid artery; LS, left subclavian artery

variable and patients may be hypertensive (50%), normotensive (35%) or hypotensive (15%). Patients may **look shocked despite an apparently normal blood pressure**. It is important to look for evidence of cardiac tamponade.

Other findings may include fever, pleural effusions (typically on the left), limb or mesenteric ischaemia and paraplegia (secondary to dissection of the anterior spinal arteries).

INITIAL INVESTIGATIONS

An electrocardiogram (ECG) is considered important, but will often be normal, show left-ventricular hypertrophy or have 'non-specific' changes. In a few patients there will be evidence of acute myocardial infarction (typically inferior) due to extension of the dissection flap into a coronary artery. Thrombolysis in this scenario is often fatal.

Almost invariably a chest X-ray is performed and it is abnormal in 60–90% of patients (Box 17.2 & Fig. 17.4). The value of the chest X-ray in the immediate management of aortic dissection is controversial, with some authorities claiming that it simply delays diagnosis; further investigations are essential for diagnostic certainty.

Box 17.2: Chest X-ray features of aortic dissection

Widening of aortic knuckle
Widening of mediastinum
Widening of descending aorta
Abnormal cardiac contour
Pleural effusion
Tracheal shift
Displacement of intimal calcification
Normal

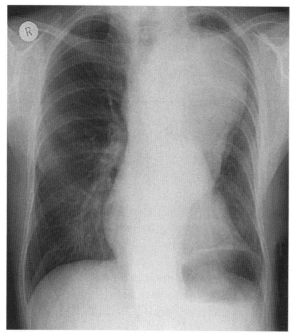

Figure 17.4
Chest X-ray of patient with large, thoracic aneurysm, secondary to trauma

Conventional biochemical tests are non-specific and often show signs of inflammation with an elevated C-reactive protein and mild leucocytosis. Raised concentrations of smooth muscle myosin heavy chain can be detected and are relatively specific to dissection, raising the possibility of biochemical diagnosis in the future.

DIAGNOSTIC INVESTIGATIONS

These comprise:

- Transthoracic (TTE) and transoesophageal echocardiography (TOE)
- Spiral computed tomography (CT)

- Magnetic resonance imaging (MRI)
- Angiography
- Intravascular ultrasound (IVUS).

The method selected will depend on the situation and local expertise. Early liaison with the local cardiothoracic centre is imperative to plan management and transfer. If the diagnosis is strongly suspected it is appropriate to arrange transfer to a specialist centre without waiting for definitive tests. Investigations must provide information in addition to confirming the diagnosis, including tear localization, the extent of dissection, and detailing involvement of the aortic valve, coronaries and branches of the aorta. No single investigation can provide all the information.

TTE is relatively insensitive for the detection of intimal flaps, particularly where the dissection commences in the descending aorta. However, it is non-invasive, quick to perform and often readily available. It can provide information on aortic valve function and determine the presence of a pericardial collection. It has a specificity of 93–96%, but its sensitivity is much lower, and it is important to stress that a normal TTE does not exclude dissection.

TOE (Fig. 17.5) overcomes many of the limitations of TTE and some studies have suggested that the sensitivity for detecting dissection is as high as 97–99%. TOE can be performed both rapidly and safely at the bedside. Important information regarding the size of the aortic root and the state of the aortic valve can be gained. Some authors argue that it should be the first-line investigation. It is important to remember, however, that the distal ascending aorta and proximal arch cannot be seen well due to the position of the trachea.

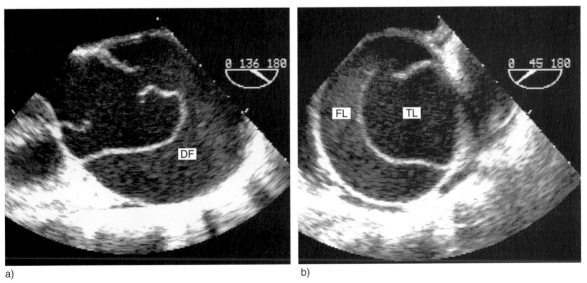

a)

b)

Figure 17.5
(a) TOE of dissection flap (DF); (b) in cross-section the true lumen (TL) and false lumen (FL) can be seen

Spiral CT is widely available, relatively quick to perform, and is both sensitive and specific. It provides no information about aortic valve function, and is limited in determining the site of dissection. It is recommended where TOE is not available as the initial investigation.

MRI is arguably the gold standard for the diagnosis of aortic dissection with sensitivities and specificities around 98%. High-quality images are obtained that can be viewed from many angles (Fig. 17.6), but it is not available in all centres and is less suitable for unstable patients.

Angiography was for many years the only accurate method of diagnosing aortic dissection. It is less sensitive than other investigations (77–87%) as false negatives can occur for a number of reasons. These include thrombosis of the false lumen and simultaneous filling of the true, and false lumens. Furthermore, there are inherent risks with any invasive procedure. It remains the gold standard for imaging the coronary arteries if this is felt to be essential pre-operatively.

IVUS can be used in conjunction with conventional angiography to overcome some of its limitations. It is particularly good at visualizing the intimal flap and delimiting the extent of the dissection. Branch involvement can be determined more easily than with TOE or CT. Older catheters lacked Doppler imaging, but this is available with newer equipment.

In summary there are a number of imaging modalities appropriate for investigating a possible case of aortic dissection. Ideally, a strategy should be agreed between district general hospitals and the local tertiary referral centre to facilitate the rapid assessment and immediate management of suspected cases.

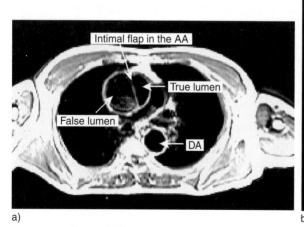

a)

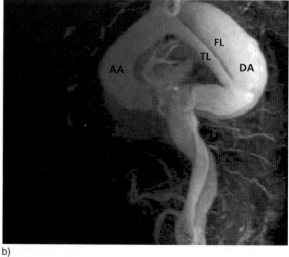

b)

Figure 17.6
(a) Magnetic resonance imaging (MRI) of aortic dissection – cross-section. Note the relatively small, compressed true lumen (TL) and the larger false lumen (FL) with thrombus within it. (b) MRI of aortic dissection – 3-D reconstruction. The full extent of the dissection can be seen. AA, ascending aorta; DA, descending aorta

IMMEDIATE MANAGEMENT

Initial medical resuscitation of the patient with aortic dissection is essential. A peripheral arterial line is preferably placed in the right arm to remain functional during surgery, unless blood pressure is significantly higher in the left arm. Speed is of the essence and transfer to theatre where required should not be delayed in an attempt to stabilize the situation.

Where the blood pressure is elevated, opiates should be used to alleviate pain. Systolic blood pressure should be lowered to around 100 mmHg or the lowest level commensurate with adequate perfusion. Short-acting intravenous beta-blockers such as labetalol and esmolol are recommended as they reduce both blood pressure and the force of left ventricular ejection. Reducing the force of left ventricular ejection (dP/dt) is important in reducing aortic wall stress. This will reduce the chances of extension and rupture. A short half-life is important as the haemodynamic situation can change rapidly. In situations where beta-blockers are contraindicated, sodium nitroprusside or calcium channel blockers are appropriate alternatives. If medical management is considered the definitive management strategy, then intravenous agents should in time be converted to suitable oral agents. Cardiac tamponade often complicates a proximal dissection and may be rapidly fatal. Pericardiocentesis has been used to stabilize patients prior to surgery, but it may provoke haemodynamic collapse and be harmful rather than beneficial. Its use should, therefore, be restricted to situations of marked hypotension or electromechanical dissociation.

DEFINITIVE MANAGEMENT

There is a general consensus as to how patients with aortic dissection should be managed (Box 17.3). For acute type A dissection surgery is considered superior to medical therapy. There are a number of surgical approaches to the repair of type A dissection beginning in

---

Box 17.3: Indications for medical and surgical therapy

Medical
Uncomplicated type B dissection
Stable chronic dissection

Surgical
Type A dissection
Type B dissection complicated by:
  Progression
  Rupture
  Marfan's syndrome
  Vital organ compromise
  Retrograde propagation into ascending aorta

the ascending aorta. Generally, after division of the aorta at the sinotubular junction, a tube graft is anastomosed to the sinotubular ridge, and the aortic valve repaired or replaced. The distal connection of the tube graft is usually made in the arch or beyond as required. There is much debate, it appears, in the management of the acutely dissected arch. Total replacement with re-anastomosis of branch vessels may be required.

Those patients suffering from acute type B dissection are at lower immediate risk and medical therapy is favoured. This is because the risks of surgery are not negligible. In particular, the risk of paraplegia is around 18%. However, these patients should still be discussed with a cardiothoracic centre, as if the distal dissection is complicated by progression, vital organ compromise, rupture, retrograde propagation into the ascending aorta, or if the patient has Marfan's syndrome then surgery is indicated. Patients with chronic dissection are managed differently, and, unless complicated, medical management is the treatment of choice for type A and B dissections.

ENDOVASCULAR TECHNIQUES

Stenting and fenestration are still relatively new techniques, but are becoming more commonly used.

Fenestration was first devised in 1990. It involves repeatedly perforating the intimal flap with a wire, thus entering the false lumen. A balloon is then used to enlarge the perforation. A more complete discussion of the precise indications for fenestration is beyond the scope of this chapter.

Stents may be used to open affected arterial branches, or stent grafts used to treat the dissection itself. Large diameter stent grafts (on average 3.5 cm), placed via the femoral artery, aim to close the site of entry into the false lumen and promote thrombosis within it (Fig. 17.7). Complications of stent-graft placement include paraplegia and stent-graft migration.

The exact role of stenting has yet to be determined, but in complicated type B dissection, where intervention is felt necessary, stent-graft placement is beginning to replace surgical intervention in experienced centres. Stents have recently been used to treat type A dissection successfully.

FOLLOW-UP

Long-term medical therapy to control hypertension is indicated for all patients. Late aneurysm rupture is far more common in patients with poorly controlled blood pressure. Blood pressure should be maintained below 135/80 mmHg. Beta-blockers are the agents of choice; calcium channel blockers such as diltiazem or verapamil are second line. Combination therapy is often required.

Approximately one-third of late deaths occur from rupture of the dissecting aneurysm, or rupture of an aneurysm at a remote site. These often occur more distally and usually arise

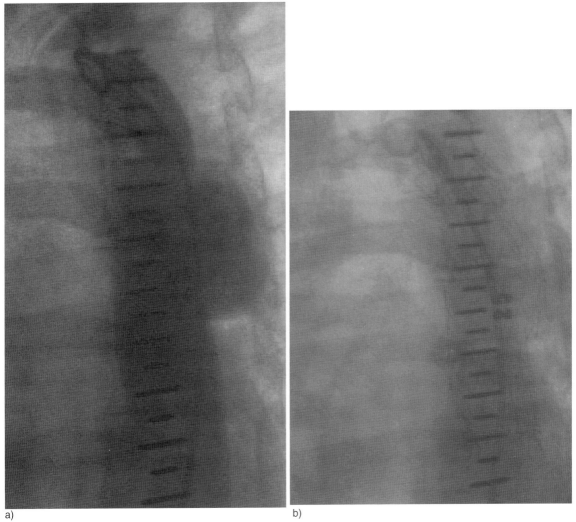

a)
b)

Figure 17.7
Descending thoracic aneurysm (a) pre- and (b) post-stent

from the residual false lumen. They typically appear around 18 months, and the majority have occurred by 2 years.

Long-term surveillance is, therefore, essential, and serial aortic imaging by TOE, CT, or MRI is recommended. MRI is the method of choice, as it is non-invasive, does not involve exposure to ionizing radiation, and can provide complete visualization of the entire aorta.

The European Society of Cardiology guidelines recommend follow-up at 1, 3, 6 and 12 months, and then yearly examinations. In an ideal world, combined medical and surgical follow-up is desirable.

MARFAN'S SYNDROME

Marfan's syndrome is a well-known multi-system disease. Most deaths used to be due to aortic rupture or heart failure. Close follow-up of patients with Marfan's combined with timely surgery has increased the life expectancy from 45 years in 1972 to 72 years in 1995.

Current recommendations advocate close monitoring of the aortic root and valve by serial echocardiography (yearly), and the use of beta-blockers (of particular benefit when the root has yet to dilate and is less than 4 cm), which reduce the rate of aortic root dilatation. A slowly enlarging aortic root should be replaced when it reaches a diameter of 5.5–6 cm. Those whose roots expand by more than 0.5 cm per year and those with a strong family history of early (<40 years) dissection should undergo surgery when the aortic root reaches 5 cm, or possibly less.

The 30-day mortality of elective repair is approximately 2%, with survival at 10 years 75%. This clearly contrasts favourably with the outcome of acute aortic dissection. Similar strategies of surveillance and management in those with aortic root dilatation secondary to other pathologies may be appropriate.

CONCLUSIONS

Acute aortic dissection is a lethal condition, which requires a high degree of clinical suspicion to diagnose. The immediate management is medical, and continued medical therapy is the mainstay for type B dissections and chronic dissection. Early surgery is generally required for those with proximal dissection. Endovascular techniques offer a promising alternative for complex type B dissection. Close long-term follow-up is essential, with frequent repeat imaging, as distal aneurysm formation is common and associated with a high risk of rupture. Patients with Marfan's syndrome are at high risk of dissection and regular monitoring of the aortic valve and root with timely intervention is essential.

Further reading

Braunwald E, Zipes D, Libby P (eds) 2001 Heart disease. A textbook of cardiovascular medicine, 6th edn. WB Saunders, Philadelphia, pp. 1431–1448

Devereux R, Roman M 1999 Aortic dissection in Marfan's syndrome. NEJM 340: 1358–1359

Erbel R, Alfonso F, Boileau C et al. 2001 Diagnosis and management of aortic dissection. Recommendations of the task force on aortic dissection, European Society of Cardiology. Eur Heart J 22: 1642–1681

Hagan P, Nienaber C, Isselbacher E et al. 2000 The International Registry of Acute Aortic Dissection (IRAD): New insights into an old disease. JAMA 283: 897–903

Nienaber C, Eagle K 2003 Aortic dissection: new frontiers in diagnosis and management. Part II: Therapeutic management and follow-up. Circulation 108: 772–778.

SELF-ASSESSMENT

Questions
a. What initial features make you suspect aortic dissection?
b. What immediate steps should you take?
c. When would you refer a patient with Marfan's for consideration of aortic root surgery?

Answers
a. Severe, tearing interscapular pain; one or more absent peripheral pulses; and shocked appearance despite normal or high blood pressure. The latter is important – patients often look acutely unwell despite no obvious focal signs.
b. The immediate aim is to decrease the risk of progression and complications, such as aortic wall rupture. Rapid control of pain with intravenous opiates will decrease sympathetic activation with its detrimental haemodynamic effects. Further blood pressure control, preferably with a short-acting intravenous beta-blocker, should be introduced ideally with intra-arterial blood pressure monitoring. The case should be discussed early with the local cardiothoracic centre.
c. Patients with a strong family history of acute dissection at a young age; patients with a rapidly enlarging aortic root; and when the aortic root reaches 5.5–6.0 cm if slowly enlarging.

Management of pulmonary embolism

18

M. Stewart

EPIDEMIOLOGY

Deep vein thrombosis (DVT) and pulmonary emboli (PE) affect 1.0 and 0.65 per 1000 respectively of the general population, mainly during, or soon after, a period of hospitalization. Each year in the UK 65 000 patients are hospitalized due to PE and 20 000 patients die as a direct consequence of the disorder. The incidence of vascular thrombotic events (VTE) increases sharply with age from 1 per 100 000 per year in childhood to nearly 1% per year over the age of 80 years. Pulmonary embolism is still the principal cause of death in 10% of all patients who die in hospital and is a contributory cause in a further 10%.

AETIOLOGY

Virchow described the classic triad of factors that predispose towards VTE:

1. Local trauma to a vessel wall
2. Hypercoagulability
3. Blood stasis.

In most patients risk factors are acquired (including major trauma):

- Recent surgery
- Immobilization
- Smoking
- Increasing age
- Obesity
- Pregnancy and the oral contraceptive pill
- Neoplasia.

Some patients have a hereditary predisposition to hypercoagulability:

- Defects in fibrinolysis
- Congenital deficiencies of antithrombin, protein C, protein S or plasminogen
- Excess procoagulant formation may be due to the prothrombin (factor II) 20210A gene defect.

Table 18.1: Procoagulant abnormalities

Procoagulant abnormality	Incidence in population	Incidence in patients with venous thrombosis	× increase in risk of venous thrombosis
Factor V Leiden	3%	20%	8–10
Prothrombin 20210A	2%	6%	2–3
High concentrations factor VIII (>1500 IU/l)	11%	25%	6
Hyperhomocysteinaemia (>18.5 µmol/l)	5%	10%	2.5–4
Protein C deficiency	0.2–0.4 %	3%	10
Antithrombin deficiency	0.02%	1%	15–20

Proteins C and S and antithrombin are the main natural inhibitors of the procoagulant system; deficiencies of these proteins may lead to excessive thrombin formation. A polymorphism in the gene for factor V (factor V Leiden) is associated with resistance to the anticoagulant action of protein C (protein C resistance). High concentrations of factor VIII, determined by blood group and hyperhomocysteinaemia are also associated with an increased risk of thrombosis (see Table 18.1).

PATHOPHYSIOLOGY

The clinical effects of PE depend on:

- the extent of pulmonary vascular obstruction
- the release of vasoactive and broncho-constricting humoral agents from activated platelets (e.g. serotonin, thomboxane A2)
- the presence of any pre-existing cardiopulmonary disease
- the age and general health of the patient.

Right-ventricular afterload increases significantly when more than 25% of the pulmonary circulation is obstructed. Initially, right-ventricular pressure rises, the right ventricle dilates, and then, as the right ventricle begins to fail, right-ventricular pressure eventually falls. An otherwise normal right ventricle is incapable of increasing pulmonary artery pressure much above 50–60 mmHg in response to sudden major obstruction of the pulmonary circulation.

Death in massive PE is a result of acute bi-ventricular failure, a fall in systemic (aortic) blood pressure and myocardial ishaemia. Left-ventricular diastolic filling is impaired due to reduced pulmonary blood flow and displacement of the interventricular septum into the left-ventricular cavity. Myocardial ischaemia results from a fall in the trans-coronary pressure gradient due to an elevation in the right heart (coronary sinus) pressure in combination with a fall in systemic blood pressure.

CLINICAL CLASSIFICATION OF PULMONARY EMBOLISM

NON-MASSIVE PULMONARY EMBOLISM

Obstruction of small distal pulmonary arteries, often resulting in parenchymal lung infarction. Many small distal emboli are asymptomatic; when symptoms occur they include:

- tachypnoea
- pleuritic chest pain
- haemoptysis.

There is usually no haemodynamic disturbance and physical examination is often normal, but may reveal tachycardia, pleural rub or mild pyrexia.

SUBMASSIVE PULMONARY EMBOLISM

Echocardiographic signs of right-ventricular dysfunction can identify a sub group of patients with non-massive PE, termed **submassive**, and who have a worse prognosis and may benefit from more aggressive therapy.

MASSIVE PULMONARY EMBOLISM

Significant obstruction of the pulmonary arteries resulting in haemodynamic compromise consisting of shock and/or hypotension (systolic blood pressure of <90 mmHg or a pressure drop of ≥40 mmHg for >15 min) if not caused by new onset arrhythmia, hypovolaemia or sepsis.

Symptoms include:

- severe dyspnoea
- dull central chest pain due to myocardial ischaemia
- tachycardia
- gallop rhythm
- raised venous pressure
- tachypnoea.

INVESTIGATIONS (see Fig. 18.1 for suggested algorithm)

ELECTROCARDIOGRAPHY

Eighty-seven per cent of patients with proven PE, will have some non-specific electrocardiogram (ECG) change, which may include:

- sinus tachycardia
- atrial fibrillation

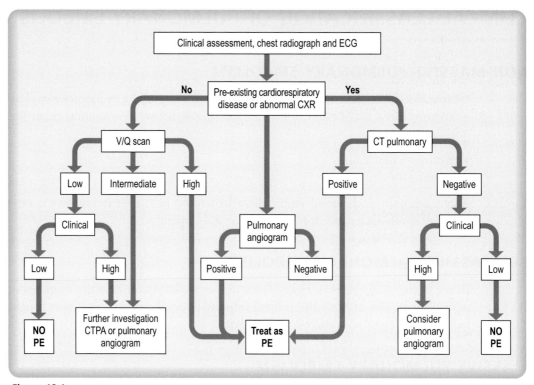

Figure 18.1
Algorithm for the investigation of suspected acute pulmonary embolism CTPA, computer tomography pulmonary angiogram; V/Q, ventilation perfusion

- T-wave changes
- ST segment abnormalities particularly in the anteroseptal leads (V1–V3).

Characteristic abnormalities including S1, Q3, T3 pattern, right bundle branch block, p pulmonale and right-axis deviation are much less common, being present in only 30% of patients with massive PE.

ECHOCARDIOGRAPHY

Right ventricular dysfunction identifies those with submassive PE without haemodynamic compromise who may benefit from thrombolytic therapy (Box 18.1). Severe right ventricular dysfunction is associated with an increased mortality in massive PE. Thrombus may rarely be seen in the right heart.

Transoesophageal echo may identify thrombus in the main pulmonary artery. If a patent foramen ovale or atrial septal defect is seen, special consideration needs to be given to the management of potential paradoxical embolism from the venous to the systemic circulation.

Box 18.1: Echocardiographic features of significant pulmonary emboli that may indicate benefit from thrombolysis

Right ventricular dilatation
Right ventricular hypokinesis
Elevated right ventricular end systolic pressure >40 mmHg
Paradoxical septal movement
Loss of inferior vena cava (IVC) collapse
Presence of thrombus in right ventricle or pulmonary artery

CHEST RADIOGRAPHY

Changes are common, but non-specific and include:

- atelectasis
- pleural effusion
- pulmonary infiltrates
- elevation of a hemidiaphragm
- dilatation of a major proximal pulmonary artery and areas of pulmonary oligaemia may suggest major arterial obstruction
- wedge-shaped opacities in the peripheral lung fields, as a result of pulmonary infarction, may occur with minor PE.

When PE is a possible diagnosis, the chest radiograph is more helpful when it suggests alternative diagnoses such as pneumonia or a pneumothorax.

ISOTOPE RADIONUCLIDE VENTILATION-PERFUSION (V/Q) LUNG SCANNING

This remains the principal investigation in suspected PE. A normal perfusion scan rules out significant PE. A reduction in perfusion associated with a ventilation/perfusion mismatch suggests PE. The clinical likelihood of PE is taken into account when interpreting the radionuclide scan, which is usually reported as indicating a low, intermediate or high probability of PE. The diagnosis of PE can be considered confirmed in patients in whom the index of clinical suspicion is high and whose isotope lung scan indicates a high probability of PE. Radionuclide scanning tends to underestimate the angiographic severity and haemodynamic disturbance of PE.

COMPUTED TOMOGRAPHY AND MAGNETIC RESONANCE SCANNING

These are increasingly being used to investigate suspected PE, especially in patients with pre-existing cardiopulmonary disease. Spiral CT angiography provides excellent identification of emboli in the main, lobar and segmental pulmonary arteries but is not able to exclude emboli beyond the subsegmental level. Coexistent pathology may be detected to provide an alternative diagnosis if PE is excluded.

Box 18.2: Conditions resulting in elevation of D-dimer

Venous thromboembolic disease
Myocardial infarction
Sepsis
Malignancy
Pneumonia
Pregnancy
Arthritis
Increased age
Renal failure

PULMONARY ANGIOGRAPHY

This remains the definitive investigation to confirm the presence of PE. It should be considered in patients with a high clinical suspicion who have had a non diagnostic radionuclide or CT scan.

D-DIMER

In conditions where thrombus is formed, plasmin-mediated proteolysis of cross-linked fibrin releases D-dimeric fragments. Increased levels of D-dimer can be identified in 99% of patients with PE proven by radionuclide lung scanning. Although elevated levels are sensitive for the presence of PE, they are not specific (see Box 18.2). A negative test can support a low clinical suspicion of PE, but a positive test cannot be used to make a diagnosis of venous thromboembolism. D-dimer assay may be useful in reducing the number of radionuclide scans in patients with a low clinical suspicion of PE.

MANAGEMENT

Management is threefold: prevention of further embolic events; therapy to support respiratory and haemodynamic function; and treatment to relieve the thrombus load and vascular obstruction.

If the patient is not haemodynamically compromised and massive PE is not suspected, low-dose molecular weight heparin may be started **before** the results of investigations are available. Supportive therapy including analgesia and oxygen should be commenced. Ventilatory support should be considered in the presence of acute respiratory failure. If haemodynamically compromised the careful use of fluids and inotropes should be considered. Fluid administration should be limited to 500 ml initially, as right ventricular function is likely to be significantly compromised and will be further impaired by over-enthusiastic fluid administration. Fluids should not be used to try to correct hypotension. Dobutamine and or dopamine may be used as inotropic agents and will improve cardiac index even if the patient is normotensive; noradrenaline may be considered if the patient is hypotensive (Fig. 18.2).

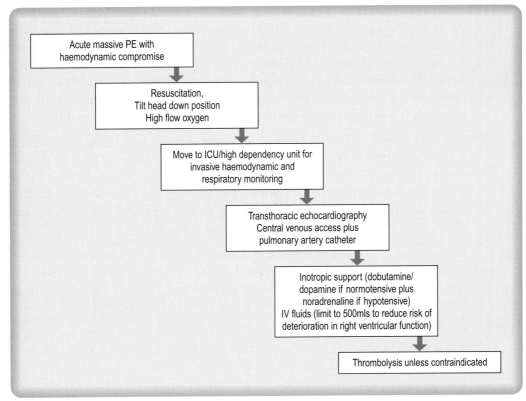

Figure 18.2
Management of acute massive PE

There are three immediate treatment options to reduce the pulmonary vascular obstruction caused by the thrombus:

1. Anticoagulation with heparin (unfractionated or low molecular weight)
2. Thrombolytic therapy
3. Pulmonary embolectomy.

The choice of treatment will depend on the severity of the PE. In the management of acute massive PE heparin should be regarded as adjunctive rather than the sole therapy; it does not reduce the immediate mortality of PE, but may reduce deaths caused by further emboli.

ANTICOAGULATION

Heparin accelerates the action of antithrombin III and prevents further fibrin deposition, allowing the body's fibrinolytic system to lyse an existing clot.

If unfractionated heparin is used in patients with DVT and PE, higher doses may be required to achieve adequate anticoagulation than in those without active thrombosis,

271

owing to the presence of high plasma concentrations of factor VIII and heparin-binding proteins. The activated partial thromboplastin time (APTT) should be kept in the range 2.0–3.0 times control values. Unfractionated heparin, 80 IU/kg, is used as a loading dose, followed by an infusion of 18 IU/kg per hour. **If unfractionated heparin is used, it is essential to ensure that a therapeutic level of anticoagulation is achieved. The APTT should be checked 6 hours after initiation and at least daily once therapeutic levels are obtained. It must be rechecked 6 hours after any alteration in infusion rate.**

Low-molecular-weight (LMWT) heparins are less prone to binding than unfractionated heparin and, therefore, resistance is unlikely. Their half-lives are longer, the dose-response is more predictable, they may cause fewer bleeding side-effects and have a lower incidence of heparin induced thrombocytopaenia. LMWT heparins are at least as effective as standard unfractionated heparin and do not require regular monitoring of anticoagulant effect (except in pregnancy, renal failure or extreme obesity).

In non-massive PE loading with an oral anticoagulant should be undertaken simultaneously. When warfarin is started during active thrombosis, the levels of protein C and protein S fall, creating a thrombogenic potential. Oral loading with warfarin should therefore be covered by simultaneous intravenous/LMWT heparin for 4–5 days.

Oral anticoagulation is given to achieve an international normalized ratio (INR) of 2.0–3.0 and is usually continued for at least 3 months if a time limited risk factor has been identified or for 6 months if the PE was an idiopathic event. For recurrent episodes of PE or if a primary coagulopathy is identified, treatment with warfarin should continue indefinitely.

THROMBOLYTIC AGENTS

These dissolve thrombi by converting plasminogen to the active agent plasmin, which degrades fibrin to soluble peptides. Controlled trials comparing thrombolytic agents with heparin have concluded that pulmonary emboli clear more rapidly with thrombolytic therapy, but their use does not alter long-term mortality in all cases of PE. In patients with massive PE with haemodynamic disturbance, thrombolysis may confer a survival benefit by reducing early mortality. Thrombolysis may also lyse potentially dangerous iliofemoral venous thrombi, which may result in further PE. Unless absolutely contraindicated, thrombolysis should be given to all patients with massive PE with haemodynamic compromise and should be considered in those with submassive PE with echocardiographic features indicating right-ventricular strain (Box 18.3 & Table 18.2).

Heparin infusion, which should not be used concurrently with streptokinase infusion, should continue on completion of thrombolysis for at least 5 days and until adequate oral anticoagulation has been achieved for at least 48 hours (the latter applies to all cases of PE).

PULMONARY EMBOLECTOMY

This may be life saving in patients severely haemodynamically compromised who may not survive the hour or two required to derive benefit from thrombolysis – early involvement of a cardiothoracic surgeon is recommended in this scenario. This may also be considered

Box 18.3: Indications for thrombolysis in pulmonary embolism

Massive pulmonary embolism (PE) with shock and haemodynamic compromise (systolic blood pressure (BP) <90 mmHg, tachycardia, fall in BP >40 mmHg for >15 min)

Consider in:
Submassive PE with right ventricular hypokinesis, elevated pulmonary artery pressures, paradoxical septal movement on echocardiogram
Extensive clot burden on computed tomography scan

Table 18.2: Thrombolysis regimes for venous thromboembolism

Agent	Regime
For pulmonary embolism	
Streptokinase	250 000 IU loading followed by 100 000 IU for 24 hours OR 1.5 million IU intravenously over 2 hours
tPA	100 mg infusion over 2 hours
Reteplase	10 mg intravenous bolus repeated after 30 mins
Urokinase	4400 IU/kg body weight loading followed by 2200 IU/kg for 12 hours
For deep venous thrombosis	
Streptokinase	250 000 IU loading followed by infusion 100 000 IU for up to 72 hours

in situations where thrombolysis may be contraindicated, or if a patient deteriorates despite its administration.

Operative mortality in those who have required cardiopulmonary resuscitation pre-operatively is greater than 50%.

If embolectomy is considered, pulmonary angiography should probably be undertaken, to demonstrate the site and extent of pulmonary arterial obstruction and, importantly, to ensure that the diagnosis is correct.

VENA CAVAL FILTERS

Following PE residual thrombus is almost always present in the deep veins. Attempts to prevent further emboli have been made by surgical interruption or plication of the inferior vena cava (IVC), but procedures involving the percutaneous insertion of devices such as filters and umbrellas are more common.

In patients considered at high risk of further emboli, in whom anticoagulation is contraindicated, or in those who have recurrent emboli despite adequate anticoagulation, an IVC filter may be beneficial in the short term. Subsequent removal of the filter within 2–4 weeks should be considered, as long-term implants are associated with complications such as thrombosis or device migration. In the acute phase of massive PE, any procedure on the IVC that reduces venous return may be potentially detrimental.

Reference

The British Thoracic Society Standards of Care Committee Pulmonary Embolism Guideline Development Group 2003 BTS guidelines for the management of suspected acute pulmonary embolism, 2003. Thorax 58: 470-484

Further reading

Guidelines on Diagnosis and Management of Acute Pulmonary Embolism. Eur Heart J 2000; 21: 1301–1336
Hirsh J, Hoak J 1996 Management of Deep Venous Thrombosis and Pulmonary Embolism. AHA Medical Scientific Statement. Circulation 93(12): 2212–2245
Reidel M 2001 Venous Thromboembolic Disease. Heart 85: 229–240 and 351–360

SELF-ASSESSMENT

Question

1. What is the potential value of newer biochemical markers?

Answer

1. Risk stratification of patients with PE may help to define treatment strategy, including the use of thrombolysis; where best to manage the patient (e.g. high-dependency unit versus ward); length of hospitalization and follow-up. Right ventricular dysfunction in pulmonary embolism is associated with adverse outcome. It has therefore been suggested that patients with submassive PE might benefit from a more aggressive therapeutic approach including thrombolysis. Echocardiography can readily identify patients with right-ventricular dysfunction, but unfortunately in the UK is not widely available out of hours. This has led on to the search for biomarkers that may identify such patients with good sensitivity and specificity and be available 24–7. In this respect troponin I and T have received most attention, with brain natriuretic peptide (BNP) also proving to be of clinical interest.

Troponin T and I

The cardiac troponins T and I are sensitive and specific markers of minor myocardial cell injury (see Ch. 8). In severe PE it is believed that right ventricular ischaemia progresses onto right ventricular dysfunction. Measurement of troponin in the setting of acute PE adds incremental prognostic value to echocardiography (normal echo and negative troponin lowest risk; elevated troponin and abnormal echo highest risk). In addition, elevation of troponins T and I is significantly associated with echocardiographically detected right ventricular dysfunction. Normotensive patients with PE and elevated troponin T levels are at high risk of complicated clinical course and premature mortality. Further studies to define the role of thrombolysis in this group are awaited. It is the authors' belief that in the meantime patients with elevated troponin and PE should be managed aggressively with meticulous monitoring in an HDU (or equivalent) setting and the pros and cons of thrombolysis be considered on an individual basis.

BNP

BNP is released from ventricular and atrial myocardium in response to increased wall stress and/or local ischaemia (see Heart failure, Ch. 12). Current data suggest that a low level of plasma BNP (below the diagnostic cut-off for chronic heart failure) may identify patients with a benign clinical course.

Pulmonary hypertension

19

G. Mikhail

INTRODUCTION

Pulmonary hypertension is a progressive disease that ultimately leads to right-ventricular failure and death. It is characterized by an elevated pulmonary artery pressure and pulmonary vascular resistance.

The incidence of primary pulmonary hypertension (PPH) is estimated to be 1–2/1 000 000/year and approximately 6% appear to be familial. There is a preponderance of females among PPH patients with a ratio of female to male varying between 1.7 and 3.5:1.

DEFINITION

Pulmonary hypertension is defined as an elevated mean pulmonary artery pressure of 25 mmHg or greater at rest or 30 mmHg with exercise. In 1998, the World Health Organization set out new guidelines for the re-classification of pulmonary hypertension (Boxes 19.1 & 19.2).

PATHOLOGY

Pulmonary arteriopathy is characterized by medial hypertrophy, intimal proliferation, concentric laminar intimal fibrosis (the latter usually arranged in a characteristic 'onion-skin' configuration), dilatation lesions, fibrinoid necrosis and plexiform lesions (Fig. 19.1). The pathogenesis of these unusual structures remains undefined. Plexiform lesions have been shown to be composed mainly of endothelial cells as well as smooth muscle cells, myofibroblasts and macrophages. They represent a mass of disorganized vessels that arise from pre-existing pulmonary arteries. The hypothesis that the development of plexiform lesions may represent a form of 'misguided angiogenesis' has been put forward.

Box 19.1: Diagnostic classification (WHO 1998)

1. **Pulmonary arterial hypertension**
   1.1 Primary pulmonary hypertension
   - Sporadic
   - Familial

   1.2 Related to:
   - Collagen vascular disease
   - HIV
   - Drugs/toxins
   - Portal hypertension
   - Persistent pulmonary hypertension of the newborn

2. **Pulmonary venous hypertension**
   2.1 Left-sided atrial or ventricular heart disease
   2.2 Left-sided valvular heart disease
   2.3 Extrinsic compression of central pulmonary veins
   2.4 Pulmonary veno-occlusive disease

3. **Pulmonary hypertension associated with disorders of the respiratory system and/or hypoxia**
   3.1 Chronic obstructive pulmonary disease
   3.2 Interstitial lung disease
   3.3 Sleep disordered breathing
   3.4 Alveolar hypoventilation disorders
   3.5 Chronic exposure to high altitude
   3.6 Neonatal lung disease
   3.7 Alveolar-capillary dysplasia

4. **Pulmonary hypertension as a result of chronic thrombotic and/or embolic disease**
   4.1 Thromboembolic obstruction of proximal pulmonary arteries
   4.2 Obstruction of distal pulmonary arteries

5. **Pulmonary hypertension due to disorders directly affecting the pulmonary vasculature**
   5.1 Inflammatory
   - Sarcoidosis
   - Schistosomiasis

   5.2 Pulmonary capillary hemangiomatosis

(Modified from Gibbs 2001)

Box 19.2: Functional assessment

A. Class I – Patients with pulmonary hypertension but without resulting limitation of physical activity. Ordinary physical activity does not cause undue dyspnoea or fatigue, chest pain or near syncope.

B. Class II – Patients with pulmonary hypertension resulting in slight limitation of physical activity. They are comfortable at rest. Ordinary physical activity causes undue dyspnoea or fatigue, chest pain or near syncope.

C. Class III – Patients with pulmonary hypertension resulting in marked limitation of physical activity. They are comfortable at rest. Less than ordinary activity causes undue dyspnoea or fatigue, chest pain or near syncope.

D. Class IV – Patients with pulmonary hypertension with inability to carry out any physical activity without symptoms. These patients manifest signs of right heart failure. Dyspnoea and/or fatigue may even be present at rest. Discomfort is increased by any physical activity.

(Modified from the New York Heart Association [NYHA] Functional Classification)

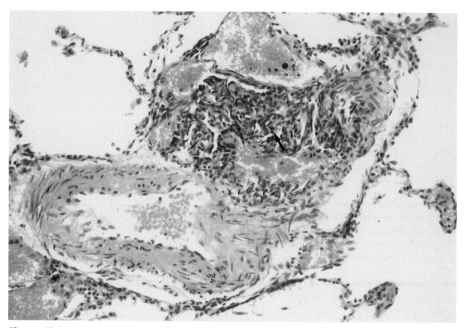

Figure 19.1
Plexiform lesion in primary pulmonary hypertension.
Plexiform lesion arising from a small muscular artery and showing a complex cellular proliferation to form tiny vascular channels (arrow). Dilated thin-walled vessels are noted around the parent vessel as well as the vessel containing the plexiform lesion (haematoxylin–eosin, ×100)

AETIOLOGY

The aetiology of PPH remains undefined. The disease can occur in a familial or sporadic form. The sporadic form of the disease may be caused by interaction between a genetic factor, possibly related to the gene encoding the familial form, with one or more triggering factors (Fig. 19.2). Such factors include:

- diet and drugs
- imbalance of vasoactive mediators
- disregulation of potassium channels
- autoimmunity
- infection
- inflammation.

The interaction between genetic and triggering factors could result in endothelial injury and vasoconstriction leading to vascular remodelling.

GENETICS

The familial form of PPH is inherited as an autosomal dominant and is associated with genetic anticipation. In this form of inheritance, there is worsening of the disease in subsequent generations. The gene for PPH has been localized to a 27-centimorgan region

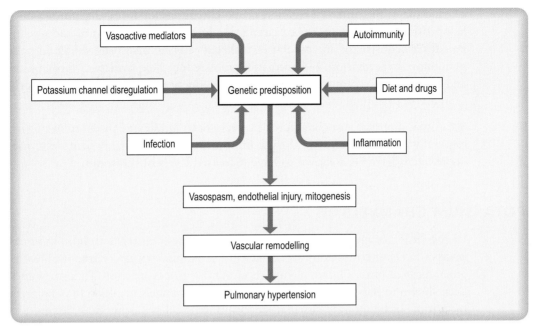

Figure 19.2
Aetiology of pulmonary hypertension. A diagrammatic illustration of the aetiology and pathophysiology of pulmonary hypertension

on chromosome 2q31-32. Both the familial and sporadic forms of PPH have been recently associated with mutations of the bone morphogenetic protein receptor type II gene (BMPR2).

DIET

There appears to be an association between appetite suppressants and the development of PPH. In the late 1960s, an epidemic of pulmonary arterial hypertension (PAH) began in Switzerland, West Germany and in Austria after the introduction of aminorex fumarate (Menocil). More recently, in Europe, a clear association was demonstrated between fenfluramine and PAH. The combination of fenfluramine and phenteramine, which is also an appetite suppressant, has also been associated with the development of pulmonary hypertension and valvular heart disease.

The use of rapeseed oil for cooking in Spain, through its illegal sale, resulted in an epidemic of pulmonary hypertension. This resulted in an acute toxic syndrome consisting of skin, gastric, neurological and pulmonary symptoms.

VASOACTIVE MEDIATORS

The tone of the pulmonary vascular tree is reliant upon a balance between vasoconstrictor and vasodilator mechanisms. An imbalance of vasoactive mediators has been demonstrated in patients with pulmonary hypertension. In such patients, there is an increase in the urinary excretion of the vasoconstrictor 11-dehydro-thromboxane B_2 and a reduction in the urinary excretion of the potent vasodilator 2,3-dinor-6-ketoprostaglandin $F_{1\alpha}$. Increased circulating levels and expression of endothelin-1, a potent vasoconstrictor, in vascular endothelial cells has also been shown in patients with pulmonary hypertension. In contrast, there is reduced expression of nitric oxide synthase and prostacyclin receptor protein as well as reductions in the enzyme prostacyclin synthase in such patients.

Serotonin, a potent vasoconstrictor, has also been implicated in pulmonary hypertension especially in association with the use of appetite suppressants. Patients who use anorexigens have been shown to have increased levels of serotonin.

POTASSIUM CHANNELS

Disregulation of potassium channels can lead to vasoconstriction. Inhibition of membrane potassium channels leads to depolarization of pulmonary artery smooth muscle cells and an increase in intracellular calcium resulting in vasoconstriction. Patients with PAH have been shown to have abnormalities of potassium channels resulting in depolarization of the membrane of pulmonary vascular smooth muscle cells. Furthermore, aminorex, fenfluramine and dexfenfluramine have been shown to inhibit potassium channels.

AUTOIMMUNITY

There are a number of associations between various autoimmune diseases and PAH. Patients with scleroderma, the CREST syndrome, dermatomyositis, rheumatoid arthritis and systemic lupus erythematosus as well as hypothyroidism have been known to develop pulmonary hypertension.

INFECTION

A viral aetiology has been previously suggested as a possible cause for the development of PAH. There is also an association with HIV and PAH.

INFLAMMATION

Various mediators of inflammation have been implicated in the pathophysiology of pulmonary hypertension. Such mediators can result in vasoconstriction and cell growth. Macrophages as well as B and T cells have been found in the vicinity of remodelled pulmonary vessels. Such cells are thought to be responsible for the release of cytokines and growth factors such as transforming growth factor (TGF)-beta, platelet derived growth factor (PDGF) and vascular endothelial growth factor (VEGF). Increased serum concentrations of interleukin 1, interleukin 6 and the chemokine MIP-1alpha in lung tissue in patients with PAH has been demonstrated. Overexpression of 5-lipoxygenase and 5-lipoxygenase activating protein (FLAP) has also been associated with PAH.

CLINICAL PRESENTATION

The onset of symptoms is usually insidious with several years elapsing before the diagnosis is actually made. Patients can present with any of the following symptoms:

- Dyspnoea
- Presyncope or syncope
- Chest pain
- Palpitations
- Haemoptysis
- Sudden death.

The physical signs in pulmonary hypertensive patients are often advanced at the time of presentation. These include:

- cyanosis
- raised jugular venous pressure
- right-ventricular heave
- loud pulmonary component of the second heart sound
- murmurs of tricuspid regurgitation and/or pulmonary regurgitation
- hepatomegaly
- ascites
- peripheral oedema.

SCREENING FOR PULMONARY HYPERTENSION

The onset of symptoms in pulmonary hypertension is insidious and the diagnosis is usually made when the disease is advanced. Patients with a suspected diagnosis of pulmonary hypertension should be referred to a specialized centre without delay. The diagnosis can then be confirmed and initiation of treatment can be made when it is most likely to be successful. The following groups of patients should be screened: 1) families with known PPH, 2) patients with HIV, 3) patients with connective tissue diseases, 4) patients with liver disease and/or portal hypertension, 5) patients with a history of appetite-suppressant drug use, and 6) patients with a history of intravenous drug abuse.

Screening should begin with a thorough history and clinical examination. Investigations should begin with an **electrocardiogram, chest radiograph** (Box 19.3) and **respiratory function tests**. Patients with suspected pulmonary hypertension should have a **transthoracic echocardiogram**. If these baseline investigations suggest a diagnosis of pulmonary hypertension, patients should be referred to a specialized centre.

Cardiac catheterization remains the gold standard for establishing the diagnosis of pulmonary hypertension. At the time of cardiac catheterization, full haemodynamic measurements should be made as well as testing for acute vasodilator response. A number of other investigations need to be carried out in order to confirm the diagnosis and to exclude secondary causes (Box 19.3).

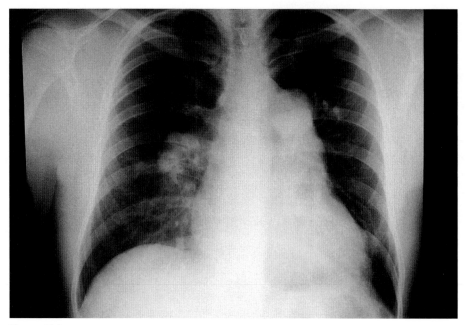

Figure 19.3
A chest X-ray of a patient with PAH. There is significant enlargement of the main pulmonary artery and of the hilar pulmonary vessels bilaterally. The peripheral parenchymal vascularity appears diminished

---

Box 19.3: *Investigations for the diagnosis of pulmonary hypertension*

Electrocardiogram
Chest radiograph
Respiratory function tests
Echocardiogram
Ventilation perfusion scan
High-resolution computed tomography (CT) scan
Contrast, helical CT scan
Pulmonary angiography
6-minute walk or incremental shuttle test
Nocturnal oxygen saturation
Respiratory function tests
Cardiac catheterization with vasodilator study
Blood tests

- Haematology
  - Full blood count
  - ESR
  - Clotting screen
  - Thrombophilia screen
  - Abnormal haemoglobin

- Biochemistry
  - Urea and electrolyte, glucose, lipids
  - Liver function tests
  - Serum ACE
  - Thyroid function

Box 19.3: (Cont'd) Investigations for the diagnosis of pulmonary hypertension

- Urine
  - Beta HCG

- Autoimmune
  - Anti-nuclear factor –   DsDNA Abs
  - Anti-centromere –   ANCA
  - Anti SCL 70, RNP, Sm, La, Ro, Jo-1 –   rheumatoid factor

- Tumour markers
  - HCG, AFP, CA-125

- Microbiology/virology
  - Hepatitis B, C status –   EBV, CMV, H simplex
  - VDRL/TPHA –   toxoplasma, aspergillus
  - HIV –   schistosomiasis, fileria

TREATMENT

MEDICAL THERAPIES

Vasodilator therapy is the mainstay of treatment in patients with PAH. Such therapy is used in an attempt to reduce pulmonary artery pressure and, thus, right-ventricular afterload. Vasodilator therapy, however, can also be associated with an increased risk to the patient and should not be used in patients with pulmonary venous hypertension. Acute vasodilator testing can help identify those patients who may respond to long-term oral vasodilator treatment. Thus, all patients should have an initial trial with short-acting vasodilator therapy (such as inhaled nitric oxide, nebulized or intravenous epoprostenol or intravenous adenosine) during right-heart catheterization. Incremental doses of any of the above mentioned agents are administered during right-heart catheterization and haemodynamic measurements are carried out at baseline and at the end of each dose. A positive response is defined as >20% reduction in mean pulmonary artery pressure or pulmonary vascular resistance without a decrease in cardiac output.

Patients who respond to acute vasodilator testing and who have a cardiac index >2.1 l/min/m², and/or mixed venous oxygen saturation >63%, and/or right atrial pressure <10 mmHg, should be commenced on calcium channel blockers such as **nifedepine** or **amlodopine**. Calcium channel blockers should be administered whilst the patient is in hospital. The dose should be uptitrated according to symptoms and with close monitoring of oxygen saturation, blood pressure and exercise tolerance. Patients who are 'non-responders' as well as those patients with a cardiac index <2.1 l/min/m², and/or mixed venous oxygen saturation <63% should be commenced on intravenous **epoprostenol** (Fig. 19.4). A number of studies have shown that patients on long-term intravenous epoprostenol therapy have improved exercise tolerance, haemodynamics and survival. Intravenous epoprostenol is usually administered via a Hickman line using a portable infusion pump. If the infusion is abruptly stopped, this can result in rebound pulmonary hypertension and death.

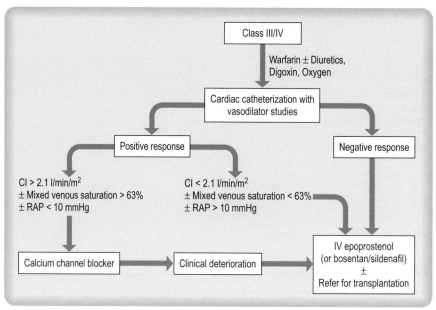

Figure 19.4
Treatment of primary pulmonary hypertension CI, cardiac index; RAP, right atrial pressure

The major drawback of intravenous epoprostenol is with the drug delivery system, including pump failure and catheter infection. Nebulized epoprostenol acts as a selective pulmonary vasodilator and has been shown to reduce the pulmonary vascular resistance in patients with pulmonary hypertension with little effect on systemic vascular resistance.

Inhaled **nitric oxide** also acts as a selective pulmonary vasodilator which is used usually in the hospital setting for the acute reduction in pulmonary artery pressure.

Warfarin has been shown to prolong survival in patients with pulmonary hypertension. In PAH there is a predisposition to thrombosis because of right ventricular failure. Furthermore, thrombotic lesions have been demonstrated in the pulmonary vascular tree.

Other medical therapies available for the treatment of PAH include **oxygen, diuretics** and **digoxin.** The latter has been shown to improve right-ventricular function in such patients and can be commenced when patients remain symptomatic whilst on medical therapy.

New therapies

More recent therapies have evolved for the treatment of patients with pulmonary hypertension. These include: intravenous or nebulized **iloprost** (a stable analogue of prostacyclin with a longer half life), subcutaneous **treprostinil** (a heat stable form of prostacyclin), **beraprost** (an oral prostacyclin analogue), oral **bosentan** (an endothelin antagonist) and oral **sildenafil** (a cGMP-specific phosphodiesterase type 5 inhibitor).

SURGICAL TREATMENT

Various therapeutic options are available for the treatment of patients with pulmonary hypertension. These include **atrial septostomy,** which, by creating a right-to-left shunt, can help to decompress the right ventricle. It is of particular benefit in patients with syncope. **Thromboendarterectomy** has also been shown to be of benefit in patients with thromboembolic pulmonary hypertension. Patients who continue to deteriorate despite medical therapy will require **heart and lung transplantation.** The 1-year survival is approximately 65–70%. Obliterative bronchiolitis, however, remains the major complication of long-term survival in lung-transplant recipients.

CONCLUSIONS AND FUTURE DIRECTIONS

Patients with PAH present with non-specific symptoms and signs, and the diagnosis is often made at the end stages of the disease. Such patients constitute a small and neglected group, who require specialized investigations and treatment. Pulmonary hypertension continues to be a challenge to the physician diagnosing and treating it.

Over recent years, various aetiological mechanisms have come to light, and newer novel therapies are now available for the treatment of this condition. Further research is clearly required in this field, which could result in the improved management of this condition.

Editors note: Developments in this rapidly advancing field are reflected in the recently published guidelines from the European Society of Cardiology, on pulmonary arterial hypertension (2004), Galié N et al.

Further reading

Abenhaim L, Moride Y, Brenot F et al. 1996 Appetite-suppressant drugs and the risk of primary pulmonary hypertension. International Primary Pulmonary Hypertension Study Group. N Engl J Med 335(9): 609–616

Barst RJ, Maislin G, Fishman AP 1999 Vasodilator therapy for primary pulmonary hypertension in children. Circulation 99: 1197–1208

Barst RJ, Rubin LJ, Long WA et al. 1996 A comparison of continuous intravenous epoprostenol (prostacyclin) with conventional therapy for primary pulmonary hypertension. The Primary Pulmonary Hypertension Study Group. N Engl J Med 334(5): 296–302

Channick RN, Simonneau G, Sitbon O et al. 2001 Effects of the dual endothelin-receptor antagonist bosentan in patients with pulmonary hypertension: a randomised placebo-controlled study. Lancet 358: 1119–1123

Christman BW, McPherson CD, Newman JH et al. 1992 An imbalance between the excretion of thromboxane and prostacyclin metabolites in pulmonary hypertension. N Engl J Med 327(2): 70–75

Galié N, Rubin LJ 2004 Pulmonary arterial hypertension: epidemiology, pathobiology, assessment and therapy. J Am Coll Cardiol 43: Suppl

Galié N, Torbicki A, Barst R et al. 2004 Guidelines on diagnosis and treatment of pulmonary arterial hypertension. Eur Heart J 25: 2243–2278

Giaid A, Saleh D 1995 Reduced expression of endothelial nitric oxide synthase in the lungs of patients with pulmonary hypertension. N Engl J Med 333(4): 214–221

Giaid A, Yanagisawa M, Langleben D et al. 1993 Expression of endothelin-1 in the lungs of patients with pulmonary hypertension. N Engl J Med 328(24): 1732–1739

McLaughlin VA, Genthner DE, Panella MM, Rich S 1998 Reduction in pulmonary vascular resistance with long-term epoprostenol (prostacyclin) therapy in primary pulmonary hypertension. N Engl J Med 338: 273–277

McLaughlin V, Hess D, Sigman J et al. 2000 Long term effects of UT-15 on hemodynamics and exercise tolerance in primary pulmonary hypertension. Eur Respir J 16: 394s

Mikhail G, Chester AH, Gibbs JSR, Borland JAA, Banner NR, Yacoub MH 1998 Role of vasoactive mediators in primary and secondary pulmonary hypertension. Am J Cardiol 82: 254–255

Mikhail G, Gibbs JSR, Richardson M et al. 1997 An evaluation of nebulized prostacyclin in primary and secondary pulmonary hypertension. Eur Heart J 18: 1499–504

Nagaya N, Uematsu M, Okano Y et al. 1999 Effect of orally active prostacyclin analogue on survival of outpatients with primary pulmonary hypertension. J Am Coll Cardiol 34: 1188–1192

Nichols WC, Koller DL, Slovis B et al. 1997 Localization of the gene for familial primary pulmonary hypertension to chromosome 2q31-32. Nat Genet 15(3): 277–280

Prasad S, Wilkinson J, Gatzoulis M 2000 Sildenafil in primary pulmonary hypertension. N Engl J Med 343: 1342–1343

Rich S 1999 Executive summary from the World Symposium on Primary Pulmonary Hypertension 1998. http://www.who.int/ned/evd/pph.htm

Rubin LJ, Badesch DB, Barst RJ 2002 Bosentan therapy for pulmonary arterial hypertension. N Engl J Med 346: 896–903

Simon J, Gibbs R 2001 Recommendations on the management of pulmonary hypertension in clinical practice. Heart 86(Suppl 1): i1–i13

Wilkens H, Guth A, Konig J et al. 2001 Effect of inhaled iloprost plus oral sildenafil in patients with primary pulmonary hypertension. Circulation 104: 1218–1222

SELF-ASSESSMENT

Questions

A 36-year-old obese woman presents with an 8-month history of increasing breathlessness. Over the last month she has had two episodes of presyncope. An electrocardiograph (ECG) performed by the GP showed right axis deviation and right-ventricular hypertrophy. A chest X-ray showed dilated proximal pulmonary arteries with peripheral prunning.

a. What is the likely diagnosis?

b. What would you like to establish from the history?

c. What other investigations would you perform?

d. How would you treat this patient?

e. What available options are there with regard to transplantation and what would be her overall prognosis following the operation?

f. She has two children and is asking whether there is a screening test available for primary pulmonary hypertension (PPH)?

Answers

a. The likely diagnosis is pulmonary hypertension. The patient is breathless, has right-ventricular hypertrophy on her ECG and has dilated pulmonary arteries on her chest X-ray.

b. This woman is obese and a history of appetite suppressant intake needs to be established. Anorexigens have been strongly associated with pulmonary hypertension. A case-control study which investigated 95 patients with PPH from Europe, demonstrated a clear association between the appetite suppressant fenfluramine and the development of PPH. The relative risk of pulmonary hypertension associated with the administration of dexfenfluramine for more than 3 months was approximately 30 and this was similar to that associated with aminorex.

c. Prompt referral to a specialist pulmonary hypertension centre is needed. The patient will need an echocardiogram to assess right-ventricular function and to estimate her pulmonary artery pressure. She will also need to undergo various imaging investigations and blood tests to exclude secondary causes of pulmonary hypertension (see Box 19.3). A cardiac catheter needs to be performed in order to establish the diagnosis. Reversibility studies using a short acting vasodilator need to be carried out at the time of right heart catheterization.

d. Treament should be commenced with warfarin and diuretic therapy. The patient may well require oxygen therapy if her saturations are <90%. Oral calcium channel blockers such as amlodipine or nifedipine can be commenced if there is a positive response to vasodilators and if the cardiac index is >2.1 l/min/m^2. In 'non-responders', intravenous prostaglandins should be administered via a Hickman line. Alternatively, treprostinil can be administered subcutaneously to avoid intravenous line infection. Oral bosentan has been shown to improve haemodynamics, exercise capacity and functional class in patients in the New York Heart Association (NYHA) Class II and III. It can be used as first-line therapy in such patients.

e. This patient can be offered either a heart–lung, double-lung or single-lung transplant depending on donor availability and on centre expertise. The overall survival at 1 year is 60%, at 5 years 40%, and at 10 years 30%. There does not appear to be a recurrence of pulmonary hypertension in the transplant recipients. However, the main cause of mortality is obliterative bronchiolitis.

f. In the familial form of PPH, the age of onset is variable and the penetrance is incomplete, such that members of families with PPH can inherit the gene as well as have progeny with PPH yet may never develop the disease. The gene for PPH has been localized to chromosome 2q31-32 and has been associated with mutations of BMPR2. It has to be explained to the patients that, although there is a screening test for BMPR2 mutations, only a proportion of those with the gene alteration actually develop the disease. Until further research is carried out, she should be advised that her children could be investigated for early signs of PPH (with ECG, chest X-ray and echo) rather than undergo genetic testing.

Pericardial disease

20

L. Blows and S. Redwood

INTRODUCTION

The pericardium is involved in many different disease processes. Acute inflammation, chronic inflammation, pericardial effusion and constriction present in different manners as a result of their different physiological and pathological effects but the aetiologies are similar. The symptoms and signs with which an individual patient presents will depend upon the relative degree of inflammation, the extent of compression by pericardial fluid and the constrictive effect of thickened pericardium on cardiac function.

The aim of this chapter is to review the aetiology, diagnosis, clinical presentation and management of various aspects of pericardial disease with emphasis on acute and chronic pericarditis, pericardial constriction and pericardial effusion.

ACUTE PERICARDITIS

This condition is caused by inflammation of the pericardium. The most common causes in the UK are Coxsackie viral infection, which can occur in epidemics, and post-myocardial infarction (see Box 20.1).

PRESENTATION

The predominant clinical feature of this condition is chest pain, however, if a significant effusion develops, the haemodynamic effects of this may give rise to the additional symptoms and signs of cardiac tamponade.

Symptoms occur as a direct result of pericardial inflammation. Sharp chest pain, which may be referred to the left shoulder if the diaphragmatic surface is involved, is prominent. The pain is typically worse on inspiration, aggravated by movement and lying down, and relieved by sitting forwards. Occasionally the pain may be epigastric only.

Associated clinical features will vary depending on the cause. Systemic features such as fever, cough, arthralgia, a rash or pruritus may be present and reflect the underlying aetiology. The clinical signs of uncomplicated acute pericarditis may be sparse but a

> **Box 20.1: Causes of acute pericarditis**
>
> Idiopathic
>
> Infections
>
> Viral, e.g. Coxsackie, Epstein–Barr virus (EBV)
>
> Bacterial
>
> Fungal
>
> Parasitic
>
> Immunological
>
> Relapsing pericarditis
>
> Post-infarction (Dressler's syndrome)
>
> Post-cardiotomy syndrome
>
> Rheumatic fever
>
> Still's disease
>
> Rheumatoid arthritis
>
> Systemic lupus erythematosus (SLE)
>
> Mixed connective-tissue disease
>
> Polyarteritis nodosum/Churg–Strauss syndrome

pericardial rub is diagnostic. This may be transient, as an effusion develops. The sound persists on breath holding and is best heard at the lower left sternal edge, leaning forward in inspiration.

INVESTIGATIONS

Investigation of this condition is aimed, firstly, at establishing the diagnosis and, secondly, to establish the aetiology. The search for an underlying cause may be extensive and fruitless. However, baseline investigations may include:

- Full blood count
- Inflammatory markers such as erythrocyte sedimentation rate (ESR) and C-reactive protein (CRP)
- Markers of myocardial necrosis – creatine kinase isomer MB (CKMB), troponin
- Urea and electrolytes
- Blood cultures and viral titres (acutely and during convalescence)
- Antistreptolysin-O (ASO) titre and throat swabs
- Autoantibody profile and complement levels
- Paul Bunnell screen
- Cold agglutinins
- Electrocardiogram (ECG) – this may provide evidence for acute pericarditis. Initially there is ST elevation. Generally, this is concave and widespread involving more than one arterial territory (Fig. 20.1). Later in the course of the condition ST depression and T wave inversion may develop indicating possible myocardial involvement.

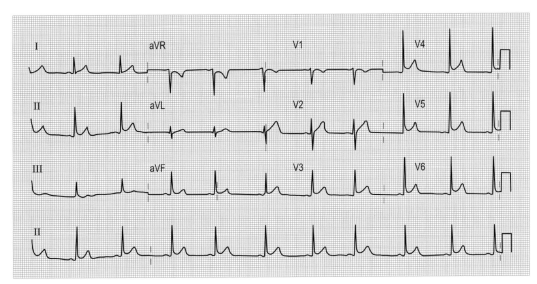

Figure 20.1
Electrocardiogram in acute pericarditis showing widespread concave ST elevation

The differential diagnosis of the ECG appearance includes early repolarization (especially in young adult males), acute early anterior myocardial infarction and acute myocarditis, emphasizing the need for a clear history.

TREATMENT

The treatment of uncomplicated acute pericarditis is generally with non-steroidal anti-inflammatory drugs (NSAIDs) (e.g. aspirin, naproxen or indomethacin) and bed rest. If severe, recurrent or in the context of connective-tissue disease, systemic corticosteroids may be of benefit and can be of dramatic benefit, but maintenance doses do not necessarily prevent relapses. For recurrent disease, colchicine is the drug of choice, in combination with NSAIDs for the acute attack.

SPECIFIC FORMS OF PERICARDITIS

Bacterial

Septicaemia or pneumonia may be complicated by purulent pericarditis. Staphylococci and *Haemophilus influenzae* account for two-thirds of cases. Treatment is with antibiotics and surgical drainage. However, the prognosis is poor and staphylococcal infection is frequently fatal.

Tuberculous

Tuberculosis is increasingly seen in immigrant populations and in those who are HIV positive and may be the result of atypical or resistant forms. This non-suppurative form of pericarditis presents with a chronic low-grade fever, especially in the evening, malaise and weight loss. Frequently pericardial aspiration of a concurrent pericardial effusion is required to make the diagnosis. This effusion is usually serous but may be blood stained. Tuberculin testing may be of use with the caveat that in acute pericarditis it may be negative. Treatment is with prolonged anti-tuberculous chemotherapy.

Uraemic

This condition is often asymptomatic, occurs in the terminal stages of uraemia, and is an indication for dialysis.

Dressler's syndrome

This can occur 2 weeks to 1 year after myocardial infarction and pericardiotomy. It is associated with antibodies against cardiac muscle. A pericardial rub, pericarditic chest pain and fever occur in up to 20% of patients post infarction.

CONSTRICTIVE PERICARDITIS

Following acute pericarditis of almost any cause, constrictive pericarditis can occur as the pericardium becomes unduly thickened, fibrosed and calcified. The heart becomes encased in a solid shell and, therefore, cannot fill properly. It may develop within a few weeks of the precipitating cause or during the next 30 years.

CLINICAL FEATURES

The systemic features associated with constrictive pericarditis may develop slowly and the diagnosis is often missed. Right-sided signs are prominent, with development of ascites, dependent oedema (often comparatively little), and hepatomegaly. Atrial fibrillation is seen in up to 30% of patients.

The jugular venous pressure (JVP) is elevated in the absence of pulmonary venous distension. The waveform has a rapid 'y' descent in contrast to pericardial tamponade because of fast early ventricular filling-Friedrich's sign (Fig. 20.2).

In addition, there are signs of impaired ventricular filling:

- Kussmaul's sign – The jugular venous pressure paradoxically rises with inspiration. This may also be present in any condition with elevated right atrial pressure including cardiac tamponade, right ventricular infarction, restrictive cardiomyopathy, and tricuspid stenosis (Fig. 20.3).
- Pulsus paradoxus – This is the result of a fall in systolic pressure on inspiration of more than 10 mmHg. The incidence of this clinical finding is variable and is reported to be present between 16% and 84% dependent on the series. This sign is not unique to constriction and is also present in cardiac tamponade, severe asthma and severe bronchitis.
- Pericardial knock – This is characteristic of constriction and is due to sudden halting of ventricular filling. It is heard in early diastole and thought to be an exaggerated early

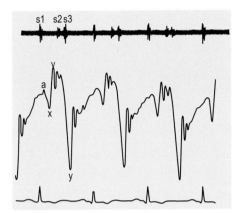

Figure 20.2
Left atrial pressure trace in constriction demonstrating the prominent 'y' descent

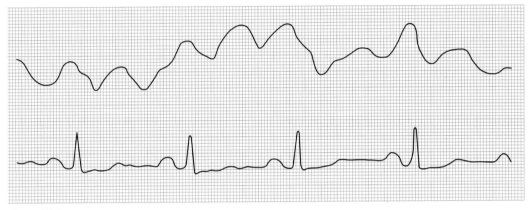

Figure 20.3
Kussmaul's sign. Elevation of right atrial pressure with inspiration

third heart sound. It may become more prominent with squatting, which increases venous return and peripheral resistance. However, this sign is thought to be present in less than 40% of cases.

A number of conditions mimic constriction and include: chronic pericardial effusion, restrictive cardiomyopathy, dilated cardiomyopathy, mitral stenosis with pulmonary hypertension and tricuspid regurgitation, hypertrophic cardiomyopathy involving right and left ventricle, and ischaemic congestive cardiac failure.

PHYSIOLOGY OF CONSTRICTION

The findings consistent with constrictive physiology reflect the late diastolic impairment in filling. In addition, the thickened pericardium fails to transmit the usual patterns of ventricular filling in relation to intra-cardiac and intra-thoracic pressures.

In normal subjects, inspiration leads to a fall in pulmonary wedge pressure because of reduced intra-thoracic pressure. However, the lowered intra-thoracic pressure is also transmitted to the pericardium and results in a fall in intra-pericardial and intra-cardiac pressure. Thus, the filling gradient is maintained throughout the cardiac cycle.

In constrictive pericarditis the pulmonary wedge pressure falls on inspiration but the intra-pericardial and intra-cardiac pressure remain high thus reducing the filling gradient of the left ventricle. In addition, the fixed intra-cardiac volume available means the ventricles cannot fill independently of each other. Filling of the right ventricle impairs filling of the left resulting in reduced cardiac output.

INVESTIGATION

The diagnosis is often delayed as the clinical signs may be subtle and the patient may be misdiagnosed with conditions such as cirrhosis or malignant disease. Establishing the diagnosis requires evaluation of the clinical signs, chest X-ray (CXR) review, transthoracic echocardiography (TTE) and right- and left-heart catheterization.

Chest X-ray

The CXR may reveal pericardial calcification (Fig. 20.4). A lateral CXR may be useful to demonstrate calcification of the atrioventricular groove, anterior right-ventricular and diaphragmatic surfaces of the pericardium.

Transthoracic echocardiography

Diagnosis of constriction using echocardiography requires a comprehensive examination with particular reference to Doppler measurements of transvalvular velocities and hepatic

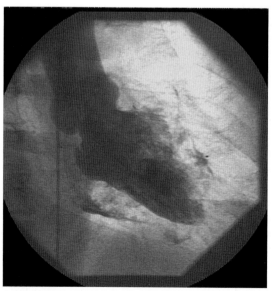

Figure 20.4
Pericardial calcification in constrictive pericarditis at fluoroscopic examination

Box 20.2: Echocardiographic diagnosis of constriction

2-D
Thickened pericardium
Normal-sized ventricles with enlarged atria
Atrial and ventricular septal bulge to left during inspiration ('septal bounce')
Dilated inferior vena cava with lack of inspiratory variation (<50%)

M-mode
Pericardial thickening
Paradoxical septal motion
Abnormal early diastolic ventricular septal motion
Rapid early and flat diastolic motion of the posterior wall of the left ventricle
Premature diastolic opening of the pulmonary valve
Mid-systolic closure of the aortic valve
Pseudo systolic anterior motion of the mitral valve
Increased 'a' wave depth of the pulmonary vein on inspiration

Doppler
Excessive (>25%) inspiratory decrease in mitral E velocity
Excessive increase in isovolumic relaxation time during inspiration
Excessive decrease in tricuspid velocity during expiration
Normal inspiratory decrease in atrial and systolic reversal of hepatic vein flow
Marked expiratory decrease in atrial and systolic reversal of hepatic vein flow

vein flow, and the change in these patterns with respiration. Findings consistent with the diagnosis are summarized in Box 20.2.

Cardiac catheterization

Right- and left-heart catheterization is usually required to confirm the diagnosis and exclude restrictive cardiomyopathy. This requires simultaneous right-ventricular, left-atrial and left-ventricular measurements. Improved diagnostic accuracy is achieved if left-atrial pressure is directly measured using trans-septal puncture. This provides instantaneous pressure recordings, avoids the effect of pressure damping, and minimizes effects of chronic lung disease, which may affect measurements if pulmonary wedge pressure is used as a surrogate.

The generalized constricting process results in elevation and equilibration of diastolic pressures in all four cardiac chambers. Early diastolic filling of the ventricle is unimpaired hence the rapid 'y' descent seen in the right atrial trace. However, filling is abruptly halted as the non-compliant pericardium limits the intra-ventricular volume during late diastole. This results in the classic dip and plateau diastolic ventricular waveform (Fig. 20.5).

Haemodynamic effects alone may not be sufficient to distinguish constriction from restriction and the change in pressures with respiration may be necessary to distinguish between the two (Table 20.1). The dissociation between intra-thoracic and intra-cardiac pressure seen in constriction results in a fall in the left-ventricular filling gradient on inspiration, which is not seen in restriction.

The interdependence of ventricular filling seen in constriction results in elevation of right-ventricular pressure and a simultaneous fall in left-ventricular pressure with inspiration.

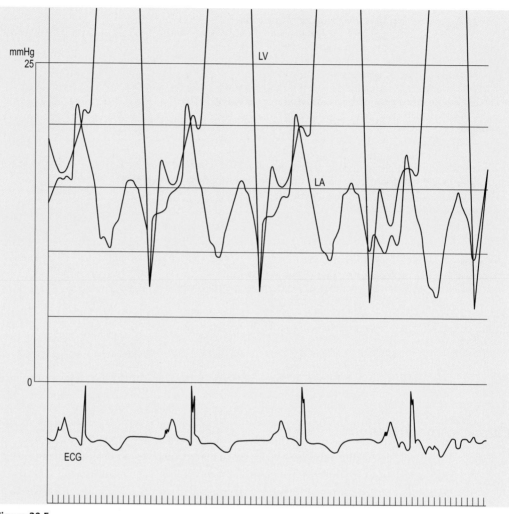

Figure 20.5
Simultaneous left-atrial and left-ventricular pressure measurement in constrictive pericarditis demonstrating dip and plateau waveforms and equalization of end diastolic pressures

Table 20.1: Characteristic features of constrictive pericarditis and restrictive cardiomyopathy at cardiac catheterization

	Constriction	Restriction
Respiratory variation in right atrial pressure	Absent	Present
Discordant left- and right-ventricular end systolic pressures with respiration	Present	Absent
Rapid and prominent 'y' descent in right atrial trace	Present	May be present
Dip and plateau waveform in diastolic ventricular traces	Present	Present
Right-ventricular systolic pressure	<55 mmHg	>55 mmHg
Right-ventricular end diastolic pressure at least one-third systolic pressure	Present	Absent

When analysing the respiratory variations of the pressure trace, the first beat after inspiration should be used, which minimizes possible confounding effects of chronic lung disease.

If the patient is in atrial fibrillation or has an irregular rhythm, fixed-rate temporary pacing will negate the effect of heart rate on pressure measurements.

Low filling pressures may mask constriction and if the left-ventricular end diastolic pressure (LVEDP) is less than 15 mmHg, 500 ml of intravenous fluid should be given. Likewise very high filling pressures may mask respiratory patterns and diuresis may be required.

Endomyocardial biopsy may be required in addition to examine for histological features of restriction.

TREATMENT

Diuretics may be of some temporary benefit in treating patients with constriction but, ultimately, the treatment of choice is pericardectomy. Negatively chronotropic agents should be avoided, as a tachycardia is often necessary to maintain cardiac output. The prognosis without surgical intervention is poor and with pericardial stripping extremely good. However, surgery itself may be associated with substantial risk because of difficulties in removing densely adherent tissue.

PERICARDIAL EFFUSION

Almost all causes of pericarditis can also induce pericardial effusion. The haemodynamic effects of the effusion reflect the rise in intra-pericardial pressure. High intra-pericardial pressure impairs filling of the right heart and as a result, compensatory movement of the inter-ventricular septum impinges on left-ventricular volume with subsequent reduction in left-ventricular stroke volume. The conditions most likely to result in tamponade are listed in Table 20.2. The diagnosis should be considered in all patients with oliguria, a low output state, and raised venous pressure failing to respond to inotropes.

Table 20.2: Causes of cardiac tamponade

Acute	Chronic
Myocardial infarction with rupture of ventricular free wall	Collagen vascular disease
Aortic dissection into pericardial space	Dressler's syndrome
Post cardiac surgery	Viral, bacterial or tuberculous pericarditis
Chest trauma	Chylous effusions
Trans-septal puncture	
Uraemia	
Malignant disease	
Acute pericarditis	

CLINICAL FEATURES

Cardiac tamponade was defined by Beck using a triad of clinical features:

1. Low arterial blood pressure
2. High venous pressure
3. Absent apex beat.

However, echocardiography has shown that even in patients without overt cardiac tamponade there may be evidence of impaired diastolic filling and, thus, the symptoms and signs associated with pericardial effusion occur on a continuum rather than an 'all or nothing' phenomenon.

A significant pericardial effusion may develop in the context of a small amount of pericardial fluid depending on the speed with which it has accumulated and the compliance of the pericardium. Patients with large effusions may be asymptomatic or else may present in extremis with emergency drainage required to prevent death. **Cardiac tamponade is, therefore, essentially a clinical diagnosis supported by echocardiographic findings.**

SYMPTOMS

Clinical features of the underlying cause may be present. Patients may complain of breathlessness, cough, hoarseness and hiccoughs as a result of local compression. They may complain of dull central chest pain, facial engorgement, abdominal and ankle swelling.

SIGNS

- Pulse – Generally the patient is tachycardic and atrial arrhythmias are common.
- Blood pressure – This is usually low. Pulsus paradoxus may be present.
- JVP – This is elevated with a sharp 'x' descent. Classically there is no 'y' descent. **Kussmaul's sign** may be present (see Fig. 20.3).
- Apex beat – This is typically impalpable.
- Heart sounds – These are usually quiet and there may be a rub, which usually disappears as the effusion increases in size.

INVESTIGATIONS

- CXR – This will reveal a large globular heart with normal pulmonary vasculature. Pulmonary vascular congestion suggests co-existent myocardial disease.
- ECG – Typically shows small voltage. Electrical alternans, varying complex size, may be present in the presence of a large effusion as the heart 'swings' in the pericardial sac.
- Echocardiography – Although an effusion may be noted on CT or MRI the most useful diagnostic tool remains echocardiography. This not only provides information as to the position and depth of the effusion but also provides information as to the

haemodynamic effects on the heart and additional myocardial disease (Figs 20.6, 20.7 & Box 20.3).

MANAGEMENT OF PERICARDIAL EFFUSIONS

Effusions causing symptoms and haemodynamic compromise should all be drained either percutaneously or surgically. Likewise, all purulent effusions require drainage. Asymptomatic patients with chronic (longer than 3 months) large effusions (>20 mm) appear to have an adverse prognosis irrespective of the aetiology. This may reflect a tendency to develop unheralded life-threatening tamponade, possibly caused by hypovolaemia, arrhythmias or further episodes of acute pericarditis. It is, therefore, recommended that these patients also undergo drainage.

In the context of acute haemodynamic compromise, intravenous fluids will 'buy time' but, ultimately, drainage is required and may be lifesaving. Intravenous fluids will increase

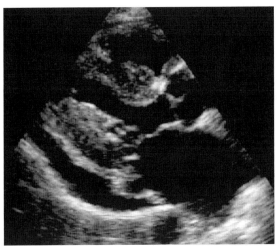

Figure 20.6
Parasternal long axis view of posterior pericardial effusion

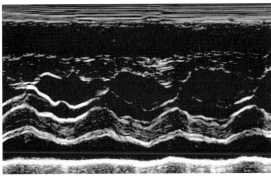

Figure 20.7
M-mode of pericardial effusion

Box 20.3: Echocardiographic diagnosis of cardiac tamponade

2-D
'Swinging' heart
Right-ventricular diastolic collapse in early diastole
Atrial collapse in late diastole and early systole
Left-ventricular diastolic collapse
Inspiratory bounce of interventricular septum towards left ventricle
Dilated inferior vena cava with lack of inspiratory collapse

M-mode
Right-ventricular compression (right-ventricular internal diastolic diameter (RVIDd) <0.7 cm)
Increased right-ventricular diastolic dimension with inspiration
Decreased left-ventricular diastolic dimension with inspiration
Decreased mitral-valve E–F slope with inspiration (<50 mm/s)
Delayed mitral-valve opening with inspiration
Decrease left-ventricular ejection time with inspiration

Doppler
Increase isovolumic relaxation time with inspiration
Tricuspid flow velocity increases by >25% on inspiration
Mitral flow velocity decreases by >25% on inspiration
Decreased (or reversed) hepatic-vein diastolic forward flow on expiration

Distinguishing an effusion from other conditions
Effusions rarely collect behind the left atrium
Effusions are seen anterior to the descending thoracic aorta
Epicardial fat pads are usually located anteriorly

---

intra-cardiac pressure above intra-pericardial pressure thus improving left-ventricular filling and cardiac output. In spite of the oliguria associated with this condition, the use of diuretics is contraindicated, as any reduction in intra-cardiac pressure results in further impairment of left-ventricular filling and a potentially catastrophic haemodynamic deterioration.

Pericardiocentesis

Drainage of pericardial effusions may be performed by inserting a pericardial drain or by creation of a pericardial window (surgically, or using balloon pericardiotomy). Effusions may be recurrent and development of a further collection after two preceding percutaneous attempts is an indication for a wide anterior pericardectomy.

In the context of palliation for recurrent malignant effusions, percutaneous creation of a pericardial window using balloon techniques may be preferable to definitive surgery. However, disruption of pericardial tumour makes any further procedure very difficult, as a form of plasticising tumour encasement subsequently may occur.

Untreated, cardiac tamponade is a lethal condition. However, the treatment itself may be associated with significant morbidity and mortality. Complications include: laceration of the liver and other intra-abdominal structures, cardiac arrhythmias, tearing of major epicardial vessels, and myocardial rupture.

Procedural monitoring

- Electrocardiogram – Connection of the exploring electrode of a unipolar electrocardiogram (V lead) to the hub of the needle may be used to characterize potentially inaccurate and dangerous positioning of the needle tip. ST segment elevation or frequent ventricular ectopic beats are associated with the breaching of, or direct contact with, the epicardium.
- Echocardiography – The safety of the procedure has improved with the use of echocardiography during the procedure, and direct ECG monitoring of the advancing needle is now unnecessary in most situations.
- Fluoroscopy – This is not essential and agitated saline as echo contrast is sufficient if there is doubt regarding needle position and fluoroscopy is unavailable.

Technique

The patient is best positioned at 45° with the chest and abdomen exposed. The patient should be draped creating a sterile field. Having instilled local anaesthetic, a needle is advanced towards the pericardium. Once pericardial fluid is reached, a guide wire is advanced into the pericardial space. A tract is then created using a dilator and the drain advanced over the wire. Obtaining heavily blood stained fluid that clots rapidly suggests the ventricular wall or a major blood vessel has been breached.

Traditionally, needle aspiration of pericardial fluid has been performed from a subxiphoid approach. In some centres, alternative routes for the aspiration of the effusion are preferred. The most common of these is the apical route. In cases of large anterior effusions, fluid may lie less than 1 cm from the anterior chest wall and a drain may easily be placed with little risk of damage to the internal mammary artery. The risk of pneumothorax, as with the subxiphoid route, is present and is maximal as the needle traverses the chest wall. In practice, the distended pericardium almost always displaces the left lung. The presence of a loculated effusion may direct aspiration from the site at which the collection is largest to minimize the risk of perforation and damage to adjacent structures.

Extensive scarring, fibrosis, or recurrent local tumour tissue may make drainage from either route impractical. In these situations, creation of a pericardial window surgically may be required. Similarly, in the weeks following cardiac surgery surgical drainage is preferred.

Following relief of acute tamponade gradual drainage of any remaining fluid over a period of hours reduces the risk of sudden collapse and low output state post aspiration. It has been shown that leaving the catheter in situ for prolonged drainage reduces the risk of reaccumulation of fluid. Rather than leaving the catheter on continuous free drainage, it has been suggested that the fluid should be taken off intermittently at 4–6 hourly intervals; this is thought to reduce the incidence of catheter blockage especially if the catheter is flushed after every aspiration.

Fluid should be sent for cytology, microbiological assessment with Ziehl–Neelsen (ZN) stain and if suspicious polymerase chain reaction (PCR) for TB.

In malignant effusions infusion of chemotherapeutic agents such as cisplatin, and in immunological conditions triamcinolone infusion into the pericardial space at the time of aspiration, have been shown to prevent recurrence.

Further reading

Hancock EW 2001 Differential diagnosis of restrictive cardiomyopathy and constrictive pericarditis. Heart 86(3): 343–349

Higano ST, Azrak E, Naeem K et al 1999 Hemodynamic rounds series II: hemodynamics of constrictive physiology: influence of respiratory dynamics on ventricular pressures. Catheter Cardiovasc Interv 46(4): 473–486

Hoit BD 2002 Management of effusive and constrictive pericardial heart disease. Circulation 105(25): 2939–2942

Myers RBH, Spodick DH 1999 Constrictive pericarditis: clinical and pathophysiologic characteristics. Am Heart J 138: 219–232

Nishimura RA 2001 Constrictive pericarditis in the modern era: a diagnostic dilemma. Heart 86(6): 619–623

Oakley CM 2000 Myocarditis, pericarditis and other pericardial diseases. Heart 84(4): 449–454

Spodick DH 2001 Pericardial disease. In: Braunwald E, Zipes DP, Libby P (eds) Heart disease: a textbook of cardiovascular medicine, 6th edn. WB Saunders, Philadelphia, pp. 1823–1831

Swanton RH 2003 Pericardial disease. In: Swanton RH (ed.) Pocket consultant cardiology, 4rd edn. Blackwell Science, Cambridge, pp. 359–369

SELF-ASSESSMENT

Questions

1. A 25-year-old man was admitted with a 5-day history of non-specific aches and pains, a slight fever and central chest pain. His electrocardiogram (ECG) shows a sinus tachycardia with widespread concave ST elevation with no reciprocal ST depression. Investigations were unremarkable except for an elevated ESR and CRP.
   a. What is the likely diagnosis?
   b. Is this condition benign?
   c. What treatment would you institute?

2. A 31-year-old man presented with a history of weight loss, exertional breathlessness and night sweats. On examination, he was found to be tachycardic with a pulse of 140 in atrial fibrillation. His blood pressure was 110/65 mmHg with a 30 mmHg paradox. His jugular venous pulse was elevated and increased on inspiration. A provisional diagnosis of cardiac tamponade was made.
   a. What echocardiographic findings would confirm this diagnosis?
   b. What is the likely aetiology?
   c. Why is 'Pulsus Paradox' a paradox?

3. A 65-year-old man, who had undergone coronary artery bypass grafting previously, presented with abdominal swelling, and increasing exertional breathlessness. On examination, his pulse was regular at 90 beats per minute, his blood pressure was 130/70 mmHg and he was comfortable lying with one pillow. The venous pressure was elevated and there was marked ascites, hepatomegaly and ankle oedema. The ECG showed no acute ischaemic changes and the chest X-ray showed a normal cardiothoracic ratio with clear lung fields.
   a. Based on this clinical information what is the differential diagnosis?
   b. How would you differentiate between these conditions?
   c. What do the waveforms in the JVP reflect in normal subjects and what pattern is seen in patients with constrictive pericarditis?

Answers

1. a. The likely diagnosis is acute pericarditis.
   b. The condition is generally benign. Myocardial involvement may occur and is strongly suggested by the presence of pulmonary oedema or cardiac arrhythmias. Pericardial effusion and cardiac tamponade may occur, necessitating pericardiocentesis.
   c. Treatment is with non-steroidal anti-inflammatory drugs for the acute attack and with colchicine if it is recurrent.

2. a. There are a number of features implying cardiac tamponade. Ventricular diastolic collapse is present and on inspiration there is delayed mitral valve opening, decreased left-ventricular ejection time, decreased mitral flow velocity, increased tricuspid flow velocity and lack of usual collapse of the dilated inferior vena cava.
   b. In view of the patient's age, and presence of night sweats, lymphoma is a strong possibility. However, TB should also be rigorously excluded.

   c. The paradox is that during inspiration, although the heart rate increases, clinically it seems to disappear.

3. a. Constrictive pericarditis, restrictive cardiomyopathy and chronic pulmonary hypertension.

   b. It may be possible to distinguish between these conditions using echocardiography. The classical appearance of amyloid heart disease, for example, may be present. However, in the absence of such a clue, distinguishing between constrictive pericarditis and restrictive cardiomyopathy requires evaluation of subtle changes in flow patterns with respiration, which may be challenging or impossible in patients with a poor echo window. It is, therefore, usually necessary to undertake right- and left-heart catheterization with evaluation of intracardiac pressures during the respiratory cycle.

   c. The 'a' wave occurs as a result of atrial systole. The 'x' descent is caused by the fall in right-atrial pressure during ventricular systole because of downward movement of the heart. The 'v' wave results from atrial filling against a closed tricuspid valve and the 'y' descent occurs during ventricular filling. In constrictive pericarditis the JVP is elevated and there is a prominent 'y' descent.

Cardiovascular co-morbidity with renal disease

21

E. Shurrab and P. A. Kalra

INTRODUCTION

Cardiovascular and renal disease frequently co-exist in patients. The relationship may be acute (e.g. sudden fall in cardiac output complicating myocardial infarction or arrhythmia may lead to ischaemic acute renal failure (ARF)) or chronic, causative (e.g. secondary 'renal' hypertensive heart disease) or co-existent within the same disease process (e.g. generalized atheromatous vascular disease). Although a comprehensive review of the relationship between disease in these two vital organ systems is beyond the scope of this chapter, particular consideration will be given to the important topics of cardiac disease complicating chronic kidney disease (CKD), screening for coronary disease in potential renal transplant recipients, and renal failure complicating cardiac investigation.

CARDIAC DISEASE IN PATIENTS WITH CHRONIC AND END-STAGE RENAL DISEASE

EPIDEMIOLOGY

Cardiovascular disease accounts for >50% of deaths in patients with CKD (glomerular filtration rate (GFR) <50 ml/min) and end-stage renal failure (ESRF) (GFR <10 ml/min, dialysis patients and those with renal transplants). After stratification for age, race and gender cardiovascular mortality is 10–20 times higher in the dialysis than general population;[1] patients with diabetic nephropathy or atheromatous renovascular disease (ARVD) are at greatest risk of cardiovascular death than those with other causes of renal failure. The main cardiac manifestations are coronary artery disease (CAD)[2], left-ventricular hypertrophy (LVH), cardiac dysfunction and chronic heart failure (CHF), valvular heart disease and arrhythmias. Other more specific cardiac diseases, such as uraemic pericarditis and infective endocarditis, are also seen in ESRF patients and will be discussed later.

Left-ventricular hypertrophy

LVH develops early in the course of renal disease and it is present in 70–80% of patients reaching dialysis.[3] Treatment of renal anaemia and blood pressure seem to improve LVH,

305

but usually without complete resolution. As some normotensive dialysis patients have LVH, usually in the form of asymmetrical septal hypertrophy, this suggests that several different factors may be involved in the pathogenesis.

Coronary artery disease

The incidence of CAD is greater in patients with renal failure than in the general population. In a study of 433 patients at the start of ESRD therapy, 14% had proven CAD and 19% angina pectoris.[3] CAD usually manifests in a more severe form (multiple vessel disease) and at a younger age than in the general population; it has even been documented in children approaching dialysis need. Calcification in the coronary lesions and vessel wall is common (Ch. 7, Fig. 7.5). The incidence is greatest in patients with diabetic renal failure. Pathogenetic risk factors for CAD in patients with CKD are discussed below.

Cardiac dysfunction

Both systolic and diastolic dysfunction are common in renal patients. In a cohort of patients reaching ESRD, 15% had systolic dysfunction and 32% left-ventricular dilatation on echocardiography.[3] Systolic dysfunction is thought to result from long-standing hypertension and CAD, whereas diastolic dysfunction may be due to LVH, myocardial fibrosis and stiffness.

Valvular calcification

Aortic and mitral valve calcification can be detected by echocardiography in, respectively, up to 50% and 40% of ESRD patients, but haemodynamically significant lesions are infrequent. However, valvular calcification is clinically important as it reflects poor calcium, inorganic phosphate and parathyroid hormone (PTH) metabolism, it gives rise to murmurs that require assessment, and it increases the risk of infective endocarditis. A mildly stenotic and calcified aortic valve can also rapidly progress to significant valvular disease, and so close monitoring is indicated.[4]

Dysrrhythmias

Up to 70% of haemodialysis patients have been documented to have arrhythmias (mostly ventricular) of which 20% may be life-threatening and require specific treatment. Predisposing factors are LVH, left-ventricular dilatation with sub-endocardial myocardial ischaemia, as well as electrolyte and acid–base disturbances. One study in a large cohort of dialysis patients showed no relationship between the frequency and severity of ventricular arrhythmia and survival,[5] although most agree that arrhythmias are not infrequently the cause of sudden death in dialysis patients.

PATHOGENESIS OF CARDIAC DISEASE IN THE PATIENT WITH CHRONIC KIDNEY DISEASE

In addition to the acknowledged risk factors for cardiovascular disease in the general population[6] there are specific abnormalities in patients with CKD that increase their vulnerability (Box 21.1). Although renal transplantation can reverse some of these risk factors (e.g. anaemia and raised PTH), patients continue to have a high cardiovascular morbidity after transplantation.

Hypertension

Hypertension is a major contributor to LVH, cardiac dysfunction and CAD of the CKD population. It is present in 80–90% of patients reaching ESRD (Fig. 21.1). Its prevalence varies according to the primary renal disease, but within a single disease category blood pressure is inversely proportional to degree of renal function. For example, hypertension is present in 40% of patients with mesangiocapillary glomerulonephritis and normal renal function but in almost 100% of those reaching ESRD, whereas only 20% of patients with chronic pyelonephritis have hypertension at presentation and 70% at ESRD.[7] In the dialysis patient, fluid overload is a unique contributor to renal-related hypertension, and some patients respond well to its control (salt and fluid restriction, diuretics or dialysis), even precluding the need for anti-hypertensive agents. The UK Renal Association has suggested target blood pressure of <140/90 mmHg or <160/90 mmHg for dialysis patients aged <60 or >60 years old, respectively. Ambulatory blood pressure monitoring (ABPM) can improve evaluation of control, and a mean arterial pressure (MAP) of <98 mmHg is targeted over a 24-hour period.

Box 21.1: Specific risk factors for cardiovascular disease in renal patients

Hyperparathyroidism
Anaemia
Hypercalcaemia and overtreatment with calcium and vitamin D
Hyperphosphataemia
Hyperhomocysteinaemia
Increased oxidative stress and endothelial cell permeability
Inflammation

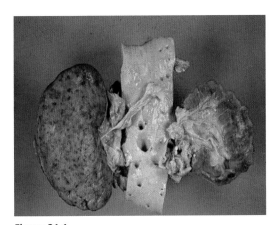

Figure 21.1
Post-mortem section through the abdominal aorta, renal arteries and the kidneys from a hypertensive patient. It shows severe atherosclerotic changes in the left renal artery and with associated renal scarring and atrophy. Even the 'normal' right kidney manifests hypertensive damage

Dyslipidaemia

Renal disease is associated with disturbances of lipid metabolism, but there is no clear link between these abnormalities and the incidence of cardiovascular disease. In a large prospective study on the survival of dialysis patients, raised serum cholesterol was associated with better survival.[8] This unexpected result probably reflected the nutritional status of these patients, as poor nutrition is associated with low cholesterol, low albumin and, in turn, poor outcome.

Hyperparathyroidism and abnormal calcium and phosphate metabolism

Secondary hyperparathyroidism is common in uraemic patients (Fig. 21.2), and is usually manifest when the creatinine clearance falls to <35 ml/min. Excessive PTH may be cardiotoxic, and dilated cardiomyopathy has been shown at echocardiography in such patients. Some studies have documented an improvement in myocardial function after parathyroidectomy. PTH receptors have been detected in the myocardium; in experimental studies, high concentrations of PTH in myocardial cell culture first lead to increased contractility and rate of contraction, and then to cell death. PTH is also associated with increased myocardial fibrosis. As mentioned previously, valvular (and vascular) calcification may frequently complicate abnormal calcium and inorganic phosphate metabolism (high phosphate levels, and increased calcium × phosphate product).

Anaemia

Anaemia is inevitable in most patients with CKD; it has many contributory factors (Box 21.2), the most important of which is the relative deficiency of erythropoietin. Anaemia is an important cause of LVH, the LV mass being directly related to the degree of the anaemia.[9] LVH increases myocardial oxygen demand, but the anaemia, per se, decreases myocardial oxygen supply with a tendency to worsen any ischaemic symptoms. Correction of anaemia is associated with some resolution of LVH and improved cardiovascular survival. Management of anaemia in renal patients depends on good nutrition, adequate dialysis, iron supplementation and the use of recombinant human

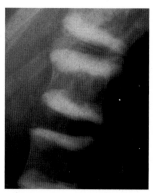

Figure 21.2
X-ray of the lumbar spine showing characteristic changes of renal bone disease ('rugger jersey' spine) as seen in patients with chronic kidney disease

erthropoietin (r-EPO). Target haemoglobin concentration is 10–12 g/dl (haematocrit >30%); the main side effect of r-EPO is hypertension, which may limit adequate dosage. Transfusions should be avoided (wherever possible) in patients likely to be transplanted, so as to avoid allo-sensitization.

Hyperhomocystinaemia

This is an independent risk factor for atherogenesis, and in ESRF its prevalence is much greater than in other populations. Homocysteine can cause endothelial injury and stimulate platelet aggregation and it has been associated with increased incidence of acute myocardial events. Although folic acid has been shown to lower serum homocysteine levels, there is no evidence that this has any long-term benefit of decreasing cardiovascular disease in uraemic patients.

Increased oxidative stress and endothelial damage

Uraemic patients have increased endothelial cell permeability, and this is an important step in the pathogenesis of atherosclerosis. It is thought to be due to the accumulation of various toxins and increased oxidative stress in uraemia.

SCREENING FOR CARDIOVASCULAR DISEASE IN PATIENTS WITH CHRONIC KIDNEY DISEASE

The majority of patients with ESRD, and many with advanced CKD in the pre-dialysis phase, will be considered as candidates for renal transplantation. Cardiovascular screening is necessary in certain CKD and ESRD sub-groups, especially as cardiac events frequently occur in the peri- and post-operative period in asymptomatic patients, with diabetics particularly at risk. In non-renal populations patients with CAD are commonly symptomatic, and so a combination of clinical assessment and well-validated non-invasive tests for reversible myocardial ischaemia (exercise tolerance testing (ETT), stress nuclear myocardial perfusion imaging (MPI) and dobutamine stress echocardiography (DSE)) are used to select patients for coronary angiography. However, ETT is a poor test in patients with ESRD, as they are often incapable of exercising adequately; resting electrocardiograph abnormalities (e.g. severe LVH) also limit interpretation. MPI has been used with variable success to predict CAD in ESRD[10,11] (e.g. sensitivity ranging from 37–92% and specificity 37–94%, compared to 90% for both parameters in the general population) and DSE is yet to be properly validated in the CKD population.

Echocardiographic detection of cardiac dysfunction (and valvular abnormalities) is an important part of the assessment of potential renal transplant recipients. Mild-to-moderate LV systolic dysfunction is not a contraindication as there is evidence of improvement in cardiac function and LVH after renal transplantation. Patients with severe cardiac dysfunction (ejection fraction <25%) are usually not considered, with the exception of those few patients suitable for combined cardiac and renal transplantation.

Screening protocols

A typical protocol will involve :

- Echocardiography in all patients
- patients stratified as high risk (Box 21.3) should undergo stress MPI. Patients with positive MPI are investigated with coronary angiography
- coronary angiography being recommended for patients with any of the risk factors listed in Box 21.4, as stress MPI has a low sensitivity for predicting CAD in diabetic nephropathy.

MANAGEMENT OF CARDIOVASCULAR DISEASE IN RENAL PATIENTS

The general management is the same as that of the general population, with attention to hypertension and dyslipidaemia control being important. Patients with CAD awaiting renal transplantation fare better if managed by coronary revascularization (rather than medical treatment); this effect is exaggerated in diabetics with ESRD. In the past retrospective studies have suggested that the revascularization procedure of choice should be coronary artery bypass grafting (CABG),[12] based upon the rate of coronary artery re-stenosis and the control of angina symptoms. Although CABG carried a higher peri-operative mortality, this may have been because patients treated with CABG tended to have more severe CAD. More recent evidence suggests that percutaneous transluminal coronary angioplasty (PTCA) may give comparable long-term results to CABG,[13] but it is

---

Box 21.3: High-risk factors for cardiovascular disease in end-stage renal disease patients being referred for renal transplant

Age >50 years
History of angina
Insulin-dependent diabetes mellitus
Chronic heart failure
Abnormal ECG (excluding LVH)

Box 21.4: High-risk factors for coronary artery disease in diabetic patients with end-stage disease being referred for renal transplant

Age >45 years
History of smoking
ST and T wave changes on ECG
Duration of diabetes >25 years

now accepted that a prospective study is required, especially comparing the outcomes of patients with similar degrees of coronary disease.

ACE-inhibitors (ACE-I) and angiotensin II receptor blockers (ARBs)

These are now strongly indicated in many patients with cardiac disease. Patients with CKD (pre-dialysis) are at risk of worsening renal function (not just those with significant bilateral renovascular disease), but such a trade off can be acceptable in patients with poor LV function. As a general rule, patients with serum creatinine levels of <200 µmol/l can be commenced on these agents, but discontinuation is usually advised if the serum creatinine levels rise by more than 20% above baseline. For those with baseline creatinine levels of >200 µmol/l, renal physician review is usually indicated, unless the renal impairment can be fully explained by obvious clinical factors (e.g. very poor cardiac output and age). Hence, in patients with severe CHF greater degrees of renal functional deterioration may be accepted, as the benefits to cardiac function and survival often outweigh these changes. In general, these agents can be used in almost all patients with renal disease provided that close monitoring of renal function is performed.

Dialysis for patients with cardiovascular disease

Haemodialysis can be detrimental to patients with advanced cardiovascular disease especially those with CHF and low blood pressure. Increased blood flow through the arteriovenous fistula will increase cardiac demand and may worsen cardiac failure and angina. A well-functioning fistula has a blood flow of about 500 ml/min, which can contribute to LVH and even predispose to cardiac failure in patients with normal cardiac function (Fig. 21.3). The extra-corporeal circulation may also increase the cardiac demand. Hence, patients with severe cardiac dysfunction, or CAD with significant angina, are better managed by peritoneal dialysis, which causes far less haemodynamic embarrassment. The decision on the best modality of dialysis will also depend on the general condition and capabilities of the patients (e.g. ability to perform peritoneal

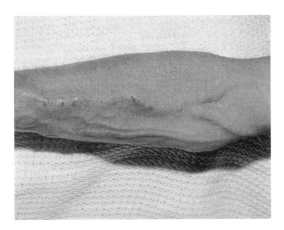

Figure 21.3
Radiocephalic arteriovenous fistula showing significant arterialization of the veins. Needling sites are clearly seen

dialysis). It may appear inappropriate to offer some patients with very severe co-morbidity (e.g. severe CHF with hypotension) any form of dialysis. Full discussion with the patient and carers is necessary in these circumstances, and management options include either no dialysis treatment or a trial of dialysis to assess tolerability and the impact upon the patient's quality of life. For patients awaiting cardiac transplant haemodifiltration may be appropriate.

CARDIOVASCULAR DISEASE IN RENAL TRANSPLANT RECIPIENTS

Cardiovascular disease is the major cause of late mortality in renal transplant recipients. In a Scandinavian study, atherosclerotic vascular disease accounted for 60% of deaths in renal transplant patients; in the 55–64 years age group, the risk of death from CAD was 6 and 20 times greater in non-diabetic and diabetic transplant recipients, respectively, than in the general population.[14] In addition to the standard risk factors for CAD, specific post-transplant abnormalities are contributory:

- Hypertension is almost universal in patients receiving calcineurin inhibitors (ciclosporin or tacrolimus) and it is made worse by steroids.
- Development of diabetes – tacrolimus is diabetogenic (in approximately 3–5% of treated patients); high-dose steroid treatment for acute rejection episodes, coupled with maintenance steroid therapy may also predispose to diabetes.

These two important atherogenic risk factors should be minimized by using the lowest possible dose of immunosuppression; there is now a trend to use steroid-free regimes. Calcium channel blockers are often appropriate for hypertension control as they ameliorate the vasoconstriction caused by ciclosporin and tacrolimus, but their combined use with ciclosporin can exacerbate gingival hypertrophy.

SPECIFIC CARDIAC COMPLICATIONS IN PATIENTS WITH RENAL DISEASE

Uraemic pericarditis

Pericarditis is a feature of very advanced uraemia (CKD or ARF). In the era before dialysis was available it was known as the 'harbinger of death', as survival was measured in days or weeks after its onset. It can be asymptomatic and detected as a pericardial rub, but it can present with chest pain, dyspnoea and hypotension if the patient is developing tamponade. It is important to diagnose, as it indicates the need to commence dialysis urgently, and this should be intensive and involve heparin-free haemodialysis in the initial stages, the latter because of the risk of haemorrhagic pericarditis, which could be fatal.

Infective endocarditis in dialysis patients

Infective endocarditis is common in patients receiving dialysis; predisposing factors are shown in Box 21.5. Diagnosis can be difficult clinically, as many renal patients already have cardiac murmurs. These are usually flow murmurs due to anaemia or the arterio-venous fistula, but valvular calcification is also common. A high index of suspicion for the diagnosis is necessary, and repeated blood cultures and echocardiography should be performed.

Treatment is the same as for non-uraemic patients, but the removal of the source of infection (e.g. long-term tunnelled haemodialysis catheters) should be performed early. Conversely, infective endocarditis in non-uraemic patients may lead to acute renal failure.

Atherosclerotic renovascular disease (ARVD)

The clinical characteristics that would suggest the presence of ARVD (Fig. 21.4) in patients with hypertension or CKD are shown in Box 21.6. There is a high prevalence of CAD in patients with ARVD, and >30% of elderly patients with CHF have ARVD,[15] which may be contributory to cardiac dysfunction; there are reports of improved cardiac

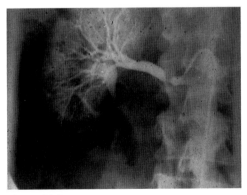

Figure 21.4
Intra-arterial digital subtraction angiography showing tight right renal artery stenosis with mild post-stenotic dilatation

function after renal revascularization. The sub-group who present with 'flash pulmonary oedema' account for a significant proportion of those ARVD patients in whom renal revascularization is considered essential (see also Ch. 15). ARVD is not an absolute contraindication to the use of ACE-I or ARBs, but one must be cautious and renal function should be checked before and after these agents are commenced. The treatment should be discontinued if the serum creatinine level rises by more than 20%. ARVD is a predictor of poor outcome after cardiac revascularization, and dialysis patients with ARVD have a very high mortality (comparable with their diabetic counterparts). The co-morbid prevalence of CAD, peripheral vascular and cerebrovascular disease in ARVD patients raises the question of which lesion should be dealt with first. At the present time there is no consensus view.

Autosomal dominant polycystic kidney disease and the heart

Autosomal dominant polycystic kidney disease (ADPKD) (Fig. 21.5) is often associated with valvular abnormalities, most commonly mitral valve prolapse, as well as LVH. Other less commonly observed valvular lesions are aortic regurgitation and tricuspid regurgitation. LVH and increased LV mass is always secondary to hypertension.

RENAL FAILURE COMPLICATING CARDIAC DISEASE

Glomerulonephritis secondary to infective endocarditis

Glomerulonephritis was a common complication (>50%) of infective endocarditis, but this has fallen to 20% of cases with the advent of antibiotics. Glomerulonephritis is more likely to occur in acute endocarditis associated with *Staphylococcus aureus*. The pathology is usually either diffuse proliferative or focal segmental proliferative glomerulonephritis (Fig. 21.6). Renal functional recovery is anticipated after appropriate duration antibiotic therapy, but occasionally pulsed steroids are necessary for crescentic glomerular disease. Renal impairment from immune complex disease should be distinguished from interstitial nephritis (usually secondary to antibiotic treatment and accompanied by eosinophilia) or from the effects of nephrotoxic drugs (e.g. aminoglycosides). With the latter, renal function usually deteriorates at initiation of

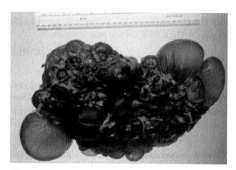

Figure 21.5
Kidney from patient with autosomal dominant polycystic kidney disease. The kidney is almost completely replaced by multiple cysts of varying size, some containing old haemorrhage

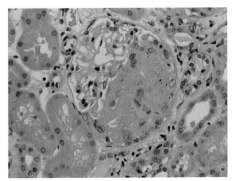

Figure 21.6
Immune complex-mediated focal segmental proliferative glomerulonephritis as seen in patients with infective endocarditis

treatment and aminoglycoside levels will be raised. However, if any uncertainty exists regarding the aetiology then renal biopsy should always be performed.

Renal failure secondary to cardiac failure

In patients with reduced cardiac output there is a decrease in the renal blood flow; the GFR is initially preserved by efferent arteriolar vasoconstriction, which maintains the glomerular hydrostatic pressure. The use of ACE-I or ARBs can abolish this compensatory mechanism, leading to a significant drop in GFR in vulnerable patients; up to 5% of all ARF admissions are thought to result from this effect.[16] Such patients have usually been exposed to high-dose loop diuretics with consequent intra-vascular volume depletion. The possibility of renovascular disease in these patients should also be borne in mind.

Contrast nephropathy and cholesterol embolization complicating cardiac catheterization

Renal impairment is likely to complicate many (>20%) cardiac catheterization procedures, but the true incidence is unknown as the majority of cases are likely to go unrecognized (e.g. discharged after day-case investigation). Contrast nephropathy is the most frequent cause, and is associated with iodinated contrast materials. These cause nephrotoxicity by several mechanisms, including vasoconstriction and direct tubular toxicity. Risk factors for contrast nephropathy are shown in Box 21.7. Several studies have investigated effective prophylaxis for the condition in those at risk (serum creatinine >140 µmol/l), and saline infusion (1 ml/kg body weight/hour) from 12 hours before to 12 hours after contrast administration is the favoured approach.[17] N-acetylcysteine in a dose of 600 mg twice daily for 2–3 days after the procedure may also be of benefit to the most vulnerable patients.[18] Compared to peri-procedure hydration alone, N-acetylcysteine with hydration significantly reduces the risk of contrast nephropathy in patients with CKD.[19] The onset of ARF is rapid (1–3 days) after contrast injury; many cases are non-oliguric, and renal functional recovery can be anticipated within 5–10 days in the majority. Conversely, ARF due to cholesterol emboli (Fig. 21.7) may develop several weeks after the catheterization procedure; it is associated with livideo reticularis, elevated C-reactive protein (CRP) and eosinophilia, and renal recovery is the exception rather than the rule.

> **Box 21.7: Risk factors for contrast nephropathy**
>
> High-contrast load
> High iodine content of contrast
> Hypovolaemia
> Diabetes
> Myeloma
> Hypercalcaemia
> Age
> Pre-existing chronic renal failure
> Hyperuricaemia
> Concurrent administration of nephrotoxic drugs
> Chronic heart failure

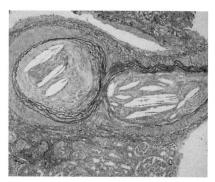

Figure 21.7
Cholesterol crystals lodged in the renal arterioles in a patient with cholesterol embolization

References

1. Coresh J, Longenecker JC, Miller ER 3rd, Young HJ, Klag MJ 1998 Epidemiology of cardiovascular risk factors in chronic renal disease. J Am Soc Nephrol 9(12 Suppl): S24–S30
2. Ikram H, Lynn KL, Bailey RR, Little PJ 1993 Cardiovascular changes in chronic hemodialysis patients. Kidney Int 24: 371–376
3. Foley RN, Parfrey PS, Harnett JD et al. 1995 Clinical and echocardiographic disease in patients starting end-stage renal disease therapy. Kidney Int 47: 186–192
4. Raine AEG 1994 Acquired aortic stenosis in dialysis patients. Nephron 68: 159–168
5. Sforzini S, Latini R, Mingardi G, Vincenti A, Redaelli B 1992 Ventricular arrhythmias and 4 year mortality in hemodialysis patients. Lancet 339: 212–213
6. Longenecker JC, Coresh J, Powe NR et al. 2002 Traditional cardiovascular disease risk factors in dialysis patients compared with the general population: the CHOICE Study. J Am Sos Nephrol 13: 1918–1927
7. Wilkinson R 1994 Renal and renovascular hypertension. In: Swales J D (ed.) Textbook of Hypertension. Blackwell, Oxford, pp. 831–857
8. Lowrie EG, Lew NL 1990 Death risk in hemodialysis patients: Predictive value of commonly measured variables and evaluation of the death rate differences between facilities. Am J Kidney Dis 15: 458–482
9. Silberberg JS, Rahal DP, Patton DR, Sniderman DR 1989 Role of anemia in the pathogenesis of left ventricular hypertrophy in end stage renal disease. Am J Cardiol 64: 222–224
10. Marwick TH, Steinmuller DR, Underwood DA, Hobbes RE, Go RT, Swift C, Braun WE 1990 Ineffectiveness of dipyridamole SPECT thallium imaging as a screening technique for coronary artery disease in patients with end-stage renal failure. Transplantation 49: 100–103
11. Schmidt A, Stefenelli T, Schuster E et al. 2001 Informational contribution of non-invasive screening tests for coronary artery disease in patients on chronic renal replacement therapy. Am J Kidney Dis 37: 56–63

12. Rinehart AL, Herzog CA, Collins AJ 1992 Greater risk of cardiac events after coronary angioplasty (PTCA) than bypass grafting (CABG) in chronic dialysis patients. J Am Soc Nephrol 3: 389

13. Agirbasli M, Weintraub WS, Chang GL et al. 2000 Outcome of coronary revascularization in patients on renal dialysis. Am J Cardiol 86: 495–499

14. Lindholm A, Albrechtsen D, Frodin L, Tufveson G, Persson NH, Lundgren G 1995 Ischemic heart disease-major cause of death and graft loss after renal transplantation in Scandinavia. Transplantation 60: 451–457

15. MacDowall P, Kalra PA, O'Donoghue DJ, Waldek S, Mamtora H, Brown K 1998 Risk of morbidity from renovascular disease in elderly patients with congestive cardiac failure. Lancet 352: 91213–91216

16. Ichikawa I, Pfeffer JM, Pfeffer HM, Hostetter TH, Brenner BM 1984 Role of angiotensin II in the altered renal function of congestive cardiac failure. Circ Res 55: 669–675

17. Friedrichsohn CB, Riegel W, Kohler H 1997 What is reliable in prevention of contrast medium-induced nephropathy? Med Klin 92: 629–634

18. Briguori C, Manganelli F, Scarpato P et al. 2002 Acetylcysteine and contrast agent-associated nephrotoxicity. J Am Coll Cardiol 40: 298–330

19. Alonso A, Lau J, Jaber BL, Weintraub A, Sarnak MJ 2004 Prevention of radiocontrast nephropathy with N-acetylcysteine in patients with chronic kidney disease: A meta-analysis of randomized, controlled trials. Am J Kidney Dis 43: 1–9

SELF-ASSESSMENT

Questions

1. A 56-year-old man presented with an 8-week history of being generally unwell and with intermittent chest pains not related to exertion. In the last week he had become progressively short of breath, and had developed nausea and vomiting. He was not taking any medications. He had no significant past medical history except that he had occasionally been told that he had a raised blood pressure, but he was never commenced on any anti-hypertensive medications. On examination he looked generally unwell, pale, with raised jugular venous pressure (JVP) and blood pressure 95/50 mmHg. Cardiac auscultation revealed a grade 2–3/6 aortic ejection systolic murmur and bilateral fine inspiratory crepitations were noted to the mid-zone of his chest. Urgent blood investigations revealed the following: Na 139 mmol/l, K 5.6 mmol/l, urea 52 mmol/l, creatinine 1075 µmol/l, Hb 8.2 g/dl, WBC 15.6 × 10⁹/l and platelets 195 × 10⁹/l.

   a. What investigations should you request that will help in the acute management of this patient?

   b. What is your differential diagnosis, and how would you reach a definite diagnosis?

2. A 72-year-old man was referred to the cardiology outpatient department with worsening exertion-related breathlessness. He was known to have ischaemic heart disease and he had had a myocardial infarction 5 years earlier. His medications included aspirin 75 mg once daily (od), amlodipine 5 mg od, isosorbide mononitrate 60 mg od, atorvastatin 20 mg od and furosemide 80 mg od. On examination he was found to have a pulse rate of 84/min regular, blood pressure 125/70, normal JVP, normal heart sounds with a pan-systolic murmur at the apex and basal bilateral inspiratory crepitations on chest auscultation. The rest of the examination was unremarkable. His clinical notes showed that he had a serum creatinine of 192 µmol/l at a clinic visit 6 months earlier.

   a. What other investigations would you request to help in the assessment and management of this patient?

   b. What would be your management plan for this patient?

Answers

1. a. This patient is unwell with advanced renal failure and fluid overload; he is breathless and hypotensive. For emergency assessment he will need:
   - arterial blood gases (ABG)
   - chest X-ray (CXR)
   - echocardiography
   - blood cultures.

ABG will help to determine the degree of hypoxia and acidosis as contributors to the dyspnoea. CXR is very important for the assessment of cardiac size and outline. An enlarged globular heart may suggest pericardial effusion and the raised JVP and hypotension could suggest tamponade which will require urgent intervention. An urgent echocardiogram should be performed to confirm the diagnosis, after which he may need insertion of a pericardial drain. He will require urgent haemodialysis, but any form of anticoagulation (heparin or warfarin) should be avoided as this may precipitate haemorrhagic pericarditis and worsen the tamponade. The CXR will also show pulmonary congestion.

Cardiac murmurs are common in uraemic patients due to anaemia, valvular calcification or fluid overload, and so they cannot be relied upon for the diagnosis of infective endocarditis. Other clinical features of the disease (splenomegaly, nail bed and skin infarcts, and retinal changes) should be sought, but echocardiography is essential. Blood cultures (and, indeed, any other cultures, e.g. mid-stream urine (MSU), sputum) are appropriate to identify an infective cause that might be leading to hypotension and septicaemia in a uraemic patient.

    b. The differential diagnosis includes:
- advanced uraemia with uraemic pericarditis and tamponade
- advanced uraemia with sepsis and septic shock
- infective endocarditis with secondary renal failure.

Further investigations are aimed at establishing the diagnosis. Ultrasound of the renal tract is essential to rule out obstructive uropathy and to assess renal size. If the kidneys are of normal size then renal biopsy should be considered to establish the exact nature of injury. If the kidneys are small in size (<8.0 cm) then it is most likely that the patient has ESRD, e.g. secondary to long standing untreated hypertension and nephrosclerosis. Other investigations should include dipstick of the urine; if there is an active urinary sediment (blood and protein) an immunology screen is recommended to establish other possible causes of renal disease such as anti-neutrophil cytoplasmic antibody (ANCA)-positive vasculitis, systemic lupus erythematosus (SLE) or multiple myeloma. Further investigations would be dictated by the findings of all the above investigations.

2. a. This gentleman presents with ischaemic heart disease and cardiac dysfunction as well as mild renal impairment. He will need assessment of his cardiovascular and renal diseases. Investigations should include:
- biochemical profile
- dipstick of the urine and 24-hour urine collection
- ultrasound of the abdomen/renal tract
- echocardiography.

Knowledge of the biochemical profile is essential to establish baseline renal function before any decision regarding further management is made. Ischaemic heart disease with left-ventricular failure (LVF) would require ACE-I or ARBs as an essential part of the management; the cause of the patient's stable CRF should be investigated in parallel. If the renal function has significantly deteriorated in the last 6 months, then he will need urgent assessment of his renal pathology before any further action is taken.

Urinary dipstick will give a pointer to the likely underlying renal disease – an active sediment (i.e. haematuria and proteinuria) would be suggestive of chronic glomerulonephritis or vasculitis, and an inactive sediment would be compatible with conditions such as nephrosclerosis or renovascular disease. Ultrasound of the kidney will again help exclude obstructive pathology and determine renal size. Bilaterally small kidneys indicate chronic renal disease, the cause of which may be difficult to establish; discrepancy in the size of the kidneys may suggest ARVD or chronic pyelonephritis. Normal-sized kidneys usually indicates the need for renal biopsy to establish the diagnosis (although this pattern may be seen in patients with very poor cardiac ouput and renal perfusion due to LV dysfunction). Echocardiography is essential for the assessment of the severity of LV dysfunction and to determine the nature of any murmurs.

Further investigation will depend on the findings of the above, e.g. haematuria and proteinuria on the urinary dipstick indicates the need for a renal immunology screen and/or biopsy, whereas obstruction seen at ultrasound requires urological referral.

b. If the renal function is unchanged compared to 6 months earlier, then it would be safe to commence this patient on small doses of ACE-I or ARBs, with a view to gradual dose increase. The renal profile should be checked 7–10 days after initiating treatment to ensure that renal function has remained stable. Any significant deterioration (e.g. creatinine increasing by >2%) should prompt investigations for underlying ARVD. The best screening test for the latter is magnetic resonance angiography (MRA), as intra-arterial angiography would have a high risk of contrast nephropathy in this patient with poor LV function and CRD.

Cerebrovascular disease and the cardiac patient

22

D. Brull and D. Holdright

INTRODUCTION

Many patients with coronary artery disease (CAD) have coexisting cerebrovascular disease, whilst others who present with stroke have incidental CAD. Both share the same cardiovascular risk factors with a common aetiology, namely atherosclerosis. Around 85% of strokes are of ischaemic origin and a fifth of these are caused by cardiogenic embolism. In view of the clinical significance of both conditions several major questions should be pondered when considering the importance of cerebrovascular disease in the cardiac patient. These will be addressed in turn. Closer working links between cardiologists and neurologists can only improve the quality of care for such patients.

PREDISPOSING FACTORS TO STROKE IN THE CARDIAC PATIENT

Numerous factors predispose to stroke, including structural heart disease, aortic atheroma and endocarditis. The consequences of CAD, such as impaired left-ventricular (LV) function and rhythm disturbance further increase stroke risk. Moreover, standard treatments for CAD may also give rise to stroke, for example following coronary artery bypass graft (CABG) or thrombolysis.

POST MYOCARDIAL INFARCTION

In addition to the risk of atrial fibrillation post myocardial infarction (MI), there is a risk of mural thrombus formation, highest following extensive anterior infarction. Neurological symptoms may develop in up to 15% patients with LV thrombus. Anticoagulation lowers this risk and is generally given for up to 6 months, covering the first 3–4 months where the risk of embolic stroke is highest. Several post-MI trials, most recently WARIS II (Warfarin, Aspirin, Reinfarction Study), have shown that those patients receiving both aspirin and warfarin (to a target International Normalized Ratio (INR) 2.8–4.2) have reduced incidence of reinfarction or stroke, but similar mortality to those on aspirin alone, at the expense of more frequent haemorrhages. Most centres only advocate warfarin for those at highest risk of stroke, in the presence of poor LV function, atrial fibrillation or documented thrombus.

Although stroke is generally an early complication, impaired LV function and development of an LV aneurysm are additional risk factors for late stroke, the risk increasing as ejection fraction falls. All patients should be screened by transthoracic echo where practical to help stratify post-MI risk, particularly following anterior MI. Whilst treatment strategies designed to reduce LV dysfunction (such as thrombolysis and early ACE inhibition) have reduced the incidence of mural thrombosis, thrombolytic (tPa more than streptokinase) and antiplatelet regimes have increased the risk of haemorrhagic stroke, particularly in the elderly, women and hypertensives.

RISK OF STROKE WITH A PATENT FORAMEN OVALE AND THE MERITS OF CLOSURE

The presence of a patent foramen ovale (PFO) has been identified as a potential risk factor for cryptogenic stroke (see Fig. 22.1 & Table 22.1), particularly when associated with an atrial septal aneurysm. Despite antiplatelet therapy the risk of recurrent stroke is approximately 2–4% over 4 years, rising to 15% in the presence of both a PFO and an

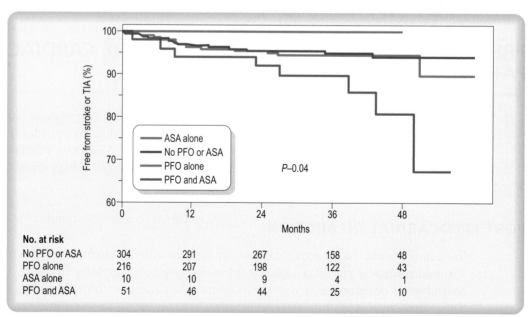

No. at risk				
No PFO or ASA	304	291	267	158	48
PFO alone	216	207	198	122	43
ASA alone	10	10	9	4	1
PFO and ASA	51	46	44	25	10

Figure 22.1
Probability that patients will remain free from recurrent stroke or transient ischaemic attack (TIA), according to the presence or absence of atrial septal abnormalities. The log-rank test was used to calculate the P value. PFO denotes patent foramen ovale, and ASA atrial septal aneurysm. After: Mas, 2001, with permission. Copyright © 2001 Massachusetts Medical Society. All rights reserved.

Table 22.1: Cryptogenic stroke and patent foramen ovale

Patient group	Management options
Isolated PFO	Aspirin 150–300 mg*
Isolated ASA	Aspirin 150–300 mg*
	Consider warfarin or PFO closure for recurrent TIA/stroke
PFO + ASA	PFO closure

* Assuming no evidence of a procoagulant state
PFO, patent foramen ovale; ASA, atrial septal aneurysm

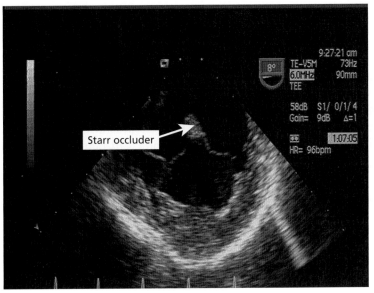

Figure 22.2
Transoesophageal image of a patient with a patent foramen ovale and Starr occluder device in situ

intra-atrial septal aneurysm. Several large prospective series have shown it is possible to close PFOs percutaneously using a variety of devices such as the Amplatzer or PFO-Star Occluder (see Fig. 22.2), with a high success rate and low rates of complications. Yet, despite recurrence rates of cerebrovascular events being as low as, or lower than, the previous series where patients were treated medically, there have been no randomized trials. In general, PFO closure is only recommended in the following situations: magnetic resonance imaging (MRI) evidence of more than one infarct in more than one cerebral territory; recurrence despite antiplatelet therapy; a clear association of symptom onset with the Valsalva manoeuvre; and in patients with a procoagulant state who are high risk for stroke recurrence.

NEUROLOGICAL COMPLICATIONS FOLLOWING PERCUTANEOUS CORONARY INTERVENTION AND CORONARY ARTERY BYPASS SURGERY

The incidence of stroke following percutaneous coronary intervention (PCI) is low (<0.5%). Factors increasing risk include old age, impaired LV function, diabetes and the use of GpIIb/IIIa inhibitors. In contrast, neurological complications following cardiac surgery account for a relatively high proportion of perioperative surgical morbidity. The incidence of stroke following CABG ranges from <1 to 6%. Risk factors include older age, previous stroke (particularly if recent, when cardiac surgery should be deferred to reduce the risk of further stroke), carotid or aortic atheroma, peripheral vascular disease, hypertension, diabetes and atrial fibrillation. Importantly, the mortality from stroke post-CABG is high (~20%), compared with 2–4% mortality for all CABG patients.

Cognitive decline primarily due to the effects of cardiac bypass has increasingly been recognized following CABG. Transient defects occur in up to 60–80% of patients, generally improving with time. Persistent cognitive defects, including disturbances of memory and attention, occur in 20–40% of patients following cardiac surgery. Recent work suggests that the improvement seen in the early months after surgery may be transient, with a later deterioration in cognitive function. Off-pump 'beating heart' coronary artery surgery without using coronary bypass offers not only the promise of reduced perioperative morbidity with a lower incidence of stroke, but also the hope of reduced incidence of cognitive decline.

COEXISTING CAROTID ARTERY DISEASE AND CORONARY ARTERY BYPASS GRAFTING: WHO SHOULD BE SCREENED?

All patients with a previous history of transient ischaemic attack (TIA) or stroke should undergo carotid ultrasound pre-CABG. Subjects shown to have severe carotid stenoses (>70%) will require further investigation using magnetic resonance imaging if further intervention is planned. Other high-risk groups requiring screening include diabetics and subjects with symptomatic peripheral arterial disease, since coexisting carotid disease is common. The presence of carotid bruits is a non-specific finding but also merits formal investigation.

Whilst **asymptomatic** carotid stenosis carries relatively low annual stroke risk (approximately 2%), **symptomatic** carotid artery stenosis carries an annual stroke risk of approximately 15%, reduced to approximately 8% per annum by antiplatelet therapy. Two multi-centre randomized controlled trials (North American Symptomatic Carotid Endarterectomy Trial; European Carotid Surgery Trialist's Collaborative Group) have demonstrated an advantage of carotid endarterectomy (CEA) and aspirin over medical therapy alone in patients with severe (>70% stenosis) symptomatic carotid stenoses. The role of surgery is unclear in patients with carotid stenosis of 50–69%, but might be

---

Box 22.1: Management guidelines for patients with carotid artery disease

Symptomatic carotid stenosis

Medical therapy
All patients should receive anti-thrombotic therapy:
Aspirin +/– dipyridamole
Clopidogrel

Endovascular therapy
Currently being evaluated
International Carotid Stent or Surgery Trial
Carotid Revascularization Endarterectomy versus Stenting Trial

Surgery: carotid endarterectomy
Patients with 70–99% stenosis, who are good surgical candidates and symptomatic within 2 years of stroke
Consider in patients with 50–69% stenosis and multiple TIAs, where the risk of stroke is greater than the predicted operative morbidity
Not indicated for <50% stenosis

Asymptomatic carotid stenosis
All patients should receive anti-thrombotic therapy:
Aspirin +/- dipyridamole
Clopidogrel
Carotid endarterectomy is not advocated

---

considered if medical therapy fails to control symptoms, and the local rate of peri-endarterectomy complications (death or stroke) is less than 3%.

Coexisting carotid disease increases the perioperative stroke risk following CABG. Significant bilateral disease increases this to about 20%. Patients with severe (>70%) symptomatic carotid stenoses who require CABG should undergo CEA provided the local surgical teams have a low rate of perioperative complications. Some centres advocate simultaneous CEA and CABG, whilst others recommend a staged procedure, operating on the more severely diseased carotid first. The severity of carotid artery disease and whether or not ipsilateral stroke has previously occurred should be considered but there are no randomized trials to guide this strategy. The role of carotid stenting in this situation is unknown. Minimally invasive and off-pump coronary artery surgery offer the prospect of fewer neurological sequelae. There are no convincing data to support the role of CEA in asymptomatic patients regardless of whether or not CABG is planned (Box 22.1).

PREVENTION AFTER STROKE: ANTIPLATELET AGENTS, STATINS, CLOPIDOGREL AND ANGIOTENSIN CONVERTING ENZYME INHIBITORS

Measures to reduce the risk of vascular events (such as blood pressure and cholesterol reduction) should be employed in all stroke patients according to the Royal College of Physicians Guidelines on stroke management. Those in atrial fibrillation have a 10–15%

risk of second stroke and this can be reduced to 5% by the use of anticoagulants. Any benefit should be offset against the risk of haemorrhage.

ANTIPLATELET AGENTS

Aspirin reduces vascular events (vascular death, non-fatal stroke and non-fatal myocardial infarction) in doses from 75–325 mg/day. There is no convincing evidence that higher doses are more effective, although side effects are more common. For every 1000 patients treated, there is an excess of 11 patients free from death and disability at 6 months, but one patient affected by cerebral haemorrhage. There is some evidence that the addition of dipyridamole to aspirin may be more effective than aspirin alone, though it is not well tolerated and should only be considered in patients who have had a stroke despite aspirin.

Data from the CAPRIE study suggest that clopidogrel is more effective than aspirin in patients with recent ischaemic stroke, MI or symptomatic peripheral vascular disease, reducing the risk of death, non-fatal MI and stroke by 8.7% compared to aspirin. The addition of clopidogrel to aspirin was investigated prospectively against clopidogrel alone in high-risk patients in the MATCH study. Results showed no advantage in combining aspirin and clopidogrel over aspirin alone. Bleeding rates were also increased with the combination.

ANGIOTENSIN CONVERTING ENZYME INHIBITORS

Many clinicians advocate the widespread use of angiotensin converting enzyme (ACE) inhibitors in subjects with significant vascular disease, on the basis of results from several large trials such as PROGRESS and HOPE.

The PROGRESS study was a randomized trial of a perindopril-based blood-pressure-lowering regimen among 6105 individuals with previous stroke or TIA. Perindopril-based therapy reduced total stroke by 28% and major vascular events by 26%. Combination therapy with indapamide resulted in a 43% reduction in stroke and 40% reduction in major vascular events. The same favourable outcomes were apparent for both normotensive (<140/85 mmHg) and hypertensive (>160/95 mmHg) patients.

The HOPE study showed, in 9297 patients with vascular disease or diabetes mellitus with ≥1 other vascular risk factor (**without** LV impairment), that treatment with ramipril was associated with a risk reduction of 25% for cardiovascular death, 20% for myocardial infarction and 32% for stroke.

LIPID-LOWERING AGENTS

Recent large-scale trials of lipid-lowering therapy in patients at risk of developing or with overt CAD have demonstrated a reduction in non-fatal stroke with treatment. In the 4S secondary prevention trial, lipid-lowering reduced the risk of non-embolic stroke and TIA by 37%. Progression of carotid wall thickening, a predictor of stroke, in asymptomatic patients and in patients with CAD is slowed when plasma low-density lipoprotein (LDL) concentrations are reduced by >25%. All patients of <75 years recovering from a stroke

Table 22.2: Trial evidence for the impact of ACE inhibitors, statins and anti-platelet therapy on stroke

	Placebo (%)	Active (%)	Relative risk reduction	P-value
PROGRESS (n = 6105)				
All cause mortality	14.6	12.9	0.88	<0.001
Cardiovascular mortality	9.2	7.7	0.84	<0.002
Stroke	6.0	4.4	0.73	<0.001
HOPE (n = 9297)				
Death/MI/CVA	17.5	13.9	0.78	<0.001
All strokes	4.9	3.4	0.68	N/A
Ischaemic stroke	3.4	2.2	0.64	N/A
CURE (n = 12 562)				
Cardiovascular death/stroke/MI	11.4	9.3	0.8	<0.001
Heart Protection Study (n = 20 536)				
All cause mortality	25.4	19.9	0.78	<0.001
Cardiovascular mortality	9.2	7.7	0.84	<0.002
Stroke	6.0	4.4	0.73	<0.001

CVA, cerebrovascular accident; MI, myocardial infarction

with carotid atheroma or with known CAD should be considered for statin treatment. There are inadequate data to guide management in older patients.

The Heart Protection Study was a randomized placebo controlled trial of simvastatin 40 mg daily in 20 000 patients with known vascular disease or diabetes aged 40–80 years who were at high risk of CAD. Over an average of 5.5 years, simvastatin reduced all-cause mortality and deaths from cardiovascular disease by 12% and 17%, together with a 27% reduction in stroke (see Table 22.2 for a summary of trial evidence).

OPTIMAL TIMING OF SECONDARY PREVENTION AFTER STROKE

Antiplatelet agents have proven to be of value within the first 48 hours after ischaemic stroke. However, lowering blood pressure within the first 72 hours of acute stroke can lead to neurological deterioration. It is generally recommended to withhold antihypertensive treatment for 72 hours in the acute setting and then cautiously add agents thereafter. In practice, this usually means 1–2 weeks after the acute event.

The benefit from lowering blood pressure is significantly greater for the prevention of stroke than for CAD. The aim is to reduce blood pressure without causing side effects, such as orthostatic hypotension (in the elderly) or deterioration in renal function (ACE inhibitors). A target blood pressure of <140/85 should be strived towards as recommended in the British Hypertension Society guidelines.

Further reading

Antithrombotic Trialists' Collaboration 2002 Collaborative meta-analysis of randomised trials of antiplatelet therapy for prevention of death, myocardial infarction, and stroke in high-risk patients. BMJ 324: 71–86

Braun MU, Fassbender D, Schoen SP et al. 2002 Transcatheter closure of patent foramen ovale in patients with cerebral ischemia. J Am Coll Cardiol 39(12): 2019–2025

CAPRIE Steering Committee 1996 A randomised, blinded, trial of clopidogrel versus aspirin in patients at risk of ischaemic events. Lancet 348: 1329–1339

Diener H-C, Bogousslavsky J, Brass LM et al. 2004 Aspirin and clopidogrel compared with clopidogrel alone after recent ischaemic stroke or transient ischaemic attack in high-risk patients (MATCH): randomised, double-blind, placebo-controlled trial. Lancet 364: 331–337

Evagelopoulos N, Trenz MT, Beckmann A, Krian A 2000 Simultaneous carotid endarterectomy and coronary artery bypass grafting in 313 patients. Cardiovasc Surg 8(1): 31–40

Hurlen M, Abdelnoor M, Smith P, Erikssen J, Arnesen H 2002 Warfarin, aspirin, or both after myocardial infarction. New Eng J Med 347(13): 1019–1022

Intercollegiate Stroke Working Party. National clinical guidelines for stroke. Second edition: June 2004. Clinical Effectiveness and Evaluation Unit, Royal College of physicians of London. ISBN 1 86016 208 8. http://www.rcplondon.ac.uk/pubs/books/stroke/stroke_guidelines_2ed.pdf

Ramsay L, Williams B, Johnston G et al. 1999 Guidelines for management of hypertension: report of the third working party of the British Hypertension Society. J Hum Hypertens 13(9): 569–592

Reversible Ischaemia Trial (ESPRIT) group 2000 Design of ESPRIT: an international randomised trial for secondary prevention after non disabling cerebral ischaemia of arterial origin. Cerebrovasc Dis 10: 147–150

Royal College of Physicians Guidelines on Stroke Management. www.rcplondon.ac.uk

Mas J-L, Arquizan C, Lamy C et al. 2001 Recurrent cerebrovascular events associated with patent foramen ovale, atrial septum aneurysm, or both. N Engl J Med 345: 1740–1746

Yusuf S, Sleight P, Pogue J, Bosch J, Davies R, Dagenais G 2000 Effects of an angiotensin-converting-enzyme inhibitor, ramipril, on cardiovascular events in high-risk patients. The Heart Outcomes Prevention Evaluation Study Investigators. N Engl J Med 342(3): 145–153

SELF-ASSESSMENT

Questions

a. Which patients with a history of recent CVA would merit transoesophageal echocardiogram (TOE) in the context of a normal transthoracic echo?

b. How should one investigate and manage a patient presenting with neurological deficit post-coronary angiography/percutaneous intervention (PCI)? When should imaging of the brain be done and is there a role for heparin or further antiplatelet agents?

Answers

a. The majority of stroke patients will have one or more identifiable 'classical' cardiovascular risk factors. Other risk factors may become apparent following careful clinical examination, such as valvular heart disease, carotid bruits and atrial fibrillation. All patients presenting with stroke proven by either computed tomography (CT) or magnetic resonance imaging (MRI) should have a routine series of screening investigations. This should include electrocardiogram (ECG), full blood count, fasting lipids and glucose, carotid and vertebral ultrasound, and transthoracic echocardiography. The broad indications for echo are summarized in Box 22.2.

TOE has a much higher sensitivity than transthoracic echo in detecting certain pathological features (such as left-atrial thrombus, patent foramen ovale (PFO), atrial septal aneurysm, left-atrial spontaneous echo contrast, valvar vegetations, ascending aorta and arch atheroma, and left-atrial appendage thrombus). TOE should be considered early in the investigation of any patient in whom there is no obvious cause predisposing them towards stroke, particularly in young patients (age <45 years) and in those with >1 stroke territory.

Transcranial Doppler (TCD) has recently been identified as a sensitive and reproducible technique to accurately detect the presence of a PFO. TCD detects microbubbles entering the middle cerebral artery territory following the intravenous injection of agitated saline. TCD allows accurate detection of a PFO in the awake patient since the Valsalva manoeuvre is easier to perform than when a patient is sedated for TOE.

b. Several mechanisms explain the cause of neurological events following either diagnostic angiography or PCI. These include dislodging large vessel atheroma, especially after difficult cannulation of the left internal mammary artery, inadvertent air or cholesterol embolization, atrial fibrillation and haemorrhage. The critical aspect in the management of such neurological events is to confirm the diagnosis by CT or MRI imaging. It is essential to exclude haemorrhagic stroke as early as possible. This is particularly important following PCI where the use of heparin and GpIIb/IIIa inhibitors often gives rise to activated clotting times in excess of 300 s, substantially increasing the risk of haemorrhage. In all cases close liaison with local neurologists is essential. A multidisciplinary approach should be taken.

In the absence of obvious cerebral haemorrhage careful heparinization with unfractionated heparin may be considered provided the area of cerebral infarction is not extensive. Aspirin can safely be continued, although the role of clopidogrel in this scenario is currently being investigated. At present thrombolytic therapy is only considered in highly specialist stroke units.

Box 22.2: Indications for using echocardiography to investigate stroke

Clinical indications
Patients of any age with abrupt occlusion of a peripheral or visceral artery
Patients <45 years with cerebrovascular event
Patients >45 years with cerebrovascular event and without evidence of cerebrovascular disease or other obvious cause
Patients for whom a clinical therapeutic decision will depend on the result of echocardiography (e.g. anticoagulation)

Transthoracic echo findings predisposing to stroke
Dilated cardiomyopathy
LV aneurysm
LV thrombus
Atrial septum
   Aneurysmal
   Patent foramen ovale
   ASD
LA dilatation + spontaneous contrast
Mitral stenosis
Mitral-valve prolapse
Vegetations
Atrial myxoma

Additional findings from transoesophageal echocardiogram
*Presence of right-to-left shunt on injection of agitated saline/contrast
Ascending aorta and arch atheroma
Thrombus in LA appendage
Low LA appendage Doppler flow velocity
Patent foramen ovale
Atrial septal aneurysm
Vegetations

*In order to clearly visualize a PFO, an intravenous injection of agitated saline should be given whilst the patient is asked to perform a Valsalva manoeuvre (transiently increasing right-atrial pressure, thus allowing right-to-left shunting of microbubbles to be seen), which can be difficult to perform during TOE. The results from TCD look more promising.

LV, left ventricle; LA, left atrium; ASD, atrial septal defect; TCD, transcranial doppler

Endocrinological disorders and cardiovascular disease

23

A. Brackenridge and D. Russell-Jones

INTRODUCTION

This chapter will concentrate on diabetes mellitus, the most common endocrinological disorder and the single disease with the greatest impact on the cardiovascular system. Thyroid dysfunction will be discussed at the end.

DIABETES MELLITUS

EPIDEMIOLOGY

Type 1 diabetes affects approximately 1% of the UK population. The prevalence of diagnosed type 2 diabetes is about 2%, but undiagnosed type 2 diabetes probably affects another 2% of the population over 40 years. The prevalence of type 2 diabetes is increasing dramatically throughout the world. This is because of the alarming increase in obesity and physical inactivity. This will have major implications with respect to cardiovascular disease.

DIABETES AND CARDIOVASCULAR DISEASE

Diabetes is a major risk factor for the development of cardiovascular disease. Up to 70% of people with type 2 diabetes will die of coronary heart disease. The risk of cardiovascular mortality in men with diabetes is two to three times higher than men without diabetes and in women the risk is three to five times higher. People with type 2 diabetes develop cardiovascular disease at a younger age and have more severe, multivessel disease. They are more likely to die following myocardial infarction in the acute phase and in the following years, they are more likely to have a further infarct and to develop left-ventricular dysfunction. Research suggests that people with diabetes are as likely to have a myocardial infarction as people without diabetes who have already had an infarct. Cardiovascular mortality is decreasing in the developed world except in people with diabetes and it is actually increasing among women with diabetes.

Type 2 diabetes is associated with a number of cardiovascular risk factors, namely obesity, hypertension and dyslipidaemia. The insulin resistance of type 2 diabetes may

331

also play a role in cardiovascular risk. This cluster of risk factors has been described as the insulin resistance syndrome, the metabolic syndrome or syndrome X, and can occur before the development of diabetes. However, these factors do not explain fully the increased cardiovascular risk seen in diabetes.

DIABETIC DYSLIPIDAEMIA

Dyslipidaemia is common amongst people with type 2 diabetes. The classic diabetic dyslipidaemia is characterized by elevated triglycerides, low high-density lipoprotein (HDL) cholesterol and elevated intermediate density lipoprotein levels. In addition, low-density lipoprotein (LDL) may also be elevated and there is an excess of a particularly atherogenic type of LDL, small dense LDL. This pattern is also seen in insulin-resistant individuals and in people with impaired glucose tolerance.

HYPERTENSION

The prevalence of hypertension in type 2 diabetes is higher than in the general population. Around 40% of people with type 2 diabetes have hypertension at 45 years and this increases to 60% by age 75 years. The presence of hypertension leads to a disproportionate rise in the risk of a cardiovascular event (Box 23.1).

The increased incidence of hypertension in diabetes is thought to be partly due to a derangement in the production of vasoconstrictor and vasodilator substances by the endothelium of blood vessels. There is a relative overproduction of vasoconstrictor substances causing a rise in vascular tone and hence blood pressure.

HYPERGLYCAEMIA

The association between microvascular complications of diabetes and hyperglycaemia has been consistently demonstrated (Box 23.2), but evidence associating hyperglycaemia and

---

Box 23.1: Mechanisms leading to hypertension in diabetes

Diabetic nephropathy
Altered sodium homeostasis
Protein glycation
Increased vascular resistance

Box 23.2: Mechanisms by which hyperglycaemia may accelerate vascular disease

Glycation of proteins
Glycation of lipoproteins
Formation of advanced glycosylation end products
Increased oxidative stress
Increased reactive oxygen species
Increased oxidized lipoproteins
Increased protein kinase C (PKC) and diacylglycerol (DAG)
Increased activation of the coagulation cascade

macrovascular disease is less persuasive. The Diabetes Control and Complications Trial (DCCT) showed significant reductions in microvascular disease with near normal glycaemia in type 1 diabetics, but did not demonstrate a significant reduction in macrovascular complications. The UK Prospective Diabetes Study (UKPDS) compared intensive blood glucose control in type 2 diabetes with standard care. There was only a borderline significant reduction in the risk of myocardial infarction in the intensively treated group, whereas there was a substantial reduction in microvascular complications.

The relative risk of macrovascular disease seems to increase with any increase in glycaemia above the normal range, whereas microvascular complications occur with more extreme hyperglycaemia. This is illustrated by the EPIC-Norfolk trial, a prospective cohort study of residents of Norfolk. In this trial glycated haemoglobin concentration (HbA1c), a measure of average blood glucose over the preceding 3 months, significantly predicted mortality from cardiovascular and other causes in men. The predictive value was stronger than that for cholesterol concentration, body mass index and blood pressure. The effect was present even at low concentrations of HbA1c, below the diabetic range suggesting a continuous relationship with cardiovascular risk rather than a threshold. The lowest death rates were in people with HbA1c less than 5%. About 70% of the population had an HbA1c between 5 and 6.9% and this group accounted for more than 80% of the excess cardiovascular mortality.

DIABETES AS A PROCOAGULANT STATE

In order to explain the associated excess cardiovascular risk diabetes has been conceptualized as a procoagulant state (Box 23.3). There is evidence that diabetes alters many factors involved in the clotting cascade (Fig. 23.1), for example increased fibrinogen and factor VII activity and decreased antithrombin III and protein C activity.

Diabetes also affects the fibrinolytic pathway. Plasminogen activator inhibitor-1 (PAI-1) is the major inhibitor of tissue plasminogen activator (tPA), which is responsible for the conversion of plasminogen to plasmin. The balance between tPA levels and PAI-1 levels determines whether clot is formed or broken down. Increased PAI-1 levels tip the balance to a procoagulant state. PAI-1 levels are increased in type 2 diabetes but normal in type 1 diabetes. They are also increased in the metabolic syndrome.

MICROALBUMINURIA

Microalbuminuria (dipstick negative albuminuria) has been established as a cardiovascular risk factor. It has been shown to be an independent predictor of stroke,

---

Box 23.3: Abnormalities leading to the procoagulant state of diabetes

Increased activity of the coagulation cascade
Decreased activity of the fibrinolytic pathway
Altered platelet function

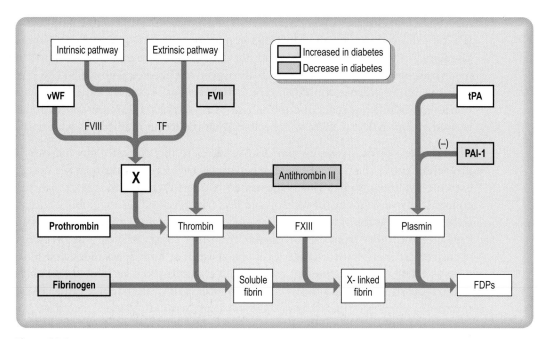

Figure 23.1
Schematic representation of the clotting cascade, resulting in the formation of fibrin and the fibrinolytic pathway, with the generation of plasmin (see text for the influence of diabetes)
vWF, Von Willebrand Factor, FVII (etc), factor seve , Fibrin degradation products; tPA, tissue plasminogen activator; PA1-1, plasminogen activator inhibitor 1; TF, tissue factor
(Adapted from Grant, 2001, with permission.)

death, myocardial infarction and chronic heart failure. It affects approximately 30% of middle-aged people with type 1 and type 2 diabetes, and 15% of a non-diabetic population of a similar age group.

ENDOTHELIAL DYSFUNCTION

Endothelial dysfunction has been suggested as the final common pathway whereby the previously discussed abnormalities cause accelerated atherosclerosis and, hence, macrovascular disease in diabetes (Fig. 23.2). Endothelial dysfunction has been demonstrated in individuals with type 2 diabetes, individuals with type 1 diabetes, especially those with microalbuminuria, and also those with impaired glucose tolerance, insulin resistance and previous gestational diabetes.

MANAGEMENT

PREVENTION OF DIABETES

It has now been shown that type 2 diabetes can be prevented. Two studies, one Finnish and one American, have targeted people with impaired glucose tolerance (and, therefore,

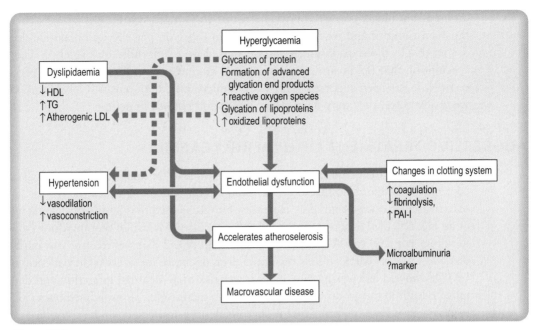

Figure 23.2
Proposed mechanism by which hyperglycaemia results in endothelial dysfunction and subsequent cardiovascular risk.

at high risk of developing diabetes). Both studies showed that an intervention consisting of dietary advice and an exercise programme decreased the proportion of people who developed diabetes by more than 50%.

TIGHT BLOOD PRESSURE CONTROL

The UKPDS showed that in the group assigned to tight control of blood pressure there was a significant reduction in death due to diabetes, stroke and heart failure. The risk of death was reduced by 24% and the risk of heart failure by 56%. The mean blood pressure in the tight control group was 144/82 mmHg compared with 154/87 mmHg in the standard care group. There was no significant difference in outcome between those treated with captopril and those treated with atenolol.

The clinical benefit of lowering systolic blood pressure by 10 mmHg and diastolic blood pressure by 5 mmHg was greater than intensive blood glucose control.

ANGIOTENSIN CONVERTING ENZYME (ACE) INHIBITORS

The benefit of ACE inhibitors has been demonstrated in people with and without diabetes post myocardial infarction, for the treatment of hypertension and for the treatment of chronic heart failure. The HOPE study demonstrated that an ACE inhibitor (ramipril) significantly lowered the risk of major cardiovascular outcomes in high-risk middle-aged and elderly patients with diabetes compared with placebo. Patients had diabetes plus at least one other risk factor (lipids, smoking, hypertension or microalbuminuria). The difference in blood pressure between groups was small (systolic fell by 1.92 mmHg in those on ramipril and rose by 0.55 mmHg in those on placebo and diastolic decreased by 3.3 mmHg in those on ramipril and decreased by 2.3 in those on placebo). This has led to speculation that the positive effects of ACE inhibitors are more than blood pressure control. It has been suggested that via a reduction in angiotensin II level, a powerful vasoconstrictor, they may have effects on endothelial dysfunction.

AGGRESSIVE TREATMENT OF HYPERGLYCAEMIA

The goal in the treatment of people with diabetes is to try and obtain as good glycaemic control as possible as no threshold has been established above which the risk of macrovascular disease markedly increases. HbA1c is used to quantify glycaemia with the aim of an HbA1C of 7% or less. In type 1 diabetes, intensive insulin therapy (four or more injections per day) can help to reach this goal. In type 2 diabetes treatment is initially with diet and exercise. Metformin is the initial drug of choice for overweight patients, as the UKPDS showed less weight gain and a lower risk of myocardial infarction and diabetes-related death in the group treated initially with metformin. Thiazolidinediones (TZDs) are a relatively new class of agents that reduce insulin resistance and can be combined with metformin. There is speculation about the possibility of cardiovascular disease prevention with TZDs due to their beneficial effects on insulin resistance and lipids, but as yet there are no prospective data.

It is increasingly recognized that insulin is often needed for the treatment of type 2 diabetes. Initiation of insulin therapy often leads to weight gain, but combining metformin with insulin can reduce this.

The DIGAMI trial showed that intensive metabolic treatment in people with diabetes with acute myocardial infarction reduced mortality by 30% at 1 year and the effect was sustained for more than 3 years in follow-up studies. Patients were treated for at least 24 hours with an insulin and glucose infusion, and then with intensive subcutaneous insulin therapy for at least 3 months.

TREATMENT OF HYPERLIPIDAEMIA

Aggressive treatment of diabetic dyslipidaemia is important in the prevention of cardiovascular disease. Because of the particular pattern of lipid abnormalities seen in diabetes treatment with fibrate drugs which have a more marked effect on triglyceride levels is often necessary. This may be the case even in patients with normal total cholesterol or LDL levels because of their adverse risk profile.

CARDIOVASCULAR INTERVENTION

People with diabetes have a poorer outcome than people without diabetes when treated with angioplasty or coronary artery bypass graft (CABG). There is some evidence that they do particularly badly with angioplasty. The BARI trial showed a significant survival benefit in people with diabetes who had CABG as the first coronary revascularization procedure compared to those who had angioplasty. This difference was not seen in the non-diabetics or in other high-risk groups. This trial was done before the use of coronary stents and GIIbIIIa antagonists was standard practice and this may improve the outlook for people with diabetes. Drug eluting stents, at least in theory, may reduce the incidence of restenosis. Long-term prospective data are now awaited.

DIABETIC CARDIOMYOPATHY

People with diabetes are recognized to be at increased risk of chronic heart failure. This is partially due to macrovascular coronary artery disease and also coronary microangiopathy. However, it is now recognized that diabetes also leads to histological changes in the cardiomyocytes, which may be relevant in the development of the cardiomyopathy of diabetes.

POLYCYSTIC OVARY DISEASE

Polycystic ovary disease (PCOS) is associated with the metabolic syndrome. The incidence of diabetes and impaired glucose tolerance is up to 30% in obese women with PCOS, and the prevalence of diabetes in older women with PCOS is up to six times greater than expected. As of yet there are no data on cardiovascular disease in these women but it is presumed that they will have a high cardiovascular risk. Interestingly, metformin is now being used as a treatment for women with PCOS and seems to have beneficial effects on ovulation and fertility. Work is also in progress using the TZDs.

THYROID DISEASE

Thyroid abnormalities are the second most common endocrinological disorder and also have effects on the cardiovascular system.

Hypothyroidism

Hypothyroidism is commonly associated with bradycardia; less common features include heart failure and pericardial effusion. It is also associated with hypercholesterolaemia. These features are reversed by treatment with thyroxine. It is important to be cautious when initiating thyroxine for people with hypothyroidism who also have ischaemic heart disease. Thyroxine can precipitate worsening angina, myocardial infarction and even death due to the resulting increase in metabolic rate and heart rate. Therefore, it should be started at a dose of 25 µg per day (or even 25 µg alternate days) and the dose increased very slowly with regular monitoring.

> **Box 23.4: Effects of amiodarone on the thyroid in euthyroid patients**
>
> Decreased peripheral conversion of T4 to T3 (40% have T4 levels above the normal range)
> Inhibition of entry of T3 and T4 into peripheral tissue
> Early increase in TSH levels (first 3 months)
> TSH often returns to normal after this

Hyperthyroidism

Hyperthyroidism leads to tachycardia and atrial fibrillation develops in 5–15%. In addition patients with sublinical hyperthyroidism (normal T3 and T4 levels but suppressed thyroid stimulating hormone (TSH)) are at increased risk of atrial fibrillation. The combination of hyperthyroidism and atrial fibrillation increases the risk of thromboembolism and patients should receive anticoagulation.

Amiodarone and thyroid disease

Amiodarone is rich in iodine and a maintenance dose of 200 mg per day results in a daily intake of iodine up to one thousand times greater than required. Therefore, amiodarone affects thyroid physiology in nearly all patients who are treated with it (Box 23.4).

Abnormal thyroid function test results without clinical symptoms increase with the duration of treatment and the dose accumulated.

Thyrotoxicosis

The reported incidence of amiodarone induced thyrotoxicosis (AIT) varies from 1 to 23%. It can be difficult to diagnose due to the increase in T4 levels seen in many patients treated with amiodarone. It is, therefore, helpful to measure the T3 level too and the diagnosis is made if the T4 and T3 levels are high, and the TSH is suppressed. It is more common in areas with low iodine intake and is usually divided into two separate forms:

1. Type I (AIT) occurs in abnormal thyroid gland for example a nodular goitre or latent Graves. The iodine load triggers increased thyroid hormone synthesis and release.
2. Type II (AIT) affects normal thyroid glands and is due to a destructive thyroiditis leading to hormone release.

Mixed forms occur too.

The management of AIT is difficult. Up to 20% of cases may spontaneously recover. However, treatment is usually recommended because of the adverse cardiological effect of thyrotoxicosis. Type I AIT may not respond to treatment with conventional drugs (carbimazole and propylthiouracil) because of the high iodine content of the thyroid. Sometimes the addition of potassium perchlorate, which inhibits iodine uptake, may be necessary.

Type II AIT responds to treatment with steroids. Carbimazole is not helpful as it decreases thyroid hormone synthesis and this condition is due to release of preformed hormone rather than synthesis. Radioactive iodine is not useful due to suppressed thyroid iodine uptake because of the high circulating levels of iodine.

Thyroidectomy may be necessary in particularly resistant cases. If possible it is best to withdraw amiodarone treatment.

Hypothyroidism

This effects between 1 and 32% of patients treated with amiodarone. It occurs more commonly in areas with high iodine intake and in people with pre-existing thyroid antibodies. It can be transient or persistent. In contrast to AIT it is easy to diagnose and treat. It is diagnosed by low T4 levels and increased TSH levels. Treatment is to discontinue amiodarone if possible and thyroxine replacement. The goal of treatment is to restore the T4 level to the high end of the normal range. In contrast to other forms of primary hypothyroidism, the TSH is not such a good guide to replacement dose.

Further reading

BARI investigators 2000 Seven year outcome in the bypass angioplasty revascularization investigation (BARI) by treatment and diabetic status. J Am Coll Cardiol 35(5): 1122–1129

Bartalena L, Bogazzi F, Martino E 2002 Amiodarone induced thyrotoxicosis: a difficult diagnostic and therapeutic challenge. Clin Endocrinol 56: 23–24

Calles-Escandon J, Cipolla M 2001 Diabetes and endothelial dysfunction: A clinical perspective. Endocrine Rev 22(1): 36–52

Colwell JA 2001 Treatment for the procoagulant state in type 2 diabetes. Endocrin Metabol Clin N Am 30(4): 1011–1030

Diabetes Control and Complications Trial Research Group 1993 The effect of intensive treatment of diabetes on the development and progression of longterm complications in insulin dependent diabetes. N Eng J Med 329: 977–986

Diabetes Prevention Program Research Group 2002 Reduction of the incidence of type 2 diabetes with lifestyle interventions or metformin. N Eng J Med 346: 393–403

Gerstein HC, Mann JFE, Yi Q et al. 2001 Albuminuria and risk of cardiovascular events, death and heart failure in diabetic and nondiabetic individuals. J Am Med Assoc 286(4): 421–426

Grant P, 2001 Insulin resistance and cardiovascular disease: redefining type 2 diabetes. British Journal of Cardiology 8(4): S1–S2

Harjai KJ, Licata AA 1997 Effects of amiodarone on thyroid function. Ann Int Med 126: 63–73

Heart Outcomes Prevention Evaluation (HOPE) Study Investigators 2000 Effects of ramipril on cardiovascular and microvascular outcomes in people with diabetes mellitus: results of the HOPE study and MICRO-HOPE substudy. Lancet 355: 253–259

Khaw K-T, Wareham N, Luben R et al. 2001 Glycated haemoglobin, diabetes and mortality in men in Norfolk cohort of European Prospective Investigation of Cancer and Nutrition (EPIC-Norfolk). BMJ 322: 1–6

Klein I, Ojamaa K 2001 Thyroid hormone and the cardiovascular system. N Eng J Med 344(7): 501–509

Malmberg K 1997 Prospective randomised study of intensive insulin treatment on long term survival after acute myocardial infarction in patients with diabetes mellitus. BMJ 314: 1512–1515

Stratton IM, Adler AI, Neil HAW et al. 2000 Association of glycaemia with macrovascular and microvascular complications of type 2 diabetes (UKPDS 35): a prospective observational study. BMJ 321: 405–412

Taylor AA 2001 Pathophysiology of hypertension and endothelial dysfunction in patients with diabetes mellitus. Endocrin Metabol Clinics N Am 30(4): 983–997

Tuomilehto J, Lindström J, Eriksson JG et al. 2001 Prevention of type 2 diabetes by changes in lifestyle among subjects with impaired glucose tolerance. N Eng J Med 344: 1343–1350

UK Prospective Diabetes Study Group 1998 Tight blood pressure control and risk of macrovascular complications in type 2 diabetes: UKPDS 38. BMJ 317: 703–713

Fitness to fly

24

M. Popplestone

INTRODUCTION

In the year 2000 over 1.6 billion passengers flew on commercial aircraft worldwide, 500 million of these travelling on international services. A significant number of passengers will be suffering from some form of chronic illness and, with the increasing age of the population and availability of long distance travel, this is likely to increase.

The impact of the aircraft cabin environment is limited in healthy individuals but may have adverse consequences in those with existing disease. In addition, the physical and psychological stresses of a long journey or unusual exotic destinations should not be underestimated.

CABIN ENVIRONMENT

Modern commercial jet aircraft fly at altitudes of up to 44 000 feet (13 400 m). The cabin pressure is controlled automatically during flight equivalent to an altitude of between 6000 and 8000 feet (1800 and 2400 m) maximum, 81 kPa (610 mmHg) to 75 kPa (560 mmHg), compared to 101 kPa (760 mmHg) at sea level.

In addition to gas expansion of up to 30%, the principle effect of the lower pressure is to reduce the partial pressure of oxygen (pO_2) (Table 24.1).

Table 24.1: pO_2 at sea level and maximum cabin altitude

| | Sea level | | 8000 feet (2400 m) | |
	kPa	mmHg	kPa	mmHg
Inspired air	19.7	148	14.4	108
Alveolar air	13.7	103	8.5	64
Arterial blood	12.6	95	7.4	56

340

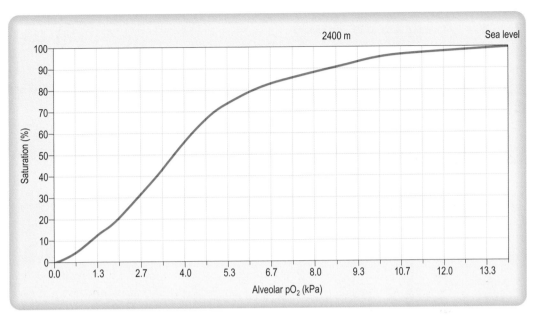

Figure 24.1
Haemoglobin oxygen dissociation curve

Individuals with normal cardio-respiratory function usually tolerate the resulting arterial oxygen saturation of around 90% without difficulty.

As the pO_2 decreases below approximately 8 kPa, haemoglobin oxygen saturation decreases to a proportionately greater extent, a phenomenon which normally facilitates oxygen delivery to the tissues (Fig. 24.1). Compensatory response is by a combination of hyperventilation and increased heart rate, which results in increased cardiac oxygen demand.

Patients who are hypoxic at sea level will, therefore, experience a greater reduction in oxygen saturation and may develop symptoms of hypoxia, including light headedness and dyspnoea. In passengers with impaired left-ventricular function or ischaemic heart disease the decreased oxygen supply combined with increased demand may result in chest pain and in the potential for cardiac decompensation.

FITNESS TO TRAVEL ASSESSMENT

There is little objective basis for fitness to fly assessment and criteria are generally based on the experience of the airline industry and are viewed as guidelines only.[1] On the basis of good clinical assessment and management most patients are fit to fly. The final decision should be a judgement, based on consideration of the impact of general factors on the individual's health as well as medical (Table 24.2) criteria.

Table 24.2: Medical fitness to fly assessment

	In all cases
Stability	No recent deterioration
Medication	Treatment optimized well in advance
Clinical examination	In good general condition Hypertension controlled
Exercise tolerance	50 metre walk on the flat or single flight of stairs without symptoms or additional oxygen
Flying history	Uneventful recent flight
	Specific conditions
Ischaemic heart disease Exercise ECG testing	A normal result or changes only at maximal exercise is reassuring but testing is not compulsory
Arrhythmias Rhythm Pacemakers and other implantable devices	Normal or well-controlled cardiac rhythm Most compatible with airport security devices (refer to manufacturers' literature and take a copy on the trip) If in doubt, request a manual security check
Chronic heart failure NYHA* Classes I and II	Fit to fly if stable
NYHA* Classes III and IV	Fit to fly with supplementary oxygen, if stable
Use of ground oxygen	Provide in flight oxygen at increased flow rate Ground oxygen requirement of 4 l/min or more, unfit to fly
Arterial oxygen saturation (breathing room air at rest)	Saturation, with no other pathology: >92%, should be fit to fly 92–95%, consider hypoxic challenge test** <92%, provide in-flight oxygen With coexisting respiratory pathology: >95%, should be fit to fly <95%, provide in flight oxygen
Blood gases (if available, need not be performed specifically as part of assessment)	Breathing room air at rest: PaO_2 >9.3 kPa (70 mmHg) should be fit to fly PaO_2 <9.3 kPa (70 mmHg) only fit to fly if stable and only with supplementary oxygen

* NYHA – New York Heart Association functional classification
**Hypoxic challenge testing (16% oxygen at sea level) has been used to assess chronic respiratory disease,[2] and could be considered in cardiac failure

CONTRAINDICATIONS TO FLYING

There are some contraindications to flying, which include:

- unstable angina
- uncontrolled heart failure
- uncontrolled arrhythmia

> **Box 24.1: General advice**
>
> **Medication**
> Medication should carry pharmacy labels
> Carry a list of drugs separately
> Carry enough for the trip and any likely delays
> Carry enough (including glyceryl trinitrate (GTN)) in hand baggage for the likely journey time
> If crossing time zones, adjust dose timings after arrival at destination
> Beware cardiac side effects and drug interactions with some antimalarial drugs
>
> **Airport wheelchairs**
> Should be requested at the time of reservation if required
>
> **E111 form**
> Entitlement to health care in Europe
> Will not cover costs of repatriation
>
> **Travel insurance**
> Should be strongly encouraged
> Full disclosure of existing conditions mandatory (to avoid invalidating policy)
> Should cover additional costs including medical repatriation
>
> **Airline clearance**
> Airline should be informed of the medical condition
> Detailed medical information may be required (the airline will provide a 'Medif' form)

- myocardial infarction within 1 week
- cardiac surgery within 10 days or with residual pleural gas
- angiography within 24 hours
- angioplasty within 3 days
- severe cyanotic congenital heart disease
- transient ischaemic attack (TIA) within 24 hours
- cerebrovascular accident (CVA) within 3 days.

Depending on circumstances, some of these may become relative rather than absolute contraindications. For example, some patients can fly home on short UK domestic routes as early as 7 days after bypass surgery.

ADVICE TO PATIENTS

Once fitness to travel has been established, the basic advice given in Box 24.1 is applicable to all patients to reduce the risk of problems occurring. If there is any doubt about fitness to fly, concerns should be discussed with the airline's medical advisor, via the airline's reservation department.

TRAVELLERS' THROMBOSIS

Studies have suggested an association between long journeys (by car, bus, rail or air) and the occurrence of deep vein thrombosis (DVT) and pulmonary embolism, particularly in those with pre-existing risk factors.

A common factor in all forms of long-distance travel is prolonged immobility, and there is no clear evidence that flying, in itself, or the aircraft cabin environment are specific additional risk factors. The magnitude of any increased risk or benefit from specific preventive measures is unknown. However, any of the following may be beneficial in patients with cardiovascular disease:

- Exercising legs, ankles and feet
- Regular walking
- Correctly fitted below-knee graduated compression stockings
- Low-molecular-weight heparin before leaving for the airport.

For those with multiple risk factors, it might be considered appropriate to discourage long-distance travel.

References

1. Air Transport Medicine Committee 1997 Medical guidelines for airline travel. Aerospace Medical Association, Virginia (www.asma.org)
2. British Thoracic Society 2002 Managing passengers with respiratory disease planning air travel: British Thoracic Society recommendations. Thorax 57: 289–304

Further reading

Ernsting J, Nicholson AN, Rainford DJ 1999 Aviation medicine, 3rd edn. Butterworth Heinemann, London
British Airways website: www.britishairways.com/health
Zuckerman JN 2001 Principles and practice of travel medicine. Wiley, New York

FREQUENTLY ASKED QUESTIONS

Questions
a. What are the arrangements for dealing with medical emergencies on board?
b. When can passengers safely undertake elective travel following myocardial infarction or bypass surgery?
c. Can timing of medication be altered to accommodate travel schedules and departure times?

Answers
a. Minimum levels of equipment and medication vary, depending on the regulatory authority, the route and the airline and it is not possible to guarantee what will be available. However, many airlines carry enhanced medical kits, which may include stethoscope, sphygmomanometer and oropharyngeal airways as well as medications such as GTN, atropine, epinephrine, lignocaine and furosemide. Some airlines also provide automatic external defibrillators (for use by cabin crew). Access to in flight medical advice from specialist ground-based organizations is increasingly available.
b. Providing there has been a good uncomplicated recovery with resumption of reasonable physical activity, flying can be contemplated as early as 3–4 weeks after the event, though it may be sensible to wait until after 6 weeks. Travel insurance will almost certainly be subject to higher premiums.
c. As far as possible, medication regimes should remain unchanged pre-flight. Diuretics can be a particular inconvenience for morning flights but are essential to avoid the prospect of decompensated heart failure occurring in flight. One solution may be to take the medication after an early arrival at the airport.

Pre-operative assessment for non-cardiac surgery

25

M. Seddon and A. Calver

PRINCIPLES

Surgical procedures are most frequently performed on older patients, and the presence of cardiovascular disease increases with age. Hence, in the patient population undergoing surgical intervention, there is the potential for significant cardiovascular morbidity and mortality. The risk for individual patients is not uniform – it is dependent on a number of patient-related and surgery-related determinants.

The role of the cardiology opinion is NOT to decide on patient fitness for surgery, but to evaluate the patient's medical status and determine whether/ how this can be optimized to minimize surgical risk. This involves recommendations regarding:

- medical management
- further necessary cardiac investigations
- risk of surgery and timing of non-emergency surgery (decided in conjunction with the surgical team)
- long-term plan (post surgery) for cardiovascular disease.

The indications for further cardiac investigations and treatments are, in general, the same as in the non-operative setting. The timing of these depends on the urgency of surgery, type of surgery, and individual patient predictors of risk. There must be a balance between need for surgery and risk.

APPROACH

PATIENT FACTORS (see Table 25.1)

History, physical examination and electrocardiogram: salient features

1. Cardiac history (particularly recent change)
2. Risk factors for ischaemic heart disease
3. Optimization of associated conditions:
   a. Anaemia
   b. Peripheral or cerebral vascular disease (higher chance of coronary disease)

Table 25.1: Patient predictive risk factors

Predictive risk	Risk factors
Major	Unstable coronary syndromes Decompensated heart failure Severe valve disease (especially aortic/mitral stenosis) Significant arrhythmias (high-grade AV block, fast supraventricular or symptomatic ventricular arrhythmias with underlying heart disease)
Intermediate	Angina Previous MI on history or Q waves on ECG Compensated/prior heart failure Diabetes Renal impairment
Minor	Elderly Rhythm other than sinus rhythm Abnormal ECG (BBB, LVH, ST changes) Previous stroke Uncontrolled hypertension (control preferably with beta-blockers) Poor functional capacity (as scored below)

AV, atrioventricular; MI, myocardial Infarction; ECG, electrocardiogram; BBB, bundle branch block; LVH, left-ventricular hypertrophy
Adapted from ACC/AHA Guidelines

    c. Diabetes (acute control, e.g. sliding scale)
    d. Renal impairment (optimize fluid status)
       i. dialysis/transplant patients should be evaluated in the same way as others
      ii. increased burden of cardiovascular disease (see Ch. 21)
     iii. consider dialysis pre-op to prevent fluid overload
     iv. liaise with renal team re immunosuppression regimen peri-operatively in renal transplant patients
4. Functional capacity in metabolic equivalents (METS)
    a. 1 MET – e.g. self-care, eat, dress, wash self, walk around house
    b. 4 METS – e.g. baking, slow ballroom dancing, walking fast, golfing with a cart
    c. 7 METS – e.g. jogging, moderate cycling, walking fast uphill
    d. 10 METS – e.g. strenuous activity

(poor = <4 METS, moderate = 4–7 METS, good = 7–10 METS, excellent = >10 METS).

Functional ability, quantified in METS, provides an indication of the patient's general level of fitness. New York Heart Association (NYHA) class (heart failure) and Canadian Cardiovascular Society (CCS) class (angina) can also be used to assess whether a patient is deemed to be in the high or intermediate risk group, on the basis of symptomatic limitation.

SURGICAL FACTORS (see Table 25.2)

Assessment of surgical risk will depend upon the exact procedure and its timing. While emergency surgery is likely to carry greater risk, this is usually offset by the escalating risks of not intervening acutely, although a brief period of stabilization may be warranted.

Table 25.2: Surgery predictive risk factors

Predictive risk	Risk factors
Major	Emergency operations Major vascular surgery Likely associated coronary disease Cardiac symptoms masked by claudication limiting exercise Increased haemodynamic stress at operation Anticipated long procedures/large blood volume loss
Intermediate	The majority of surgical procedures
Minor	Breast surgery Dermatology and superficial operations Endoscopic procedures

Adapted from ACC/AHA Guidelines

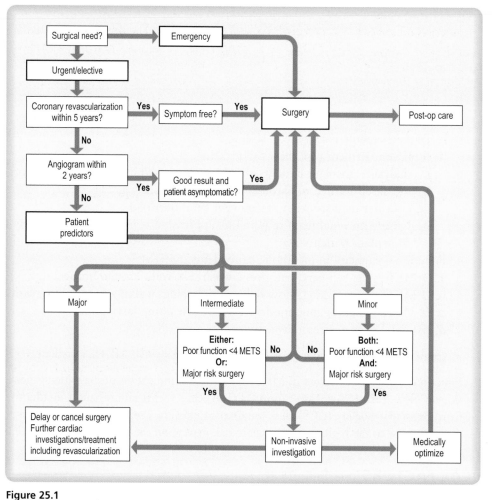

Figure 25.1
An algorithm taking into account the patient and surgical predictive risk factors described, to help guide the management of patients with coronary artery disease. Adapted from the algorithm suggested in the ACC/AHA guidelines.

Ischaemic heart disease (see Fig. 25.1)

Patients who have been revascularized and do not have symptoms can proceed to surgery. The workup for those whose coronary anatomy is not known depends on patient- and surgery-related factors. Those with major patient risk factors should, ideally, have their surgery postponed. In patients with intermediate or minor patient risk factors, the decision to investigate further will depend on their functional status and the type of surgery that is planned.

Non-invasive investigation

A completely normal electrocardiogram (ECG) suggests the probability of significant, structural heart disease is low. Left bundle branch block (LBBB) or left-ventricular hypertrophy (LVH) and strain are predictors of increased risk in intermediate/high-risk patients.

Figure 25.1 indicates which patients should be further investigated. In most ambulatory patients, the test of choice is an exercise test (ETT), which gives an indication of functional capacity and detects myocardial ischaemia. The onset of myocardial ischaemia at low exercise workloads (e.g. <6 mins) is associated with significantly increased risk of perioperative and long-term cardiac events and warrants further investigation with angiography. However, ETT has a number of limitations. Many patients are unable to exercise to target heart rate due to non-cardiac factors such as leg claudication, joint problems or lung disease. In those with resting ECG abnormalities (such as LBBB or LVH) an ETT is less helpful. In such patients stress echocardiography or perfusion imaging are useful alternatives.

Perfusion imaging results correlate with cardiac risk: a reversible perfusion defect predicts perioperative events while a fixed defect relates to long-term cardiac morbidity.

In stress echocardiography, the presence of a new wall-motion abnormality is a reliable indicator of increased perioperative risk (those with a greater degree of abnormality and/or wall motion abnormality at low workload being at greater risk).

Results of non-invasive tests dictate whether or not the patient requires angiography +/− intervention prior to surgery.

Intervention and optimization

If the patient has a pre-operative angiogram that favours bypass surgery long term, revascularization should be carried out before high- or intermediate-risk elective surgery.

If the patient requires a pre-operative percutaneous intervention (indications as for non-operative setting) surgery should be timed for 4 weeks post procedure, to allow completion of anti-platelet therapy after percutaneous intervention and reduce the chances of stent thrombosis.

Post myocardial infarction (MI), it is advisable to delay surgery 6 weeks where feasible.

In terms of pre-operative medical optimization, a growing literature suggests a significant benefit of beta-blockade in reducing peri-operative cardiac morbidity and mortality. Since most benefit has been seen in high-risk patients, it has been suggested that beta-blockers be used in any patient with ischaemic heart disease (history of angina or MI, positive exercise test or Q waves on ECG), cerebrovascular disease, insulin-requiring diabetics, those with chronic renal impairment and any patient undergoing high-risk surgery. Consideration should also be given to patients with more than one conventional risk factor for ischaemic heart disease (hypertension, diabetes, cholesterol, smoker and/or age >65 years). The optimal timing for starting beta-blockers and length of treatment is not fully known. Medical optimization also includes control of cardiac risk factors such as hypertension and diabetes (e.g. sliding scale).

Heart failure

Peri-operative risk increases with increasing NYHA class of heart failure. Patients in overt pulmonary oedema should be stabilized with the same medical measures as in the non-operative setting. In those whose surgery cannot wait, invasive haemodynamic monitoring is required. A pre-operative transthoracic echocardiogram (TTE) is recommended for patients with decompensated or deteriorating heart failure, and those with stable heart failure without cardiac evaluation in the previous 2 years. Screening all patients pre-operatively is not recommended.

The aim should be to optimize heart failure treatment and stabilize the patient on an ACE-inhibitor and a beta-blocker.

Severe valve disease

Valve disease predisposes to peri-operative heart failure, endocarditis and arrhythmias. Patients with severe aortic stenosis or mitral stenosis need valve replacement as a priority. On the whole, patients tolerate chronic regurgitant valve disease much better.

In patients with previous mild or moderate valve disease, a TTE should be performed if there has been no evaluation in the previous 2 years. A TTE is mandatory for any newly detected murmur considered not to be innocent.

All patients with valve disease require prophylaxis against endocarditis at the time of surgery.

Patients with prosthetic valves must have a regimen in place for peri-operative anticoagulation. The ACC/AHA and British Society of Haematology suggest discontinuation of warfarin 72 hours prior to routine non-cardiac surgery. Major surgical procedures require INR <1.5, and anticoagulation must be maintained with heparin, which should be continued until 6 hours before and started 6–12 hours after operation, where surgically feasible. Oral anticoagulation can usually be restarted 1–2 days post surgery. The exact timings are different for each individual case, and require close liaison between the cardiology and surgical teams.

Atrioventricular (AV) block

Indications for a temporary pacing wire peri-operatively are the same as those for a permanent system in the non-operative setting (see Ch.14).

Arrhythmias

- Atrial fibrillation – Control heart rate (beta-blockers or amiodarone > calcium channel blockers > digoxin). A combination of antiarrhythmics may be needed. Stop warfarin (if urgent, use vitamin K and fresh frozen plasma). Indications for DC cardioversion are as for the non-operative setting.
- Supraventricular tachycardias – Control heart rate/maintainance of sinus rhythm. Consider ablation pre-operatively.
- Ventricular ectopics, couplets, non-sustained ventricular tachycardia (VT) – Treat if associated with ongoing ischaemia. Peri-operative risk relates to the underlying heart disease rather than the arrhythmia itself.
- Sustained VT – Treat as for non-operative setting.

Implantable cardioverter defibrillators (ICDs), pacemakers (PPMs)

Devices should be evaluated pre-operatively for the following:

- Patient's intrinsic rhythm
- Device settings/battery status
- Is the patient pacing dependent? What is the threshold?

They may need reprogramming (e.g. increase in the basic rate in sick patients due for major surgery).

ICDs should be turned off immediately pre-operatively and on immediately afterwards to prevent any unwanted shocks.

SURVEILLANCE FOR PERI-OPERATIVE MYOCARDIAL INFARCTION

Look for symptoms, signs and evidence of cardiovascular dysfunction, including ECG change and troponin release. Symptoms of peri-operative MI may be masked by anaesthesia and analgesia.

Peri-operative MI has a high mortality rate. ST elevation myocardial infarction (STEMI) cannot be thrombolysed immediately post-operatively. Percutaneous coronary intervention (PCI) can be considered but adjunctive therapy, such as IIb/IIIa inhibitors, may predispose to bleeding. The decision as to whether PCI is appropriate will need to be made between cardiologist and surgeon on an individual basis. Most peri-operative MIs are non-STEMIs (NSTEMIs). Maximize conventional medical management (see Ch. 7) and consider angiography at a later date. The follow-up of these patients should be as for any other post-infarct patient.

POST-OPERATIVE HEART FAILURE

Patients with poor LV function are predisposed to decompensation. Most cases are due to excessive fluid resuscitation, and this responds well to conventional therapy. However, this scenario is best avoided by judicious use of fluids, careful fluid balance and invasive monitoring in appropriate cases. A new ischaemic event, arrhythmia, or low haemoglobin post-operatively may precipitate decompensation and should be treated aggressively.

LONG-TERM MANAGEMENT

The peri-operative consultation is a good opportunity to evaluate the patient's cardiovascular status and to protect the patient in the long term from future cardiac events. This may involve risk-factor management, further cardiac investigations, and outpatient follow-up.

Further reading

Auerbach AD, Goldman L 2002 Beta-blockers and reduction of cardiac events in noncardiac surgery: scientific review. JAMA 287(11): 1435–1444

Chassot PG, Delabays A, Spahn DR. 2002 Preoperative evaluation of patients with, or at risk of, coronary artery disease undergoing non-cardiac surgery. BJA 89(5): 747–759

Davison P, Ali MJ, Davison P, Pickett W et al. 2000 ACC/AHA guidelines as predictors of postoperative cardiac outcomes. Can J Anaes 47(1): 10–19

Eagle KA, Berger PB, Calkins et al. 2002. ACC/AHA guideline update for perioperative cardiovascular evaluation for noncardiac surgery. American College of Cardiology/American Heart Association Task Force on Practice Guidelines (Committee to Update the 1996 Guidelines on Perioperative Cardiovascular Evaluation for Noncardiac Surgery). 105: 1257–1267.

Gohlke-Barwolf C 2000 Anticoagulation in valvular heart disease: new aspects and management during non-cardiac surgery. Heart 84(5): 567–572

Goldman L, Caldera DL, Nussbaum SR et al. 1997 Multifactorial index of cardiac risk in noncardiac surgical procedures. NEJM 297: 845–850

Mangano DT 1990 Perioperative cardiac morbidity. Anaesthesiology 72: 153–184

Reginelli JP, Mills RM 2001 Non-cardiac surgery in the heart failure patient. Heart 85(5): 505–507

Atrial fibrillation and anticoagulation

26

T. R. Betts

INTRODUCTION

Atrial fibrillation (AF) affects 2–5% of the general population over 60 years of age. It induces a hypercoagulable state that becomes more pronounced as episodes lengthen. It can be found in 15% of all stroke patients and 2–8% of patients with transient ischaemic attacks. Atrial fibrillation confers a fivefold increased risk for stroke (an overall rate of 4.5% per year). The risk of thromboembolism is related to coexistent cardiovascular disease. The annual risk of 'lone' AF in those under 60 years is 1.3%, whereas the annual risk in those with a prior stroke may be 10–12%.

RISK FACTORS FOR THROMBOEMBOLIC STROKE

Risk increases with age, hypertension, diabetes, previous stroke or transient ischaemic attack and poor left-ventricular (LV) function. Multiple risk factors have an additive effect. A history of previous stroke or transient ischaemic attack confers an almost threefold increase in future stroke risk (12% vs 4.5% if no prior history). Echocardiographic risk factors include moderate-to-severe LV dysfunction, the presence of spontaneous contrast, left-atrial thrombus and aortic atheroma. Meta-analysis of published trials has indicated that left-atrial size is not a strong independent predictor for thromboembolic events. Moderate-to-severe mitral regurgitation may actually decrease the risk of stroke, as does regular alcohol use.

There is no evidence of a difference in annual stroke rate between patients with paroxysmal or persistent AF. The thromboembolic risk with atrial flutter is somewhere in between that of sinus rhythm and AF. In one large study, compared with sinus rhythm the stroke risk of AF was 1.6 and that of atrial flutter was 1.4. Until evidence is available, it seems prudent to treat patients with atrial flutter as if they had AF.

TREATMENT OPTIONS

ANTICOAGULATION WITH WARFARIN

Meta-analysis suggests an overall 60% reduction in stroke risk with warfarin for both primary and secondary prevention (absolute risk reduction of 3% per year for primary prevention and 8% for secondary prevention; numbers needed to treat (NNT) for 1 year to prevent one stroke are 33 and 13). The greatest benefit of warfarin therapy is in those patients with previous thromboembolic events, where it reduces the recurrence rate from 12% to 4%. In patients with additional risk factors for stroke, adjusted dose warfarin (INR 2.0–3.0) has consistently been shown to be superior to antiplatelet therapy. With adjusted-dose warfarin, the risk of haemorrhagic stroke is increased from 0.1% to 0.3% per year. In most clinical trials, bleeding complications were seen in patients with an INR >3.0. The only indication for INRs higher than 3.0 is the presence of a mechanical heart valve. The risk of recurrence is not time dependent, therefore, anticoagulation should be continued indefinitely.

EFFECT OF ANTIPLATELET THERAPY

Aspirin reduces the relative risk of thromboembolism by 20% with a 1.5% absolute risk reduction for primary and 2.5% for secondary prevention (NNT for 1 year to prevent one stroke are 66 and 40 respectively). Aspirin may actually prevent the smaller, non-cardioembolic strokes seen in elderly patients, which tend to be less disabling. Trials have used varying doses, although anything less than 100 mg would appear to be the most prudent choice. In comparison, warfarin is three times more effective than aspirin at reducing thromboembolic complications.

COMBINATION THERAPY WITH ASPIRIN AND WARFARIN

Low-dose warfarin and aspirin is no better that aspirin alone and is not as good as adjusted-dose warfarin. Adjusted-dose warfarin and aspirin results in more bleeding complications, without additional benefit.

CARDIOVERSION AND RHYTHM-CONTROL STRATEGIES

Left-atrial stunning occurs after both pharmacological and electrical cardioversion. There is a 1–5% risk of stroke following cardioversion. There is no firm evidence that restoration of sinus rhythm reduces stroke risk. Guidelines suggest that if atrial fibrillation or atrial flutter has been present for more than 48 hours' duration, warfarin treatment with an INR of 2.0–3.0 for 3 weeks before and 4 weeks after cardioversion is the minimum requirement. Anticoagulation should be continued indefinitely in those with multiple risk factors for recurrence. If urgent cardioversion is needed, intravenous heparin should be administered, followed by warfarin. Following cardioversion, typically only

30–50% of patients remain in sinus rhythm by 1 year. Data from recent trials comparing rhythm-control to rate-control strategies have shown that strokes occurred with equal frequency in the rate-control and rhythm-control groups (1% per year) and were mainly in patients who had stopped warfarin. These trials have indicated that stroke often occurs in the presence of sinus rhythm, suggesting that many patients presumed to have had sinus rhythm successfully restored and maintained may actually continue to experience paroxysms of atrial fibrillation (which may be clinically silent) and are vulnerable to thromboembolism once their anticoagulation has been discontinued.

STOPPING ANTICOAGULATION FOR SURGICAL PROCEDURES

Consensus opinion is that in patients without mechanical valves, it is safe to stop warfarin for up to 1 week without heparin cover. In high-risk patients, or if warfarin needs to be discontinued for more than 1 week, heparin should be considered.

WHO TO TREAT

Those at greatest risk have the most to benefit and many high-risk patients are elderly with additional co-morbidity. Unless contraindicated, warfarin should be prescribed to all patients over 60 years of age who have additional risk factors for thromboembolism, including hypertension, a previous thromboembolic event, heart failure and/or moderate-to-severe LV dysfunction on echo, diabetes, rheumatic heart disease (mitral stenosis) or hypertrophic cardiomyopathy. For those patients under the age of 60 with 'lone' (no obvious cause and normal cardiac structure) AF, the absolute risk reduction with warfarin may be so low that the slight increase in bleeding offsets any benefit. In this situation, aspirin is usually prescribed. Patients under 60 years with additional risk factors, and those over 75 years without additional risk factors should be assessed on an individual basis, with warfarin therapy being the preferred option. In patients aged between 60 and 75 years without additional risk factors, aspirin is an acceptable option. The evidence for warfarin therapy in the presence of coronary artery disease (CAD) and thyrotoxicosis is less clear and should probably be used only in those over the age of 60.

CAVEATS

The evidence for anticoagulant therapy in patients with AF has been gathered through many randomized controlled trials. Such trials are usually well planned with stable, frequently monitored patients. Patients at high risk of bleeding are usually excluded. Trial participants tend to be younger than the average clinical practice patient. In the real world, effective INR control may be more challenging, reducing the benefit and increasing bleeding complications. In addition, most published trials have a 1–2 year follow-up period, whereas, in reality, patients need lifelong anticoagulation.

FUTURE DIRECTIONS

Trials are currently underway to examine the role of newer antiplatelet agents. For patients in whom anticoagulation is contraindicated, a transcatheter closure device that is percutaneously delivered into the left-atrial appendage is under development.

Further reading

ACC/AHA/ESC 2001 ACC/AHA/ESC guidelines for the management of patients with atrial fibrillation. Circulation 104(17): 2118–2150

Lip GYH, Hart RG, Conway DSG 2002 ABC of antithrombotic therapy: antithrombotic therapy for atrial fibrillation. BMJ 325: 1022–1025

Index